MEDICAL
WORD FINDER
SECOND EDITION

Compiled by

George Willeford, M.D.

Parker Publishing Company, Inc.

West Nyack, N.Y.

Library of Congress Cataloging in Publication Data

Willeford, George.
  Medical word finder.

   1. Medicine--Terminology. 2. Spellers. 3. Medical
libraries--Directories. I. Title. [DNLM: 1. Diction-
aries, Medical. W13 W698m]
R123.W47 1976   610'.1'4   76-11781
ISBN 0-13-573519-X

PRINTED IN THE UNITED STATES OF AMERICA

Why This Second Edition?

The *Medical Word Finder* was originally compiled with the thought that no future revisions or additions would be necessary. It was intended to help medical and paramedical personnel deal with the spelling and syllabication of unfamiliar terms. The First Edition served this purpose well.

Eight years have passed and I have changed my mind about the need for a new edition. Why? Many new terms have been introduced into the medical field; new specialities have emerged; lists of drugs have increased, and so on.

With this in mind, I mailed questionnaires to purchasers of the First Edition. I was pleasantly surprised at the percentage of returns of these questionnaires. Overwhelmingly, users said that the Word Finder had made medical transcriptions much easier. As a result of user recommendations, many new features have been added to this new edition.

A list of commonly used prescription abbreviations has been included. Lists of commonly used drugs with both generic and proprietary names were added. The popular section of phonetically spelled terms has been enlarged, and many new terms have been added to the alphabetical section.

The section on widely used medical abbreviations has been enlarged and reorganized for easier and more accurate usage. A list of well over one hundred commonly misspelled medical words are conveniently printed in a special section at the back of the book.

With the expansion of old sections and additions of new material, this edition should increase your accuracy and make your work easier and less frustrating. I hope you will enjoy using the Word Finder as much as I have enjoyed preparing it.

George Willeford, M.D.

Acknowledgement

My sincere thanks go to Edie Anderson,
whose help made this revision possible.

How to Use This Book

The *Medical Word Finder* was compiled to provide medical, dental and allied personnel with a compact, easy-to-use guide to the spelling, syllabication and accentuation of frequently used medical terms.

The first printing in 1967 was well received by medical records librarians, medical secretaries and associated personnel. This second edition is a revision based on usage and suggestions gleaned from questionnaires sent at random to many original users.

With the additions to all sections, the *Medical Word Finder* promises to be a more valuable resource in effectively handling the ever growing stacks of medical paper work.

SECTION I is an alphabetical list of important prefixes and suffixes found in medical words.

SECTION II is an alphabetical list of current medical and paramedical terminology. The listings are accentuated to help you with pronunciation; they are syllabicated (divided) for you to aid in transcription.

SECTION III lists the phonetic spelling of "problem" words in alphabetical order. Many secretaries, transcribers and others who use medical vocabulary often run across words unfamiliar to them. This section lists these "problem" words phonetically (e.g., *new mo'ni a*), then gives you the correct spelling (e.g., *pneumonia*).

SECTION IV lists alphabetically most arteries, veins, muscles, diseases, syndromes, tests, surgical incisions, dental surfaces and descriptive positions, i.e., anatomical.

This section will save you time if you will familiarize yourself with its contents and remember to refer to it when applicable (e.g., when transcribing an operative procedure for a limb amputation, the names of several muscles will need to be properly spelled).

SECTION V lists abbreviations frequently used in medical transcription and prescription writing.

SECTION VI is comprised of alphabetical lists of frequently prescribed pharmaceuticals—both generic and proprietary names. These are correctly spelled, accentuated and syllabicated.

SECTION VII is a list of recognized medical specialities with a definition of each one.

SECTION VIII is a list of medical libraries arranged alphabetically by state. Should the need to request information from these facilities arise, a call or letter to the appropriate medical librarian should produce the desired result.

SECTION IX contains two tables of potentially important information: a conversion table of weights and measures—metric to apothecary—and an obstetrical table used to determine the expected date of confinement.

SECTION X is a special section of troublesome medical words, showing how to spell them correctly, and grouped here for quick reference.

SYLLABIC ACCENTUATION: The heavy or primary accent is marked by a single accent mark ('). The secondary accent is indicated by two accent marks (").

GEORGE WILLEFORD, M.D.

Contents

Why This Second Edition? 3

How To Use This Book 5

SECTION I

List of Prefixes and Suffixes 9

SECTION II

Alphabetical Word List 17

SECTION III

Phonetically Spelled Word List 298

SECTION IV

Alphabetical List of:

    Arteries 330
    Veins 333
    Muscles 336
    Diseases 341
    Syndromes 348
    Commonly Performed Tests 354

Contents

Surgical Incisions .373
Dental Surfaces 374
Descriptive Positions, i.e., Anatomical 375

SECTION V

Often Used Word Abbreviations 376
Often Used Prescription Abbreviations 386

SECTION VI

Commonly Prescribed Pharmaceuticals—Generic Names . . . 388
Commonly Prescribed Pharmaceuticals—Proprietary Names . .394

SECTION VII

List of Recognized Medical Specialites 400

SECTION VIII

List of Major Medical Libraries 403

SECTION IX

Conversion Tables, Metric To Apothecary 484
Obstetrical Table To Determine Date of Confinement 486
179 Troublesome Medical Words . . . and How To Spell Them
    Correctly 488

SECTION I
LIST OF PREFIXES AND SUFFIXES

PREFIX	MEANING
a-, an-	not, without, absence of
ab-	away from
abdomino-	relating to the abdomen
acou-	relating to hearing
acro-	relating to the extremities
acromio-	relating to the shoulder
ad-	motion toward, adherence
adeno-	relating to a gland
adipo-	relating to fat, fatty
andro-	relating to man or male
angio-	relating to blood vessels
ante-	before in time or position
antero-	before, in front of
anti-	against
argento-	denoting silver
arterio-	relating to arteries
arthro-	relating to joints
auri-	relating to the ear
auto-	self
bacillo-	related to the bacillus
bacterio-	related to bacteria
bi-	two
bili-	related to bile or the bile-producing system
bio-	related to life
brachio-	denoting the arm
brachy-	short
brady-	slow
bronchio-, broncho-	related to the bronchial system
calcaneo-	related to the heel
calori-	pertaining to heat
cardio-	related to the heart
cephalo-	related to the head
cervico-	related to the neck of the body or an organ
cheilo-	related to the lips
cholo-	pertaining to bile or gall

chondrio-	related to gristle, cartilage
chromato-	related to color
chrono-	pertaining to time
chylo-	related to chyle
circum-	around
cleido-	related to the collarbone
colo-	related to the colon
colpo-	pertaining to the vagina
condylo-	pertaining to a joint
contra-	against or opposite
copro-	related to feces
coraco-	pertaining to the coracoid process of the scapula
corneo-	related to the cornea
cortico-	related to the cortex
costo-	related to the rib
cranio-	related to the cranium
cryo-	pertaining to cold
cuti-	skin
cysto-	pertaining to the bladder
dacryo-	relating to tears or lacrimal glands
dactylo-	relating to fingers, toes
de-	away, not
duodeno-	relating to the duodenum
dys-	difficult or painful
e-	out, without
ecto-	outer
ectro-	congenital absence
endo-	within, internal
entero-	denoting the intestine
epi-	upon, over, outside
erythro-	denoting red blood cells
esophago-	pertaining to the esophagus
eu-	normal
ex-	beyond, from, without
extra-	outside of
gastro-	pertaining to the stomach
glosso-	pertaining to the tongue
gluco-	denoting glucose

hemato-	pertaining to blood
hepato-	pertaining to the liver
hidro-	pertaining to sweat
humero-	pertaining to the humerus
hyper-	excessive, abnormal
hypo-	lack, deficiency, below, less
hystero-	pertaining to the uterus
ileo-	pertaining to ileum
ilio-	pertaining to ilium
in-	into, in, within, on
in-	not
infra-	below, beneath, within
inter-	between, among
intra-	in or within
ischio-	pertaining to ischium or hip
iso-	same; in biology, from a different organism of the same species
jejuno-	pertaining to jejunum
juxta-	near
kerato-	pertaining to the cornea
labio-	pertaining to the lips
laryngo-	pertaining to the larynx
leio-	smooth
lieno-	pertaining to the spleen
lipo-	pertaining to fat
litho-	pertaining to stone
lumbo-	lumbar
macro-	large, enlarged
mal-	bad
masto-, mast-	pertaining to the breast
medio-, medi-	middle
mega-, meg-	enlarged, large
melano-, melan-	relating to melanin
mento-	pertaining to the chin
metro-	pertaining to the uterus
micro-, micr-	small
mono-, mon-	one
multi-	many, much
myo-	pertaining to muscle

myxo-, myx-	pertaining to mucus
naso-	pertaining to the nose
nephro-, neph-	pertaining to the kidney
neuri-	pertaining to a nerve
non-	not
occipito-	occipital
oculo-	pertaining to the eye
odonto-	pertaining to a tooth
oligo-	scant
omo-	pertaining to the shoulder
omphalo-	pertaining to the umbilicus
onco-	pertaining to tumor
oophoro-	pertaining to the ovary
ophthalmo-	pertaining to the eye
opto-	pertaining to vision
orchio, orchi-	pertaining to the testes
oro-	pertaining to the mouth
osteo-	pertaining to bone
oto-	pertaining to the ear
ovi-	pertaining to ovum
oxy-	denoting oxygen
pachy-	thick
palato-	pertaining to the palate
pan-	all
para-	beyond, beside
peri-	about, near, around
perineo-	denoting the perineum
pharyngo-	pertaining to the pharynx
phlebo-	denoting vein
phono-	sound or voice
photo-	light
pilo-, pil-	denoting hair
plano-	flat
plasmo-	pertaining to plasma
platy-	flat, broad
pleuro-	pertaining to the pleura
pneumo-	air, lung
poly-	many, much
post-	after

postero-	posterior
pre-	before
pro-	for, before
procto-	pertaining to the anus or rectum
pseudo-	false
psycho-	pertaining to the mind
psychro-	cold
pubo-	pertaining to the pubis
pulmo-	pertaining to the lung
pyelo-	pertaining to the larger collecting ducts of the kidney
pyloro-	pertaining to the pylorus
pyo-	denoting pus
rachio-	pertaining to the spine
re-	again
recto-	rectal
retro-	behind, backward
rhino-	pertaining to the nose
sacro-	pertaining to the sacrum
salpingo-	pertaining to the auditory or uterine tube
sarco-	denoting flesh
scapulo-	pertaining to the scapula
sclero-	hard
sclero-	denoting the sclera
semi-	half
sero-	denoting serum
sialo-	denoting saliva
skeleto-	pertaining to the skeleton
spleno-	pertaining to the spleen
steato-	denoting fat
sterno-	pertaining to the sternum
sub-	beneath
super-	above, upon
supra-	above
syn-	with, together
tachy-	fast
tarso-	pertaining to the ankle or instep
temporo-	pertaining to the temple
teno-	denoting tendon

thoraco-	pertaining to the thorax
thyro-	pertaining to the thyroid
tracheo-	pertaining to the trachea
trans-	across
tricho-	denoting hair
uretero-	pertaining to the ureter
utero-	pertaining to the uterus
vaso-	denoting blood vessels
vesico-	pertaining to the bladder
vulvo-	pertaining to the vulva
xantho-	yellow

SUFFIXES

SUFFIX	MEANING
-ad	in the direction of
-ase	an enzyme
-blast	a formative or germ cell
-cele	a tumor, cavity or hernia
-cyte	a cell
-dynia	pain
-ectomy	surgical removal
-graphy	X-ray examination
-itis	inflammation of
-lytic	causing lysis of
-oid	like
-ology	the study or science of
-oma	tumor-like nodule or swelling
-opia, -opy	a defect of the eye
-opsia, -opsy	a condition of vision
-optosis	a falling of
-orraphy	the closure of by suturing
-orrhagia	hemorrhage
-orrhea	excessive flow or secretion
-osis	a state, condition
-oscopy	visual examination of, using an illuminated instrument
-ostomy	establishment of an opening to the outside of the body or lumen of another hollow organ
-otomy	incision into
-pathy	disease of
-pexy	fixation of
-phobia	fear of
-phrenia	mental disorder
-plasty	plastic surgery of
-poietic	producing
-schisis	cleft or fissure of
-scope	instrument for visual examination
-scopy	seeing or examining
-tome	instrument for cutting
-tomy	a cutting operation

a ban'don ment
ab ap'i cal
ab"ap tis'ton
a bar"og no'sis
ab"ar tic'u lar
a ba'si a
a ba'sic
a bate'
a bate'ment
ab ax'i al
ab do'men
ab dom'i nal
ab dom"i no an te' ri or
ab dom"i no cen te'sis
ab dom"i no hys"ter ec'to my
ab dom"i no hys"ter ot'o my
ab dom"i no per"i ne'al
ab dom"i no pos te' ri or
ab dom"i nos'co py
ab dom'i nous
ab dom"i no ves'i cal
ab du'cens
ab du'cent
ab duct'
ab duc'tion
ab duc'tor
ab er'rant
ab"er ra'tion
ab"er rom'e ter
a be"ta lip"o pro tein e'mi a
a bey'ance
ab'i ent
ab"i et'ic
a"bi o gen'e sis
a"bi o'sis
a bi o troph'ic

a"bi ot'ro phy
ab ir'ri tant
ab ir"ri ta'tion
ab"lac ta'tion
ab late'
ab la' ti o
ab la'tion
a bleph'a ry
a blep'si a
ab'lu ent
ab nerv'al
ab neu'ral
ab nor'mal
ab nor mal'ity
ab o'ral
a bort'
a bor'ti cide
a bor'tient
a bor"ti fa'cient
a bor'tin
a bor'tion
a bor'tion ist
a bor'tive
a bor'tus
a bra'chi a
a bra"chi o ceph'a lus
a bra'chi us
a'brade
ab ra'sion
ab ra'sive
ab ra'sor
ab"re ac'tion
a'brin
a bro'si a
ab rup'ti o
ab'scess

ab scis'sa
ab scis'sion
ab'sence
ab''sen tee'ism
ab'sinthe
ab'sinth ism
ab'so lute
ab sorb'
ab sor'bance
ab sor''be fa'cient
ab sorb'ent
ab sorp''ti om'e ter
ab sorp'tion
ab''sorp tiv'i ty
ab'sti nence
ab strac'tion
a bu'li a
a bu'lic
a bu''lo ma'ni a
a buse'
a but'
a but'ment
a ca'cia
a cal''ci co'sis
a''cal cu'li a
a camp'si a
a can''thes the'si a
a can'thi al
a can'thi on
a can''tho a mel''o blas to'ma
a can'tho cytes
a can''tho cy to'sis
a can'thoid
a can''tho ker''a to der'mi a
ac''an thol'y sis
ac''an tho'ma
a can''tho pel'vis
ac''an tho'sis
ac''an thot' ic

a can'thu lus
a cap'ni a
a cap'su lar
a car'di a
a car''di o he'mi a
a car''di o ner'vi a
a car''di o tro'phi a
a car'di us
ac''a ri'a sis
a car'i cide
ac'a rid
Ac''a ri'na
ac''a ro der''ma ti'tis
ac'a roid
ac''a ro pho'bi a
a car'pi a
a car'pous
a''cat a la'si a
a cat''a ma the'si a
ac''a tap'o sis
ac''a tas ta'si a
ac''a thex'i a
ac a thex'is
a cau'dal
ac cel'er ate
ac cel''er a'tion
ac cel'er a''tor
ac cel'er in
ac cel''er om'e ter
ac cen'tu a''tor
ac cep'tor
ac''ces so'ri us
ac ces'so ry
ac'ci dent
ac''ci den'tal ism
ac cli ma'tion
ac cli''ma ti za'tion
ac cli'ma tize
ac com''mo da'tion

ac couche'ment
ac''cou cheur'
ac''cou cheuse'
ac''cre men ti'tion
ac cre'ti o cor'dis
ac cre'tion
ac crit'i cal
ac cu'mu la''tor
a''ce nes the'si a
a cen''o cou'ma rol
a cen'tric
a ceph''a lo bra'chi a
a ceph'a lo cyst''
a ceph'a lus
a ceph'a ly
a cer'' a to' sis
a cer'bi ty
a cer''bo pho'bi a
a ces'o dyne
a''ces to'ma
ac''e tab'u lar
ac''e tab''u lec'to my
ac''e tab'u lo plas''ty
ac''e tab'u lum
ac'e tal
ac''et al'de hyde
ac''et am in'o phen
ac''et an'i lid
ac''et ar'sone
ac'e tate
ace''ta zol am'ide
a ce'tic ac'id
ac''e tim'e ter
ac''e to a ce'tic
ac''e tom'e try
ac'e tone
ac''e to ne'mi a
ac''e to nu'ri a
a ce'tum

ac'e tyl
ac''e tyl cho'line
a cet'y lene
a cet''y li za'tion
ac''e tyl sal''i cyl'ic
ach''a la'si a
ache
a chei'li a
a chei'ri a
a chei'rus
a chieve'ment
A chil'les
a chil''lo bur si'tis
a chil''lo dyn'i a
ach''il lor'rha phy
ach''il lot'o my
a''chlor hy'dri a
ach''lu o pho'bi a
a cho'li a
ach''o lu'ri a
ach''o lu'ric
a chon''dro pla'si a
a''chon dro plas'tic
a'chor
a chre''o cy the'mi a
a chro'a cyte
a chro'ma cyte
a''chro ma'si a
a'chro mate
a''chro mat'ic
a chro'ma tin
a chro'ma tism
a chro''ma tol'y sis
a chro'ma to phil''
a chro''ma top'si a
a chro''ma to'sis
a chro'ma tous
a chro''ma tu'ri a
a chro'mi a

a chro′mic
a chro″mo der′mi a
a chro″mo trich′i a
a chros′tic
Ach″ro my′cin
a chyl″a ne′mi a
a chy′li a
a cic′u lar
ac′id
ac′id al bu′min
ac″id am″in u′ri a
ac″i de′mi a
ac′id-fast″
a cid″i fi ca′tion
a cid′i fy
ac″i dim′e ter
ac′id ism
a cid′i ty
a cid′o cyte
ac″i do cy″to pe′ni a
ac″i do cy to′sis
a cid′o phil″
ac″i doph′i lism
ac″i do re sist′ant
ac″i do′sis
ac″i dot′ic
a cid′u late
ac″i du′ri a
ac″i du′ric
ac′i ni
ac″i no tu′bu lar
ac′i nus
ac′la sis
a clas′tic
ac mas′tic
ac′me
ac′ne
ac′ne form
ac ne′mi a

ac ni′tis
a coe′li a
a co′lous
a co′mi a
a con′a tive
a con″u re′sis
ac″o re′a
a co′ri a
a cor′mus
a cou″es the′si a
ac″ou la′li on
a cou′me ter
a cou met′ric
a cou′me try
ac″ou oph′o ny
a cou′si a
a cous′ma
a cous′tic
a cous″ti co pho′bi a
ac quired′
ac′ral
a cra′ni a
a cra′ni us
a cra′ti a
a crat″u re′sis
ac′rid
ac″ri fla′vine
ac″ro ag no′sis
ac″ro ar thri′tis
ac″ro as phyx′i a
ac″ro a tax′i a
ac′ro blast
ac″ro ceph al′ic
ac″ro ceph″a lo syn″dac tyl′i a
ac″ro ceph′a ly
ac″ro con trac′ture
ac″ro cy″a no′sis
ac″ro der″ma ti′tis

ac'ro dont
ac''ro dyn'i a
ac''ro e de'ma
ac''ro ger'i a
ac''rog no'sis
ac''ro hy''per hi dro'sis
ac''ro hy'po ther''my
ac''ro ker''a to'sis
ac''ro ma'ni a
ac''ro mas ti'tis
ac''ro me gal'ic
ac''ro meg'a loid ism
ac''ro meg'a ly
ac''ro mel al'gi a
a cro'mi al
a cro''mi o cla vic'u lar
a cro''mi o cor'a coid
a cro''mi o hu'mer al
a cro'mi on
a cro''mi o tho rac'ic
a crom'pha lus
ac''ro my co'sis
ac''ro my''o to'ni a
ac''ro neu rop'a thy
ac''ro neu ro'sis
ac'ro nyx
ac''ro pa ral' y sis
ac''ro par es the'sia
ac''ro pa thol'o gy
a crop'a thy
ac''ro pho'bi a
ac''ro pig men ta'tion
ac''ro pig men ta'ti o
 re tic''u lar'is
ac''ro pos thi'tis
ac''ro scle ro'sis
ac' rose
ac'ro some
ac''ros tel al'gi a

ac''ro ter'ic
a crot'ic
ac'ro tism
ac''ro tro''pho neu ro'sis
a cryl'ic
act
ACTH
Ac'thar
ac'tin
ac tin'ic
ac tin'i form
ac'tin ism
Ac''ti no ba cil'lus
ac''ti no der''ma ti'tis
ac tin'o gen
ac tin'o graph
ac''ti nol'o gy
ac tin'o lyte
ac''ti nom'e ter
Ac''ti no my'ces
ac''ti no my ce'tin
ac''tin o my'cin
ac''ti no my co'ma
ac''ti no my co' sis
ac''ti no my cot'ic
ac''ti no my'co tin
ac''ti no neu ri'tis
ac''ti no phy to'sis
ac''ti nos'co py
ac''ti no ther'a py
ac'tion
ac'ti vate''
ac''ti va'tion
ac'ti va''tor
ac'tive
ac tiv'i ty
ac''to my'o sin
ac'tu al
a cu''es the'si a

a cu'i ty
a cu'mi nate
ac'u pres"sure
ac'u punc"ture
a'cus
ac"u sec'tor
a cus'ti cus
a cute'
a cute'ness
a cu"ti cos'tal
a cy"a nop'si a
a cy"a not'ic
a cy'cli a
a cy'clic
a"cy e'sis
ac'yl
a cys'ti a
a dac'ry a
a dac'tyl
a dac tyl'i a
a dac'tyl ism
a dac'tyl ous
ad"a man'tine
ad"a man"ti no car"ci no'ma
ad"a man"ti no'ma
ad"a man'to blast
Adam's ap'ple
ad"ap ta'tion
a dapt'er
ad"ap tom'e ter
ad'at"om
ad ax'i al
ad'der
ad'dict
ad dic'tion
Addis' meth'od
Ad'di son ism
ad di'tion
ad du'cent

ad duct'
ad duc'tion
ad duc'tor
a de"lo mor'phous
a del'pho site
ad"en al'gi a
ad'e nase
ad"en as the'ni a
ad"en drit'ic
ad"en ec'to my
ad"en ec to'pi a
A'den fe'ver
a de'ni a
a den'i form
ad'e ni'tis
ad"e no ac"an tho'ma
ad"e no a me"lo blas to'ma
ad"e no an"gi o sar co'ma
ad"e no car"ci no'ma
ad'e no cele
ad"e no cel'lu li'tis
ad"e no chon dro'ma
ad"e no chon"dro sar co'ma
ad"e no cys to'ma
ad"e no fi bro'ma
ad"e no fi"bro sar co'ma
ad"e no gen'e sis
ad"e nog'e nous
ad"e no hy"per sthe'ni a
ad"e no hy poph'y sis
ad'e noid
ad"e noi dec'to my
ad'e noid ism
ad'e noi di'tis
ad"e no lei"o my"o fi bro'ma
ad"e no li po'ma
ad"e no li po"ma to'sis
ad"e no log"a di'tis
ad"e no lym phi'tis

ad″e no lym′pho cele
ad″e no lym pho′ma
ad″e no′ma
ad″e no ma la′ci a
ad″e no′ma toid
ad″e no′ma tome
ad″e no ma to′sis
ad″e nom′a tous
ad′e no mere
ad″e no my″o hy per pla′si a
ad″e no my o″ma to′sis
ad″e no my o′ma
ad″e no my″o me tri′tis
ad″e no my″o sar co′ma
ad″e no my o′sis
ad″e no myx″o chon″dro
  sar co′ma
ad″e no myx o′ma
ad″e no myx″ɔ sar co′ma
ad″e non′cus
ad″e nop′a thy
ad″e no phar″yn gi′tis
ad″e no phleg′mon
ad″e no sal″pin gi tis
ad″e no sar co′ma
ad″e no sar″co rhab″
  do my o′ma
ad″e no scle ro′sis
ad′e nose
a den′o sine
ad″en o sin″e tri phos′phate
ad″e no′sis
ad′e no tome
ad″e not′o my
ad″e no vi′rus
ad′e nyl
a der′mi a
a der″mo gen′e sis
a der″mo tro′phi a

ad here′
ad her′ent
ad he′sion
ad he″si ot′o my
ad he′sive
a″di ac tin′ic
a″di ad″o cho ki ne′sis
a di″a pho ret′ic
a″di as′to le
a″di a ther′mic
Ad′ie pu′pil
ad′i ent
ad′i po cele″
ad″i po cel′lu lar
ad′i po cere″
ad″i po fi pro′ma
ad″i pol′y sis
ad″i po ne cro′sis
ad″i po pex′is
ad″i po pex′y
ad′i pose
ad″i po′sis
ad″i po si′tis
ad″i pos′i ty
ad″i po″so gen′i tal
ad″i po su′ri a
a dip′sa
a dip′si a
ad′i tus
ad just′ment
ad jus′tor
ad′ju vent
ad lib
ad me′di al
ad″mi nic′u lum
ad mix′ture
ad na′sal
ad′nate
ad nau′se am

ad ner'val
ad nex'a
ad nex'al
ad"nex i'tis
ad nex"o gen'e sis
ad"o don'ti a
ad"o les'cence
ad o'ral
ad or'bit al
ad re'nal
ad re"nal ec'to my
Ad ren'a lin
ad ren"al in e'mi a
ad ren'al in u'ri a
ad re'nal ism
ad re"na li'tis
ad'ren arch'e
ad"ren er'gic
Ad'ren ine
ad ren"o cor'ti cal
ad ren"o cor"ti co mi met'ic
ad ren"o cor"ti co tro'pic
ad ren"o cor"ti co tro'pin
Ad re'no-cor'tin
ad re"no gen'i tal
ad re'no gram
ad re"no lyt'ic
ad ren"o meg'a ly
ad ren'o pause
ad re"no tox'in
ad ren'o trope
ad ren"o tro'pic
ad ren"o tro'pin
ad"re not'ro pism
a"dri a my'cin
a dro'mi a
ad sorb'
ad sor'bate
ad sorb'ent

ad sorp'tion
ad sorp'tive
ad ster'nal
ad ter'mi nal
ad tor'sion
a dult'
a dul'ter ant
a dul'ter ate
a dul"ter a'tion
ad vance'
ad vance'ment
ad"ven ti'ti a
ad"ven ti'tious
a"dy na'mi a
a"dy man'ic
A e'des   Ae gyp'ti
ae'quum
a'er ate
a er a'ted
a'er at or
a"er a'tion
a er e'mi a
a"er en"do cor'di a
a"er en"ter ec ta'si a
aer'i al
a"er if'er ous
a'er i form"
a"er o an a"er o'bic
A"er o bac'ter
a'er obe
a"er o'bic
a"er o bi ol'o gy
a"er o bi'o scope
a"er o bi o'sis
a"er o bi ot'ic
a'er o cele"
a"er o col'pos
a"er o cys'to scope
a"er o cys tos'co py

a″er o″don tal′gi a
a″er o don′ti a
a″er o duc′tor
a″er o dy nam′ics
a″er o em′bo lism
a″er o em″phy se′ma
a″er o gas′tri a
a′er o gen″
a″er o gen′e sis
a″er o gen′ic
a′er o gram″
a″er og′ra phy
a″er o hy drop′a thy
a″er o i″on i za′tion
a″er o i″on o ther′a py
aer′o lin
a″er o mam mog′ra phy
a″er o med′cine
a″er om′e ter
a″er o neu ro′sis
a″er op′a thy
a′er o pause″
a″er o per″i to ne′um
a″er o pha′gi a
a′er o phil″
a″er o pho′bi a
a′er o phore″
a′er o phyte″
a″er o pi e″so ther′a py
a″er o ple thys′mo graph
a″er o pleu′ra
a′er o scope″
a″er os′co py
a″er o si la oph′a gy
a″er o si″nus i′tis
a er o′sis
a′er o sol″
a′er o spo″rin
a″er o stat′ics

a″er o tax′is
a″er o ther″a peu′tics
a″er o ther″mo ther′a py
a″er o ti tis me′di a
a″er o to nom′e ter
a er o trop′ic
a er ot′ro pism
a″er o tym′pa nal
a″er o u re′thro scope
ae ru′go
Ae scu la′pi us
aes thet′ic
aes′tus
a fe′brile
a fe′tal
af′fect
af fect″a bil′i ty
af′′fec ta′tion
af fec′tion
af fec′tive
af′′fec tiv′i ty
af fec″ti mo′tor
af′fer ent
af fil″i a′tion
af fi′nal
af′′fir ma′tion
af′flu ent
af′flux
af fu′sion
a fi″brin o gen e′mi a
aft′er birth″
aft′er brain
aft′er care″
aft′er cat″a ract
aft′er cur″rent
aft′er damp″
aft″er dis charge′
aft′er ef fect″
aft′er gild″ing

aft'er hear"ing
aft'er im"age
aft'er im pres"sion
aft'er pains"
aft'er per cep"tion
aft'er po ten'tial
aft'er sen sa"tion
aft'er sound"
aft'er stain"
aft'er taste"
aft'er treat"ment
aft'er vi"sion
a func'tion
a"ga lac'ti a
ag"a lor rhe'a
a gam'ete
a gam'ic
a gam"ma-glob"u lin e'mi a
a gam"o cy tog'o ny
a gam"o gen'e sis
ag"a mog'o ny
a gam'o spore
a gan"gli o'nic
a'gar
a gas'tric
a gas"tro neu'ri a
a gen'e sis
ag"e ne'si a
ag"e net'ic
a gen"i o ce pha'li a
a gen'i tal ism
a gen"o so'mi a
a gen"o so'mus
a'gent
a"ge ra'si a
a geu'si a
ag'ger
ag glom'er ate
ag glu"ti na'tion

ag glu'ti nin
ag"glu tin'o gen
ag glu'ti noid
ag glu'tin o phore"
ag"glu tin'o scope
ag'gre gate
ag"gre ga'tion
ag gres'sin
ag gres'sion
ag'i tat"ed
ag"i ta'tion
a"gi ta'tor caud'ae
ag"i to graph'i a
ag"i to pha'si a
a glan'du lar
a glau cop'si a
ag'li a
a"glo mer'u lar
a glos'si a
a glos"so sto'mi a
a glos'sus
ag"lu ti'tion
a gly ce'mi a
a gly ce'mic
a gly"co su'ria
a gly"co su'ric
ag na'thi a
ag na"tho ceph'a lus
ag'na thus
ag ne'a
ag"no gen'ic
ag no'si a
ag"om phi'a sis
a gon'ad ism
ag'o nal
a go'ni a
ag'o nist
ag'o ny
Ag'or al

ag''o ra pho'bi a
a gram'ma tism
a gran'u lo cyte''
a gran''u lo cy'tic
a gran''u lo cy to'sis
a gran''u lo plas'tic
a gran''u lo'sis
a graph'i a
ag'ri us
ag''ro ma'ni a
ag''ryp not'ic
a'gue
a''gyi o pho'bi a
a gy'ri a
a hyp'ni a
aich''mo pho'bi a
ail'ing
ail'ment
ain'hum
air my e log'ra phy
air'way''
a kar'yo cyte
ak''a thi'si a
a ker''a to'sis
ak''i ne'si a
ak''i ne'sis
a kin''es the'si a
ak''i net'ic
a'la
al'a bas''ter
a''lac ta'si a
a la'li a
a lal'ic
al'a nine
a lan'tic
a las'trim
a la'tus
al'ba
Al ba my'cin

Albers-Schönberg dis ease'
al bes'cent
al'bi cans
al''bi du'ri a
al'bi nism
al bi'no
al''bo ci ne're ous
Albright-McCune-Sternberg
   syn'drome
al''bu gin'e a
al''bu gi ni'tis
al bu'go
al bu'min
al bu'mi nate
al bu''mi nif'er ous
al bu''mi nim'e ter
al bu''mi nog'e nous
al bu'mi noid
al bu''mi nol'y sin
al bu''mi nom'e ter
al bu'mi nose
al bu''min u ret'ic
al bu''mi nu'ri a
al bu'mo scope
al''bu mo su'ri a
Al''ca lig'e nes fe cal'is
al cap''to nu'ri a
al'che my
Alcock's ca nal'
al'co hol
al'co hol ase
al'co hol ate
al''co hol'a ture
al''co hol'ic
Al''co hol'ics A non'y mous
al'co hol ism
al''co hol om'e ter
al''co hol''o phil'i a
al''co hol u'ri a

al″co hol′y sis
al″co me′ter
Al dar′sone
al′de hyde
al′dol ase
al dos′ter one
Aldrich's test
a lec′i thal
al″eu ke′mi a
al″eu ke′mic
a lex′i a
a lex′in
al′gae
al″ge don′ic
al ge′si a
al ge′sic
al″ge sim′e ter
al get′ic
al′gid
al″gi o mo′tor
al″gi o mus′cu lar
al″go gen′e sis
al″go gen′ic
al″go lag′ni a
al gom′e ter
al″go pho′bi a
al′gor
al′go spasm
al′i ble
a′lien ist
al′i ment
al″i men′ta ry
al″i men ta′tion
al″i men″to ther′a py
al″i na′sal
al″i phat′ic
al′i quot
al″i sphe′noid
al″ka le′mi a

al″ka les′cent
al′ka li
al″ka lim′e ter
al′ka line
al″ka lin′i ty
al′ka lin ize
al″ka li nu′ ri a
al″ka li pe′ni a
al″ka li ther′a py
al′ka lize
al″ka lo′sis
al″ka lot′ic
al″ka lo ther′a py
al kap″to nu′ri a
al′kyl
al ky′nol
al″la ches the′si a
al lan″to cho′ri on
al lan″to en ter′ic
al lan″to gen′e sis
al lan toi″do an gi op′a gous
al lan′to in
al lan′tois
al lax′is
al″le gor″i za′tion
al lele′
al lel″o cat″a lyt′ic
al le′lo morph
al lel″o tax′is
al len′the sis
al′ler gen
al ler gen′ic
al ler′gic
al′ler gid
al′ler gin
al′ler gist
al″ler gi za′tion
al″ler go der′mi a
al″ler go′sis

al'ler gy
al''li ga'tion
al''li ga''tor for'ceps
Allis for'ceps
al lit''er a'tion
al''lo che'zi a
al''lo cor'tex
al''lo er'o tism
al lom'e try
al''lo mor'phism
al''lo mor'pho sis
al'lo path
al lop'a thy
al loph' a sis
al'lo plasm
al''lo plas'tic
al'lo plas''ty
al''lo psy'che
al''lo psy'chic
al''lo ryth'mi a
al'lo some
al''lo ste''a to'des
al''lo syn ap'sis
al'lo therm
al lo to'pi a
al lot''ri o don'ti a
al lot''ri o geu'si a
al''lo tri'o lith
al lot''ri oph'a gy
al ot''ri u'ri a
al'lo trope
al''lo troph'ic
al''lo trop'ic
al lox'an
al'loy
all'spice''
al'lyl
al'mond
a lo'chi a

Al'o e ve'ra
a lo'gi a
al''o pe'ci a
al'pha
al''pha to coph'er ol
al pho'sis
al'ter ant
al''ter a'tion
al'ter a tive
al''ter e'go ism
Al''ter na'ri a
al''ter na'tion
al'ter na''tor
al'ti tude sick'ness
al'um
a lu'mi num
a lu'si a
Alvarez, Walter C.
al've at ed
al''ve o la'bi al
al ve'o lar
al ve'o late
al''ve o lec'to my
al ve'o li''
al''ve o lin'gual
al've o li'tis
al ve''o lo cla'si a
al ve''o lo con dyl'e an
al ve''o lo den'tal
al ve''o lo la'bi al
al ve'o lon
al ve ol'o plas''ty
al ve''o lo sub na'sal
al''ve o lot'o my
al ve'o lus
al vi'no lith
al'vus
a lym''pho cy to'sis
al''ys o'sis

Alz'hei mer's dis ease'
a mal'gam
a mal'gam ate
a mal''gam a'tion
a man'i tin
a mas'ti a
am''a tho pho'bia
am'a tive ness
am''au ro'sis
am''au rot'ic
am''a xo pho'bi a
am''bi dex ter'i ty
am''bi dex'trous
am''bi lat'er al
am''bi le'vous
am''bi o'pi a
am''bi sex'u al
am biv'a lence
am biv'a lent
am'bi vert
am''bly a cou'si a
am''bly chro ma'si a
am'bly ope
am''bly o'pi a
am'bly o scope''
am'bo cep''tor
Am bro'si a
am'bu lance
am'bu la to''ry
am bus'tion
a me'ba
a me'bic
am''e bi'a sis
a me'bi cide
a me'bid
a me'bo cyte
a me'boid
a me'boid ism
am e bo'ma

am''e bu'ri a
a mei o'sis
am el'e ia
a mel''i fi ca'tion
a mel'o blast
a mel''o blas to'ma
am''el o blas''to sar co'ma
am''e lo gen'e sis
a me'lus
a me'ni a
a men''o ma'ni a
a men''or rhe'a
a men'si a
a'ment
a men'ti a
am''er is'tic
a me''si al'i ty
a''me thop'ter in
a me'tri a
a me''tro he'mi a
am''e tro'pi a
am''i an'thoid
am''i an tho'sis
a''mi cro'vic
a mi'cron
a mi''cro scop'ic
a mic'u lum
am'ide
am'i din
a mi'do
a mi''do py'rine
A'mi gen
a mim'i a
a mine'
a mi'no ac'id
a mi'no a''cid u'ri a
am''i no cen te'sis
a mi''no phyl'line
A''min op'te rin

a mi″no py′rine
a mi″no sal″i cyl′ic
a mi″no su′ri a
a″mi to′sis
am i tot′ic
ami″tryp′ty lene
am′mo nate
am mo′ni a
am″mo ni′a cal
am mon″i fi ca′tion
am mo′ni um
am mo″ni u′ri a
am″mo ther′a py
am″ne mon′ic
am ne′si a
am′ni a
am″ni o cho′ri al
am″ni o em″bry on′ic
am″ni o gen′e sis
am″ni og′ra phy
am′ni on
am″ni or rhe′a
am″ni ot′ic
am″ni o ti′tis
am′ni o tome
am″ni ot′o my
am″o bar′bi tal
a moe′ba
a mok′
a mo ral′i a
a mor′phic
a mor′phin ism
a morph′ism
a mor′phous
amp
am per′age
am′pere
am phet′a mine
am″phi ar thro′sis

am′phi as″ter
Am phib′i a
am phib′i ous
am″phi blas′tic
am″phi blas′tu la
am″phi chro′ic
am″phi coe′lous
am″phi cra′ni a
am′phi cyte
am′phi des′mic
am″phi di″ar thro′sis
am″phi er′o tism
am″phi gas′trula
am″phi gen′e sis
am″phi ge net′ic
am phig′o ny
am″phi kar′y om
am″phi mix′is
am″phi mor′u la
Am″phi sto′ma ta
am′phi tene
am′phi the″a ter
am phit′ri chous
Am pho cil′lin
am″pho di plo′pi a
Am′pho jel
am′pho lyte
am phor′ic
am″pho ril′o quy
am″pho roph′o ny
am″pho ter′ic
am″pho ter′i cin
am pho ter′ism
am″pli fi ca′tion
am′pli fi″er
am′pli tude
am′poule
am′pul
am pul′la

am pul'lar
am pul'lu la
am'pu tate
am''pu ta'tion
am''pu tee'
a mu'si a
am''y cho pho'bi a
am''y dri'a sis
a my''e len ceph'a lus
am''y e'li a
a my'el in a''ted
a my'e lus
a myg'da lase
a myg'da loid
a myg''da loid ec'to my
a myg'da lo lith
a'myl
am''y la'ceous
am'yl ase
a myl'o gen
am'y loid
am''y loi do'sis
am''y lol'y sis
am''y lo lyt'ic
am'y lon
am''y lo pec'tin
am''y lop'sin
am'yl ose
am''y lu'ri a
a my''o es the'si a
a my''o pla'si a
a my''o sta'si a
a my''o stat'ic
a my''o tax'i a
a my''o to'ni a
a my''o tro'phi a
a my''o tro'phic
A'my tal
a myx'i a

a myx''or rhe'a
an''a bio'sis
an''a bi ot'ic
an''a bol'er gy
a nab'o lin
an ab'o lism
an''a camp'tics
an''a ce''li a del'phous
an''a cid'i ty
a nac'li sis
a na clit'ic
an ac'me sis
a nac''ro a'si a
a nac'ro tism
an''a cu'si a
an''a de'ni a
an''a did'y mus
an''a dip'si a
an'aer obe
an aer o'bic
an''aer o bi'ase
an''aer o bi o'sis
an''aer o gen'ic
an''a go'ge
an''a gog'ic
an''a lep'sis
an''a lep'tic
an''al ge'si a
an''al ge'sic
an''al ge'sist
an''al ler'gic
an'a log
a nal'o gy
a nal'y sand
a nal'y ses
a nal'y sis
an'a lyst
an''a lyt'ic
an'a ly''zer

an''am ne'sis
an''am nes'tic
an am''ni ot'ic
an''a mor'pho sis
an an''a ba'si a
an an''a phy lax'is
an an''as ta'si a
a nan cas'ti a
an an'dri a
an an''gi o pla'si a
an an''gi o plas'tic
an''a pau'sis
an''a pei rat'ic
an''aphal''an ti'a sis
an'a phase
an a'phi a
an''a pho re'sis
an''a pho'ri a
an aph''ro dis'i a
an aph''ro dis'i ac
an''a phy lac'tic
an''a phy lac'tin
an''a phy lac'to gen
an''a phy lac'toid
an''a phyl''a tox'in
an''a phy lax'is
an''a pla'si a
an''a plas mo'sis
an''a plas'tic
an'a plas''ty
an''a ple ro'sis
an''a poph'y sis
an''a rith'mi a
an ar'thri a
an''a sar'ca
an''a sar'cous
an''a stal'sis
a nas'ta sis
an''as tig mat'ic

a nas'to mose
a nas''to mo'sis
a nas to mot'ic
a nas''to mot'i ca
an''a tom'ic
an''a tom'i cal
a nat'o my
an''a tox'in
an''a tro'pi a
an au'di a
an''a vac'cine
an''a ven'in
an'chor age
an'chy lops
an''co ne'us
an'co noid
An''cy los'to ma
an''cy los''to mi'a sis
an''dra nat'o my
an''dri at'rics
an''dro blas to'ma
an''dro ga lac''to ze'mi a
an''dro gam'one
an'dro gen
an''dro gen'e sis
an''dro gen'ic
an drog'e nous
an'dro gyne
an drog'y nism
an drog'y ny
an'droid
an''dro ma'ni a
an''dro mor'phous
an''droph'i lous
an''dro pho'bi a
an dros'ter one
a ne'de ous
an''e lec trot'o nus
a ne'mi a

a ne′mic
an″e mom′e ter
a ne″mo pho′bi a
an en″ce pha′li a
an″en ce phal′ic
an″en ceph′a lus
an″en ceph′a ly
an en′ter ous
an ep′i a
an ep″i plo′ic
an″er ga′si a
an′er gy
an′er oid
an″e ryth″ro blep′si a
an″e ryth′ro cyte
an″e ryth″ro pla′si a
an″e ryth rop′si a
an es″the ki ne′sis
an″es the′si a
an es″the sim′e ter
an″es the″si ol′o gist
an″es the″si ol′o gy
an″es thet′ic
an es′ the tist
an es′the tize
an es′trum
an″e to der′ma
an eu′ploid
a neu′ri a
an′eu rin
an′eu rysm
an eu rys′mal
an″eu rys mec′to my
an″eu rys′mo graph
an″eu rys′mo plas″ty
an″eu rys mor′rha phy
an″eu rys mot′o my
an″eu tha na′si a
an frac″tu os′i ty

an frac′tu ous
an gei′al
an″gi ec′ta sis
an″gi ec tat′ic
an″gi ec′tid
an″gi ec′to my
an″gi ec to′pi a
an″gi i′tis
an gi′na
an gi′nal
an′gi noid
an′gi nous
an gi″no pho′bi a
an′gi o blast″
an″gi o blas to′ma
an″gi o car′di o gram″
an″gi o car″di o graph′ic
an″gi o car″di og′ra phy
an″gi o car″di op′a thy
an″gi o cav″er no′ma
an″gi o cav″ern ous
an″gi o chei′lo scope
an″gi o cho li′tis
an″gi o chon dro′ma
an″gi o der′ma pig″men to′sum
an″gi o der′ma
an″gi o der″ma ti′tis
an″gi o dys tro′phi a
an″gi o e de′ma
an″gi o el″e phan ti′a sis
an″gi o en″do the″li o′ma
an″gi o fi″bro blas to′ma
an″gi o fi bro′ma
an″gi o gen′e sis
an″gi o gli o′ma
an″gi o gli o″ma to′sis
an″gi og′ra phy
an″gi o hy″per to′ni a
an″gi o hy″po to′ni a

an'gi oid
an''gi o ker''a toi di'tis
an''gi o ker''a to'ma
an''gi o li po'ma
an'gi o lith''
an''gi ol'o gy
an''gi o lu'poid
an''gi ol'y sis
an''gi o'ma
an''gi o ma la'ci a
an''gi o ma to'sis
an''gi o meg'a ly
an''gi om'e ter
an''gi o my''o lip o'ma
an''gi o my o'ma
an''gi o my op'a thy
an''gi o my''o sar co'ma
an''gi o neu rec'to my
an''gi o neu ro'ma
an''gi o neu''ro my o'ma
an''gi o neu ro'sis
an''gi o neu ro'tic
an''gi o no'ma
an''gi o pa ral'y sis
an''gi o pa re'sis
an''gi op'a thy
an''gi o pla'ni a
an'gi o plas''ty
an''gi o pneu mog'ra phy
an''gi o poi e'sis
an''gi o poi et'ic
an'gi o pres''sure
an''gi or'rha phy
an''gi or rhex'is
an''gi o sar co'ma
an''gi o scle ro'sis
an'gi o scope''
an''gi o sco to'ma
an''gi o'sis

an''gi o spasm''
an''gi o stax'is
an''gi o ste no'sis
an''gi os''te o'sis
an''gi o stron''gy li'a sis
an''gi o tel''ec ta'si a
an''gi o ten'ic
an''gi o ten'sin
an''gi o ti'tis
an''gi ot'o my
an''gi ot'o nase
an''gi o ton'ic
an''gi ot'o nin
an'gi o tribe''
an''gi o troph'ic
an'gle
an'gor
ang'strom
an''gu la'tion
ang'u lus
an''he do'ni a
an hem''a to poi e'sis
an he''ma to'sis
an he''mo lyt'ic
an''hi dro'sis
an''hi drot'ic
an hy'drase
an''hy dra'tion
an''hy dre'mi a
an hy'dride
an hy'drous
an''hyp no'sis
a ni''a ci no'sis
an''i an'thi nop sy
an ic ter'ic
an id'e us
an'i line
a ni lin'gus
an'il ism

a nil'i ty
an'i ma
an'i mal
an"i mal'cule
an"i mas'tic
an"i ma'tion
an'i ma tism
an'i mism
an'i mus
an'i"on
an'i on"ic
an"i rid'i a
an"is ei kom'e ter
an"i sei ko'ni a
an i"so chro ma'si a
an i"so chro mat'ic
an i"so co'ri a
an i"so cy to'sis
an i"so dac'ty lous
an i'so dont
an i"so ga mete'
an"i sog'a my
an"i sog'na thous
an i"so me'li a
an i"so me'ri a
an i"so me tro'pi a
an i"so me trop'ic
a nis"o my'cin
an"i so'pi a
an"i so sphyg'mi a
an"i sos then'ic
an i"so ton'ic
an"i so tro'pic
an"i sot'ro py
an"i su'ri a
a"ni trog'e nous
an'kle
an"ky lo bleph'a ron
an"ky lo chei'li a

an"ky lo col'pos
an"ky lo dac tyl'i a
an"ky lo don'ti a
an"ky lo glos'si a
an'ky lose
an"ky losed
an 'ky lo'sis
an'ky lo tome
an"ky lot'o my
an'la ge
an neal'
an nec'tent
An nel'i da
an'nu lar
an'nu late
an'nu lose
an"nu lo spi'ral
an'nu lus
an"o chro ma'si a
a no"ci as so"ci a'tion
a no"ci cep'tor
a no"ci the'si a
a"no coc cyg'e al
an o'dal
an'ode
an"o der'mous
an"o don'ti a
an"o don'tous
an'o dyne
an"o dyn'i a
an"o e'si a
an"o et'ic
a noi'a
a nom'a lo scope
a nom'a lous
a nom'a ly
a no'mi a
an o'mous
an"o nych'i a

a non'y ma
an"o op'si a
a"no per"i ne'al
A noph'e les
an"o phel'i cide
an"o phel'i fuge
an"o pho'ri a
an"oph thal'mi a
an"oph thal'mos
an o'pi a
a'no plas ty
an op'si a
an or'chi a
an or'chism
an or'chus
a"no rec'tal
a"no rec'to plas"ty
a"no rec'tic
an"o rex'i
an or gas'my
an"or thog'ra phy
an"or tho'pi a
an"or tho'sis
a'no scope
an os'mi a
an'os'mic
an o"sog no'si a
a"no spi'nal
an"os to'sis
an o'ti a
an"o tro'pi a
an o'tus
a"no ves'i cal
an ov'u lar
an ov'u la to"ry
an"ox e'mi a
an ox'i a
an ox'ic
an'sa

an'sate
an'ser ine
an'si form
an'ta buse
ant ac'id
an tag'o nism
an tag'o nist
an tag"o nis'tic
ant al'ka line
ant"aph ro dis'i ac
an"te au'ral
an"te bra'chi al
an"te bra'chi um
an"te ci'bum
an"te cu'bi tal
an"te cur'va ture
an"te flex'ion
an"te hy poph'y sis
an"te-mor'tem
an"te na'ri al
an"te na'tal
An'te par
an'te par'tum
an te'ri or
an"ter o dor'sal
an"ter o ex ter'nal
an'ter o grade"
an"ter o in fe'ri or
an"ter o in te'ri or
an"ter o in ter'nal
an"ter o lat'er al
an"ter o me'di an
an"ter o pa ri'e tal
an"ter o pi tu'i tar y
an"ter o pos te'ri or
an"ter o su pe'ri or
an"te ver'sion
an'te vert ed
ant he'lix

ant″hel min′tic
an the′ma
ant″hem or rhag′ic
an″tho pho′bi a
an′thra cene
an′thra coid
an″thra co ne cro′sis
an″thra co sil″i co′sis
an″thra co′sis
an′thrax
an″thro po gen′ic
an′thro poid
an″thro pol′o gy
an″thro pom′e ter
an″thro pom′e try
an″thro po mor′phic
an″thro poph′a gy
an″thro po phil′ic
an″thro po pho′bi a
an″thro po so″ma tol′o gy
ant″hyp not′ic
an″ti ac′id
an″ti ag glu′ti nin
an″ti ag gres′sin
an″ti al′bu mate
an″ti al bu′min
an″ti a lex′in
an″ti am″bo cep′tor
an″ti am′yl ase
an″ti an″a phy lax′is
an″ti a ne′mi a
an″ti a ne′mic
an″ti an′ti bod″y
an″ti ar″ach nol′y sin
an″ti ar thrit′ic
an″ti bac te′ri al
an″ti bi o′sis
an″ti bi ot′ic
an″ti bi′o tin

an″ti blas′tic
an″ti bod″y
an″ti bra′chi al
an″ti bra′chi um
an″ti car cin′o gen
an″ti car′di um
an″ti car′i ous
an″ti ca thex′is
an″ti cath′ode
an″ti ceph′a lin
an″ti chei rot′o nus
an″ti chol in er′gic
an″ti cho″lin es′ter ase
an″ti chro mat′ic
an″ti co ag′u lant
an″ti col la′gen ase″
an″ti com′ple ment
an″ti con cep′tive
an″ti con cus′sion
an″ti con vul′sant
an″ti con vul′sive
an′ti cus
an″ti cu′tin
an″ti di″a bet′ic
an″ti di″ar rhe′al
an″ti di″u re′sis
an″ti di″u ret′ic
an″ti do′tal
an′ti dote
an″ti drom′ic
an″ti dys″en ter′ic
an″ti e met′ic
an″ti en′zyme
an″ti fe′brile
An″ti fe′brin
an″ti fer′ment
an″ti fi″bri no ly′sin
an″ti fi bro″ma to gen′ic
an″ti fun′gal

an″ti ga lac′tic
an′ti gen
an ti gen′ic
an″ti ge nic′i ty
an″ti he′lix
an″ti he″mo lyt′ic
an″ti he″mo phil′ic
an″ti hem″or rag′ic
an″ti hem″or rhoi′dal
an″ti hi drot′ic
an″ti his′ta mine
an″ti his′ta min ic
an″ti hor′mone
an″ti hy″a lu ron′i dase
an″ti hy drop′ic
an″ti in fec′tive
an″ti ke″to gen′e sis
an″ti li′pase
an″ti lip fa no′gen
an″ti lu et′ic
an″ti lym′pho cyte
an″ti lyt′ic
an″ti ma lar′i al
an″ti men or rhag′ic
an′ti mere
an″ti me tab′o lite
an″ti me tor′pi a
an′ti mo″ny
an″ti my cot′ic
an″ti nar cot′ic
an″ti neu ral′gic
an″ti neu rit′ic
an tin′i on
an″tin va′sin
an″ti o be′sic
an″ti o don tal′gic
an″ti op′so nin
an″ti ox′i dant
an″ti par″a lyt′ic

an″ti par″a sit′ic
an″ti pep′sin
an″ti pep′tone
an″ti per″i od′ic
an″ti per″i stal′sis
an″ti phag″o cyt′ic
an″ti phlo gis′tic
an″ti phlo gis′tine
an′ti phone
an″ti phthi′ri ac
an″ti plas′min
an″ti plas′tic
an″ti pneu″mo coc′cic
an tip′o dal
an″ti pro throm′bin
an″ti pro′ton
an″ti pru rit′ic
an″ti py″o gen′ic
an″ti py re′sis
an″ti py ret′ic
an″ti py′rine
an″ti py″rin o ma′ni a
an″ti ra′bic
an″ti ra chit′ic
an″ti ren′nin
an″ti re tic′u lar
an″ti rhe′o scope
an″ti rheu mat′ic
an″ti-Rh se′rum
an″ti ri″bo fla′vin
an″ti ri′cin
an″ti sca bet′ic
an″ti scor bu′tic
an″ti sep′sis
an″ti sep′tic
an″ti sep′tol
an″ti se′rum
an″ti si al′a gogue
an″ti si al′ic

an''ti so'cial
an''ti spas mod'ic
an''ti spas'tic
an''ti spi''ro che'tic
an''ti ster'num
an''ti strep''to coc'cic
an''ti strep''to dor'nase
an''ti strep''to he''mo ly'sin
an''ti strep''to ki'nase
an''ti strep''to ly'sin
an''ti su''dor if ic
an''ti syph''i lit'ic
an''ti the'nar
an''ti throm'bin
an''ti throm''bo plas'tin
an''ti tox'i gen
an''ti tox'ic
an''ti tox'in
an''ti trag'i cus
an''ti tra'gus
an''ti tris'mus
an''ti trope
an''ti tryp'sin
An'ti tus'sin
an''ti tus'sive
an''ti ty'phoid
an''ti u're ase
an''ti ve ne're al
an''ti ven'in
an''ti vi'ral
an''ti vi rot'ic
an''ti vir'u lin
an''ti vir'us
an''ti vi'ta min
an''ti viv''i sec'tion
an''ti viv''i sec'tion ist
an''ti xen'ic
an''ti xe''roph thal'mic
an''ti xe rot'ic

an''ti zy mot'ic
ant''lo pho'bi a
an'tral
an trec'to my
an tri'tis
an''tro at''ti cot'o my
an'tro cele
an''tro na'sal
ant'ro phose
an'tro scope''
an tros'to my
an''tro tym pan'ic
an'trum
An tu'trin-S
a nu'cle ar
an u'ri a
an u'ric
an u'rous
a'nus
a nus i'tis
an'vil
anx i'e ty
a or'ta
a''or tal'gi a
a or'tic
a or''ti co pul'mo na ry
a or''ti co re'nal
a''or ti'tis
a''or tog'ra phy
a or''to il'i ac
a''or tot'o my
a pal''les the'si a
a pan'cre a
a pan'dri a
ap''an thro'pi a
a par''a lyt'ic
ap''ar thro'sis
a pas'ti a
ap''a thet'ic

ap'a thism
ap'a thy
ap'atite
a pei"ro pho'bi a
a pel'lous
a per'ri ent
a pe"ri od'ic
a per"i stal'sis
a per'i tive
Apert's syn'drome
ap"er tom'e ter
ap"er tu'ra
ap'er ture
Apeu vi'rus
a'pex
a"pex car'di o gram
Apgar score
a pha'gi a
a pha'ki a
a pha'kic
aph"a lan'gi a
aph"al ge'si a
a phan'i sis
a pha'si a
a pha'si ac
a phelx'i a
a phe'mi a
a phem'ic
aph"e pho'bi a
aph'e ter
a"phil an'thro py
a pho'ni a
a phon'ic
a'phose
a phra'si a
aph"ro dis'i a
aph"ro dis'i ac
aph"ro dis'i o ma'ni a
aph"ro ne'si a

aph'tha
aph thenx'i a
aph thon'gi a
aph tho'sis
aph'thous
a"pi cec'to my
ap"i ci'tis
ap"i co ec'to my
ap"i co lo'ca tor
ap"i col'y sis
a"pi o ther'a py
a"pi pho'bi a
a pis"i na'tion
a"pla cen'tal
ap"la nat'ic
a pla'si a
a plas'tic
a pleu'ri a
ap'ne a
ap neu"ma to'sis
ap neu'mi a
ap neu'sis
ap"o cam no'sis
ap"o car"te re'sis
ap"o chro mat'ic
ap"o clei'sis
ap'o crine
ap"o de"mi al'gi a
a po'di a
ap"o fer'ri tin
a pog'a mous
a pog'a my
ap"o mix'is
ap"o mor'phine
ap"o myt to'sis
a pon"eu ror'rha phy
a pon"eu ro'sis
a pon"eu ro si'tis
ap"o neu rot'ic

a pon"eu rot'o my
a pon'i a
a poph'y sate
a po phys'eal
a poph'y sis
a poph"y si'tis
ap"o plas'mi a
ap"o plec'ti form
ap'o plex"y
a pop nix'is
ap"or rhip'sis
a po'si a
ap"o sid'er in
ap"o si'ti a
ap"o sit'ic
ap'o some
a pos'po ry
a pos'ta sis
a pos'thi a
a poth'e car"ies
a poth'e car"y
ap"ox e'me na
ap"ox e'sis
ap"pa ra'tus
ap pend'age
ap"pen dec'to my
ap pen"di ce'al
ap pen'di ces"
ap pen"di ci'tis
ap pen"di clau'sis
ap pen'di co lith"
ap pen"di cos'to my
ap"pen dic'u lar
ap pen'dix
ap"per cep'tion
ap"per son"i fi ca'tion
ap'pe tite
ap'pe ti"zer
ap'pla nate

ap'pli ca"tor
ap"po si'tion
ap proach'
ap prox'i mal
ap prox'i mate
ap prox"i ma'tion
a prac"tog no'si a
a prax'i a
A pres'o line
a proc'ti a
a proc'tous
a"pro sex'i a
a"pro so'pi a
ap sel"a phe'si a
ap"si thy'ri a
ap sych'i a
ap ty'a lism
a'pus
a py'e tous
a py'rene
a"py ret'ic
a"py rex'i a
a"py rex'i al
aq'ua
a quat'ic
Aq'ua phor
aq'ue duct
a'que ous
Ar'a bic
a rach"i don'ic ac'id
A rach'ni da
A rach'nid ism
a"rach ni don'ic
ar"ach ni'tis
a rach"no dac'ty ly
a rach'noid
a rach noid'al
a rach'noid ism
a rach"noi di'tis

a rach'noid-u re''ter os'to my
A'ra len
ar bo're al
ar''bo res'cent
ar''bor i za'tion
ar'bor vi'tae
ar''bo vi'rus
arc
ar cade'
ar ca'num
ar'cate
arch
ar cha'ic
ar''che go'ni um
ar chen'ter on
ar''che o ki net'ic
ar che py'on
ar'che type
ar''chi a'ter
ar'chi coele
ar''chi gas'tru la
ar''chi neph'ron
ar''chi pal'li um
ar''chi tec ton'ic
ar'cho plasm
ar chu'si a
ar''ci form
arc ta'tion
ar'cu ate
ar''cu a'tion
ar'cus
a're a
ar''e a'tus
a''re flex'i a
a''re gen''er a'tion
ar''e na'ceous
ar''e na'tion
ar'ene
a''re no vi'rus

a re'o la
a re'o lar
ar gam''bly o'pi a
ar'ge ma
ar gen'taf fin
ar''gen taff i no'ma
ar gen'tic
ar gen'to phile
ar gen'tous
ar''gil la'ceous
ar'gi nase
ar'gi nine
ar'gon
Argyll Robertson
ar gyr'i a
ar gyr'ic
Ar'gy rol
ar gy'ro len tis
ar gy'ro phile
ar''gy ro'sis
a rhin''en ce pha li'a
Arias-Stella phe''nom'e non
ari''bo fla''vi no'sis
a ris''to gen'ic
Aristotle
a rith''mo ma'ni a
ar'ky o chrome''
arm
ar''ma men tar'i um
ar mil'la
arm'pit''
Arnold-Chiari syn'drome
ar''o mat'ic
ar rec'tor
ar rest'
ar''rhe no blas to'ma
ar''rhe no'ma
ar''rhe not'o ky
ar rhin''en ce pha'li a

ar rhin'i a
ar rhyth'mi a
ars a man'di
ar'se nate
ar'se nic
ar sen'i cal
ar sen"i co der'ma
ar se'ni ous
ar'se nite
ar"se no ther'a py
ars phen'a mine
ar'te fact
ar ter'en ol
ar ter'i al
ar te"ri al i za'tion
ar te"ri arc'ti a
ar"te ri'a sis
ar te"ri ec'ta sis
ar te"ri ec'to my
ar te"ri ec to'pi a
ar te"ri o cap'il lar"y
ar te"ri o fi bro'sis
ar te'ri o gram"
ar te'ri o graph"
ar te"ri og'ra phy
ar te"ri o'la
ar te'ri ole
ar te'ri o lith"
ar ter"i o li'tis
ar te"ri o"lo ne cro'sis
ar te"ri o"lo scle ro'sis
ar te"ri o lo scle rot'ic
ar te"ri o ma la'ci a
ar te"ri o ne cro'sis
ar te"ri op'a thy
ar te"ri o pla'ni a
ar te"ri o plas'tic
ar te"ri o plas'ty
ar te"ri o pres'sor

ar te"ri o punc'ture
ar te"ri o re'nal
ar te"ri or'rha phy
ar te"ri or rhex'is
ar te"ri o scle ro'sis
ar te"ri o scle rot'ic
ar te'ri o spasm"
ar te"ri o ste no'sis
ar te"ri os to'sis
ar te"ri o strep'sis
ar te'ri o tome"
ar te"ri ot'o my
ar te"ri o ve'nous
ar te"ri o ver'sion
ar"te ri'tis
ar'ter y
ar thral'gi a
ar thral'gic
ar threc'to my
ar"thre de'ma
ar"thres the'si a
ar thri'tes
ar thrit'ic
ar thrit'i des
ar thri'tis
ar'thro cele
ar"thro cen te'sis
ar"thro chon dri'tis
ar"thro cla'si a
ar thro de'sis
ar thro'di a
ar"thro dyn'i a
ar"thro dyn'ic
ar"thro dys pla'si a
ar"thro em py e'sis
ar"thro en dos'co py
ar"thro er ei'sis
ar throg'ra phy
ar"thro gry po'sis

ar''thro ka tad'y sis
ar'thro lith''
ar''thro li thi'a sis
ar throl'o gy
ar throl'y sis
ar throm'e ter
ar thron'cus
ar throp'a thy
ar'thro phyte
ar''thro plas'tic
ar'thro plas''ty
ar'thro pod
ar''thror rha'gi a
ar'thro scope
ar thros'co py
ar thro'sis
ar'thro spore
ar thros'to my
ar''thro tro'pi a
ar'throus
Arthus re ac'tion
ar tic'u lar
ar''tic u lar'is ge'nus
ar tic'u late
ar tic''u la'ti o
ar tic''u la'tion
ar tic'u la''tor
ar tic'u lus
ar'ti fact
ar''ti fi'cial
ar''y ep''i glot'tic
ar'yl ene
ar''y te''no ep''i glot'i cus
a ryt'e noid
ar''y te''noi dec'to my
ar''y te''noi di'tis
ar''y te noi'do pex''y
ar''y vo cal'is
as''a fet'i da

as''a phi'a
a sar'ci a
as bes'tos
as''bes to'sis
as''ca ri'a sis
as car'i cide
As'ca ris
as cend'ing
Aschheim-Zondek test
Aschoff nod'ule
as ci'tes
as cit'ic
As''co my ce'tes
a scor'bate
a scor'bic ac'id
a se'mi a
a sep'sis
a sep'tic
a sex'u al
ash
Asherman's dis ease'
a''si a'li a
a so'cial
a so'ma
a so'ni a
asp
as''pal a so'ma
as par'a gin
as par'a gin ase
as par'tic
a spas'tic
a''spe cif'ic
as''per gil'ic
as''per gil'lin
as''per gil lo'ma
as per''gil lo'sis
As''per gil'lus
a sper mat'ic
a sper'ma tism

45

a sper"ma to gen'e sis
a sper'mi a
a sper'mous
as phyx'i a
as phyx'i ant
as phyx'i ate
as pid'i um
as'pi rate
as"pi ra'tion
as'pi ra"tor
as'pi rin
a spo"ro gen'ic
a spo'rous
a spor'u late
as sault'
as say'
as sim'il ate
as sim"i la'tion
as so"ci a'tion
as'so nance
as'sue tude
a sta'si a
as tat'ic
a ste"a to'sis
as'ter
a ster"e og no'sis
as te'ri on
as"ter ix'is
a ster'nal
a ster'ni a
as'ter oid
as the'ni a
as then'ic
as"the no bi o'sis
as"the no co'ri a
as"the no ge'ni a
as"the nol'o gy
as"the nom'e ter
as"the no pho'bi a

as"the no'pi a
as"the no sper'mi a
as"the nox'i a
asth'ma
asth mat'ic
as'ti ban
a stig'ma graph
as"tig mat'ic
a stig'ma tism
as"tig mom'e ter
a stig'mo scope
a stom'a tous
a sto'mi a
as trag'a lar
as trag"a lec'to my
as trag'a lus
as'tral
as"tra pho'bi a
as trin'gent
as'tro blast
as"tro blas"to-as"tro cy to'ma
as"tro blas to'ma
as'tro cytes
as"tro cy to'ma
as trog"li o'ma
as'troid
as"tro pho'bi a
as'tro sphere
a styph'i a
a stys'i a
a"syl la'bi a
a sy'lum
a"sym bo'li a
a"sym met'ric
a"sym met'ri cal
a sym'me try
a sym'phy tous
a"symp to mat'ic
as"ymp tot'ic

a syn′chro nism
a syn′cli tism
a syn′de sis
a″syn ech′i a
as″y ner′gi a
as″y ner′ gic
a syn′er gy
a″syn e′si a
as″y no′di a
a″syn tax′i a dor sa′lis
a sys″tem at′ic
a sys′to le
a″sys to′li a
a″sys tol′ic
A′ta brine
at″a bri no der′ma
a tac′tic
a tac′ti form
a″tac til′i a
at ar ac′tic
At′ar ax
at″a rax′ic
a tav′i cus
at′a vism
a tax″a pha′si a
a tax′i a
a tax′i a graph″
a tax′ic
a tax″i o pho′bi a
At′ e brin
at″e lec′ta sis
at″e lec tat′ic
a tel″en ce pha′li a
a te″li o′sis
at″e lo car′di a
at″e lo ceph′a lous
at″e lo chei′li a
at″e lo chei′ri a
at″e lo en″ce pha′li a

at″e lo glos′si a
at″e log nath′i a
at″e lo mit′ic
at″e lo my e′li a
at″e lo po′di a
at″e lo pro so′pi a
at″e lo ra chid′i a
at″e lo sto′mi a
at″e pho′bi a
a the′li a
ath″er o gen′e sis
ath″er o′ma
ath″er o″ma to′sis
ath″er om′a tous
ath″er o″scle ro′sis
ath′e toid″
ath″e to′sis
ath″e tot′ic
a thi″a min o′sis
a threp′si a
a thy′mi a
a thy′mic
a thy re o′sis
at lan″to ax′i al
at lan″to bas i lar′is in ter′nus
at lan″to ep″i stroph′ic
at lan″to-oc cip′i tal
at′las
at lod′y mus
at mom′e ter
at′mos phere
at″mos pher′ic
a to′ci a
at′om
a tom′ic
at″o mic′i ty
at″om i za′tion
a to′ni a
a ton′ic

at′o ny
at′o pen
a top′ic
a top″og no′si a
at′o py
a tox′ic
a tre′mi a
a tre′si a
a tre′sic
a tre″to ceph′a lus
a tre″to cor′mus
a tre″to cys′ti a
a tre″to gas′tri a
a tre″to le′mi a
a tre″to me′tri a
at″re top′si a
a tret″or rhin′i a
a tre″to sto′mi a
a tret″u re′thri a
a′tri a
a′tri al
at″ri cho′sis
at′ri chous
a″tri o sep″to pex′y
a″tri o ven tric′u lar
a″tri o ven tric″u lar′is
a′tri um
at″ro pho der′ma
at″ro pho der″ma to′sis
at′ro phy
at′ro pine
at′ ro pin ism
at ro″pin i za′tion
at′ro pin ize
at″tar
at ten′tion
at ten′u ate
at ten′u at ed
at ten″u a′tion

at′tic
at″ti co an trot′o my
at″ti co mas′toid
at″ti cot′o my
at′ti tude
at ton′i ty
at trac′tion
at tri′tion
a typ′i cal
au″di mu′tism
au″di o ep″i lep′tic
au″di o gen′ic
au di o gram″
au″di ol′o gist
au″di ol′o gy
au″di om′e ter
au″di o met′ric
au″di om′e try
au″di o vis′u al
au di′tion
au′di tive
au″di tog no′sis
au″di to psy′chic
au′di to″ry
au″di to sen′so ry
Auerbach plex′us
aug′ment
aug″men ta′tion
aug na′thus
au″lo pho′bi a
au′lo phyte
au′ra
au′rae
au′ral
Au″re o my′cin
au′ric
au′ri cle
au ric′u lar
au ric″u la′re

au''ric u lar'is
au ric''u lo fron tal'is
au ric''u lo tem'po ral
au ric''u lo ven tric'u lar
au'ris
au'rist
au ro''ra pho'bi a
au''ro ther'a py
au'rous
aus'cu late
aus cult'
aus''cul ta'tion
aus''cul'ta to ry
au'ta coid
au te'cious
au te me'si a
au'tism
au tis'tic
au''to ac''ti va'tion
au''to ag glu''ti na'tion
au''to ag glu'ti nin
au''to al''go lag'ni a
au''to a nal'y sis
au''to an''am ne'sis
au''to an''ti bi o'sis
au''to an' ti bod''y
au''to an'ti gen
au''to au'di ble
au'to blast
au''to ca tal'y sis
auto cat'al yst
au''to ca thar'sis
au toch'tho nous
au toc'la sis
au'to clave
au''to con''den sa'tion
au''to con duc'tion
au''to cy''to tox'in
au''to di ges'tion

au''to ech''o la'li a
au''to ech''o prax'i a
au''to ec''ze ma ti za'tion
au''to e mas''cu la'tion
au''to e rot ic
au''to er ot'i cism
au''to er'o tism
au''to fel la'ti o
au tog'a mous
au tog'a my
au''to gen'ic
au tog'e nous
au'to graft''
au'to graph''
au''to he mol'y sis
au''to he''mo ther'a py
au''to hy drol'y sis
au''to hyp no'sis
au''to hyp not'ic
au''to hyp'no tism
au''to im mune'
au''to im mun''i za'tion
au''to in fec'tion
au''to in fu'sion
au''to in oc''u la'tion
au''to in tox'i cant
au''to in tox''i ca'tion
au''to i''so ly'sin
au''to kin e'sis
au tol'o gous
au tol'y sate
au tol'y sin
au tol'y sis
au''to lyt'ic
au'to lyze
au''to mat'ic
au tom'a tin
au tom''a tin'o gen
au tom'a tism

au tom"a ti za'tion
au"to mat'o gen
au tom'a ton
au"to my"so pho'bi a
au"to ne phrec'to my
au"to no ma'si a
au"to nom'ic
au ton'o mous
au"to-oph thal'mo scope
au'to-ox"i da'tion
au top'a thy
au"to pha'gi a
au"to phil'i a
au"to pho'bi a
au"to pho"no ma'ni a
au toph'o ny
au'to plast
au'to plas'tic
au'to plas"ty
au"to pneu"mo nec'to my
au"to pro tol'y sis
au'top sy
au"to psy'che
au"to psy'chic
au"to psy cho'sis
au"to ra'di o gram
au"to ra'di o graph
au"to ra"di og'ra phy
au"to re in fu'sion
au"to sen"si ti za'tion
au'to site
au"to som'al
au'to some
au"to sug ges'tion
au"to syn'de sis
au"to syn noi'a
au tot'o my
au"to top ag no'si a
au"to trans form'er

au"to trans fu'sion
au"to trans"plan ta'tion
au'to troph
au"to vac"ci na'tion
au"to vac'cine
aux an'o gram
aux"a nog'ra phy
aux e'sis
aux et'ic
aux"o bar'ic
aux"o car'di a
aux'o chrome
aux'o cyte
aux'o drome
aux om'e ter
av'a lanche
a val'vu lar
a vas'cu lar
a vas"cu lar i za'tion
a ve'nin
A ven'tyl
av'er age
A'ver tin
a'vi an
a vid'i ty
a vir'u lent
a vi"ta min o'sis
a vo ca'li a
Avogadro's law
av"oir du pois'
a vul'sion
ax"an thop'si a
ax"i a'tion
ax if'u gal
ax il'la
ax'ill ary
ax'is
ax"o den drit'ic
ax"o fu'gal

ax'oid
ax"o lem'ma
ax om'e ter
ax'on
ax'o neme"
ax"o nom'e ter
ax"on ot me'sis
ax op'e tal
ax' o plasm"
Ayerza's dis ease'
a yp' ni a
a ze' o trope
az'ide
az'ine
az"o ben'zene
az"o car'mine

az'o dyes
a zo"o sper'mi a
az"o pro'te in
az o ru'bin
az"o te'mi a
Az"o to bac'ter
az"o tom'e ter
az"o tor rhe'a
az"o tu'ri a
az'ure
a zu'ro phile"
az"y go ag'na thus
a"zyg og'raphy
az'y gos
a zy'mi a
a zym'ic

B

Babinski, sign
ba'by
bac'ci form
bac'il lar"y
bac"il le'mi a
ba cil'li
ba cil'li form
ba cil"lo my'cin
ba cil"lo pho'bi a
bac"il lu'ri a
ba cil'lus
ba"ci tra'cin
back'ache"
back'bone"
back'ward ness
bac"te re'mi a
bac te'ri a
Bac te"ri a'ce ae
bac te ri cid'al
bac te'ri cide

bac"te ri ci'din
bac'te rid
bac ter"i o chlor'o phyll
bac te"ri o ci'din
bac te"ri oc'la sis
bac te"ri o er'y thrin
bac te"ri o flu"o res'cin
bac te"ri o gen'ic
bac te"ri o he"mo ly'sin
bac te'ri oid
bac te"ri o log'ic
bac te"ri ol'o gist
bac te"ri ol'o gy
bac te"ri o ly'sin
bac te"ri ol'y sis
bac te'ri o phage
bac te"ri o phag'ic
bac te"ri o pha gol'o gy
bac te"ri o pho'bi a
bac te"ri o pro'te in

bac te"ri op'so nin
bac te"ri os'co py
bac te"ri os'ta sis
bac te'ri o stat"
bac te"ri o stat'ic
bac te"ri o ther a peu'tic
bac te"ri o ther'a py
bac te"ri o tox'ic
bac te"ri o tox'in
bac te"ri o trop'ic
bac te"ri ot'ro pin
Bac te'ri um
bac te"ri u'ri a
bac'ter oid
Bac"ter o'i des
baf' fle
ba"gas so'sis
Ba hi'a ul'cer
Baker's cyst
BAL
bal'ance
ba lan'ic
bal'a nism
bal"a ni'tis
bal"a no chlam"y di'tis
bal'a no plas"ty
bal"a no pos thi'tis
bal"a no pre pu'tial
bal"a nor rha'gi a
bal"an or rhe'a
bal"an ti di'a sis
Bal"an tid'i um
bal'a nus
bald'ness
Bal'four
bal'ism
bal lis"to car'di o gram
bal lis"to car'di o graph
bal lis"to pho'bi a

bal lonne ment'
bal loon'ing
bal lotte ment'
balm
bal"ne ol'o gy
bal"ne o ther'a py
bal'sam
band'age
Bandl's ring
Bang's dis ease'
ban'minth
ban'thine
Banti's dis ease'
Banting
bar"ag no'sis
barb
bar'ba
bar"bar a la'li a
bar'bi tal
bar'bi tone
bar bit'u rate
bar"bi tu ric
bar'bi tu rism
bar bo tage'
bar"es the'si a
bar"es the"si om'e ter
bar"i to'sis
ba'ri um
bar'ley
barn
bar"o cep'tor
bar"o don tal'gi a
bar"og no'sis
bar'o graph
bar"o ma crom'e ter
ba rom'e ter
bar o met'ric
bar"o pho'bi a
bar'o scope

ba ros'min
bar"o tal'gi a
bar"o ti'tis
bar"o trau'ma
bar'ren ness
bar'ri er
Bartholin's gland
bar"tho lin i'tis
bar"to nel lo'sis
bar"y la'li a
bar"y pho'ni a
ba'sal
bas"cu la'tion
bas'cule
base
base'ment
bas-fond
ba"si al ve'o lar
ba"si bran'chi al
ba"si chro'ma tin
ba sic'i ty
ba"si cra'ni al
ba sid'i o phore"
ba sid'i o spore"
ba sid'i um
ba"si fa'cial
ba"si hy'al
ba'si lar
ba"si lat'er al
ba sil'ic
ba sil"o breg mat'ic
ba sil"o men'tal
ba sil"o pha ryn'ge al
ba"si na'sal
ba"si o al ve'o lar
ba"si oc cip'i tal
ba'si on
ba'si o tribe"
ba'si o trip"sy

ba"si pho'bi a
ba"si pre sphen'oid
ba"si rhi'nal
ba'sis
ba"si sphe'noid
ba"si syl'vi an
ba"si tem'po ral
ba"si ver'te bral
bas'ket
ba'so phil
ba"so phil'i a
ba"so phil'ic
ba soph'i lism
ba"so pho'bi a
ba"so pho'bic
ba'so plasm
bas"si net'
bath
bath"es the'si a
bath"o pho'bi a
bath"y car'di a
bath"y chro'mic
bat"o pho'bi a
bat'ta rism
bat'ter ed
bat'ter y
baux'ite
BCG
bead'ed
beam
beat
bed'bug"
bed'fast"
Bednar's aph'thae
bed'pan"
bed'rid"den
bed'sore"
be ha'vi or"ism
bel

bel'che
bel 'la don'na
bel len'gol
bel lones'
bel'ly
bel'ly ache"
bel"o ne pho'bi a
Ben'a dryl
Bence-Jones's pro'te in
Bender-Gestalt
bends
Benedict's re a'gent
be nign'
benz'a thine
ben'ze drine
ben'zene
ben'zi dine
ben'zo ate
ben zo'ic
ben'zo ic ac'id
ben'zo in
ben'zyl
Ber'i-Ber'i
be ryl"li o'sis
be ryl'li um
bes"ti al'i ty
be'ta
be'ta cism
be'ta ine
be"ta to'pic
be'ta tron
be'tel
be'va tron
bev'el
be'zoar
bi ax'i al
bib'li o clast"
bib"li o klep"to ma'ni a
bib"li o ma'ni a

bib"li o pho'bi a
bib"li o ther'a py
bi cap'i tate
bi car'bon ate
bi car'di o gram
bi'ceps
bi chlo'ride
bi chro'mate
bi cil'lin
bi cor'nate
bi cus'pid
bi dac'ty ly
bi"e lec trol'y sis
bi'fid
bi fo'cal
bi for'min
bi'fur cate
bi"fur ca'tion
bi gem'i nal
bi gem'i ny
bi'labe
bi lat'er al
bile
bil"har zi'a sis
bil'i ar"y
bi lig'u late
bil"i hu'min
bil"i neu'rine
bil'ious
bil'ious ness
bil"i pha'in
bil"i ru'bin
bil"i ru"bi ne'mi a
bil'i ru"bin-glo'bin
bil"i ru"bi nu'ri a
bil"i ther a'py
bil"i u'ri a
bil"i ver'din
Billroth op"e ra'tion

bi lo'bate
bi loc'u lar
bil'ron
bi man'u al
bi'na ry
bi na'sal
bin au'ral
bind'er
Binet's test
bin oc'u lar
bi'o as say"
bi"o aut og'ra phy
bi'o blast
bi"o chem'i cal
bi"o chem'is try
bi'o chrome
bi"o dy nam'ic
bi"o-e lec"tric'i ty
bi"o flav'o noids
bi"o gen'e sis
bi og'en ous
bi"o ki net'ics
bi'o lac
bi o log'ic
bi"o log'i cal
bi ol'o gist
bi ol'o gy
bi"o lu"mi nes'cence
bi"o math"e mat'ics
bi"o me chan'ics
bi om'e ter
bi om'e try
bi"o mi cros'co py
bi'o phore
bi"o pho tom'e ter
bi"o phys'ics
bi op'la sis
bi'op sy
bi'ose

bi"o sta tis'tics
bi"o syn'the sis
Biot's breath'ing
bi ot'ic
bi'o tin
bi'o type
bi"o ty pol'o gy
bip'a ra
bi par"a sit'ic
bi"pa ri'e tal
bip'a rous
bi'ped
bip'e dal
bi pen'ni form
bi po'lar
bi"po lar'i ty
bi"po ten"ti al'i ty
bi"re frac'tive
bi"re frin'gence
bi rhin'i a
bi ri'mose
birth
birth'mark"
birth rate
bi sex'u al
bis fe'ri ous
bis il'i ac
bis is'chi al
bis'muth
bis mu'thi a
bis"muth o'sis
bis'sa
bis"sy no'sis
bis'tou ry
bi sul'fide
bi sul'fite
bite'wing
bi thi'o nal
Bitot's spots

bit'ters
bi tu'men
bi''u ret're ac'tion
biv'a lence
bi va'lent
bi'valve''
bi ven'ter
black'damp''
black'head''
black'leg''
black'out''
black'tongue''
blad'der
Blalock, Alfred
blas te'ma
blas'tin
blas'to chyle
blas'to coele
blas'to cyst
blas'to derm
blas'to disk
blas''to gen'e sis
blas tog'e ny
blas''to ki ne'sis
blas tok'o lin
blas tol'y sis
blas to'ma
blas tom''a to gen'ic
blas'to mere
Blas''to my'ces
Blas''to my ce'tes
blas''to my co'sis
blas''to neu'ro pore
blas'to pore
blas'to sphere
blas'to spore
blas tot'o my
blas'tu la
bleb

bleed'er
blen''noph thal'mi a
blen''nor rha'gi a
blen''nor rhe'a
bleph''ar ad''e ni'tis
bleph'a ral
bleph''a rec'to my
bleph''ar e de'ma
bleph''ar e lo'sis
bleph'a rism
bleph''ar it'is
bleph''a ro ad''e ni'tis
bleph''a ro ad''e no'ma
bleph''a ro ath''er o'ma
bleph''a ro blen''nor rhe'a
bleph''a ro chal'a sis
bleph''a ro chrom''hi dro'sis
bleph''a ro clei'sis
bleph''a roc'lo nus
bleph''a ro col''o bo'ma
bleph''a ro con junc''ti vi'tis
bleph''a ro di as'ta sis
bleph''a ro dys chroi'a
bleph''a ro me las'ma
bleph'a ron
bleph''a ron'cus
bleph''a ro pa chyn'sis
bleph''a ro phi mo'sis
bleph''a roph ry plas'tic
bleph''a roph'ry plas'ty
bleph''a ro phy'ma
bleph'a ro plast''
bleph'a ro plas''ty
bleph''a ro ple'gi a
bleph''a rop to'sis
bleph''a ro py''or rhe'a
bleph''a ror'rha phy
bleph'a ro spasm''
bleph''a ro sphinc''ter ec'to my

bleph'a ro stat"
bleph"a ro ste no'sis
bleph"a ro sym'phy sis
bleph"a ro syn ech'i a
bleph"a rot'o my
bleph"so path'i a
blight
blind'ness
blink'ing
blis'ter
bloat
blood
blow'fly"
Bodansky's meth'od
bod'y
Boeck's sar'coid
boil
bo lom'e ter
bo'lus
bon'a mine
bo'rate
bo'rax
bor"bo ryg'mus
bor'der
bo'ric ac'id
bo'ron
Bor re'li a
bot'a ny
bot'fly"
both'ri oid
both'ri um
bot'ry oid
bot"ry o my co'sis
bot'u li form
bot u li'nus
bot'u lism
bou"gie'
bouil"lon'
bour'bo nac

bour donne ment'
bo'vine
bow'el
bow'leg"
brace
bra'chi a
bra'chi al
bra"chi al'gi a
bra"chi a'lis
bra'chi form
bra"chi o cyl lo'sis
brach"i o ra"di al'sis
bra"chi ot'o my
bra'chi um
brach"y car'di a
brach"y ce pha'li a
brach"y ce phal'ic
brach"y chei'li a
brach"y chei'rous
brach"y dac tyl'i a
brach"y glos'sal
brach"y glos'si a
brach"yg nath'ous
brach"y ker'kic
brach"y me tap'o dy
brach"y mei o'sis
brach"y morph'ic
brach"y mor'phy
brach"y pel'lic
brach"y pha lan'gi a
brach"y po'dous
brach"y pro sop'ic
brach"y rhin'i a
brach"y rhyn'chus
brach"y skel'ic
brach"y staph'y line
brach"y sta'sis
brach"y u ran'ic
brad"y ar'thri a

brad"y aux e'sis
brad"y car'di a
brad"y crot'ic
brad"y di as'to le
brad"y glos'si a
brad"y ki ne'si a
brad"y ki net'ic
bra"dy ki'nin
brad"y la'li a
brad'y lex'i a
brad"y pha'si a
brad"y phre'ni a
brad"y pne'a
brad"y pra'gi a
brad"y prax'i a
brad"y rhyth'mi a
brad"y tel"e o ki ne'sis
Braille, Louis
brain
bran'chi al
branch'ing
bran"chi o gen'ic
bran"chi og'e nous
bran"chi o'ma
bran'chi o mere"
bran"chi om'er ism
bran'dy
brawn'y
Braxton Hicks's con trac'tion
break'bone" fe'ver
breast
breast'bone
breath
breath'ing
breech
breg'ma
breg mat'ic
breg mat"o dym'i a
brev"i col'lis

brev"i lin'e al
bridge
bridge'work"
bri'dle
bright'ness
bril'liance
broach
Broadbent's sign
Broca, Pierre
Brodie's ab'scess
bro'mate
bro"ma tom'e try
bro"ma to ther'a py
bro"ma to tox'in
brom"hi dro'sis
bro'mide
bro'mine
bro'min ism
bro'mism
bro"mo cre'sol green
bro"mo der'ma
bro"mo hy"per hi dro'sis
bro"mo ma'ni a
bro"mo men"or rhe'a
bro"mo phe'nol blue
bro"mo selt'zer
bro"mo thy'mol blue
brom"sul'pha lein
bronch ad"e ni'tis
bron'chi
bron'chi al
bron"chi ec'ta sis
bron"chi o gen'ic
bron chi'o lar
bron'chi ole
bron"chi o lec'ta sis
bron"chi o li'tis
bron chit'ic
bron chi'tis

bron'cho cele''
bron''cho con stric'tor
bron''cho dil''a ta'tion
bron''cho di la'tor
bron''cho e de'ma
bron''cho e soph''a ge'al
bron''cho e soph''a gol'o gy
bron''cho e soph''a gos'co py
bron''cho gen'ic
bron'cho gram
bron chog'ra phy
bron'cho lith
bron''cho li thi'a sis
bron chol'o gy
bron''cho mo ni li'a sis
bron''cho mo'tor
bron''cho my co'sis
bron chop'a thy
bron choph'o ny
bron'cho plas''ty
bron''cho pleu'ral
bron''cho pneu mo'ni a
bron''cho pneu''mo ni'tis
bron''cho pul'mo na ry
bron chor'rha phy
bron''chor rhe'a
bron'cho scope
bron chos'copy
bron'cho spasm
bron''cho spi''ro che to'sis
bron''cho spi rog'ra phy
bron''cho spi rom'e ter
bron''cho spi rom'e try
bron''cho ste no'sis
bron chos'to my
bron chot'o my
bron''cho ve sic'u lar
bron'chus
bron''to pho'bi a

Brown-Séquard, Charles E.
Bru cel'la
bru''cel ler'gen
bru cel'lin
bru''cel lo'sis
bruc'ine
Brudzinski's re'flex
bruise
bruisse ment'
bruit
brux'ism
brux''o ma'ni a
bryg'mus
bu'bo
bu''bon ad''e ni'tis
bu''bon al'gi a
bu bon'ic plague
bu bon'o cele
bu bon'u lus
bu car'di a
buc'ca
buc'cal
buc'ci na''tor
buc''co ax'i al
buc''coc clu'sal
buc''co cer'vi cal
buc''co dis'tal
buc''co fa'cial ob'tu ra''tor
buc''co gin'gi val
buc''co la'bi al
buc''co lin'gual
buc''co me'si al
buc''co na'sal
buc''co na''so pha ryn'ge al
buc''co pha ryn'ge al
buc''co phar yn'ge us
buc''co pulp'al
buc''co ver'sion
buc'cu la

Buerger's dis ease'
bu'fa gins
buff'er
bug'gery
bulb
bul''bo cav''er no'sus
bul''bo nu'cle ar
bul''bo spon''gi o'sus
bul''bo u re'thral
bulb'ous
bul''bo ven tric'u lar
bul'bus
bul'bus ar te''ri o'sus
bul'bus cor'dis
bu le'sis
bu lim'i a
bu lim'ic
bull'ae
bul la'tion
bun'dle
bun'ion
bun''ion ec'to my
bu'no dont
buph thal' mi a

bur
bu ret'
burn
bur'nish er
bur'row
bur'sa
bur sat'tee
bur sec'to my
bur si'tis
bur'so lith
bur sop'a thy
bur sot'o my
bu''ta bar'bi tal
bu'ta caine''
bu''ta di ene
bu'tane
but'ter
but'tock
but'tress
bu'tyl
bu tyr'ic
bu'tyr oid
bys''si no'sis
bys'soid

C

ca ca'o
ca chec'tic
ca chet'
ca chex'i a
cach''in na'tion
ca''chou'
cac''o de mo'ni a
cac'o dyl
cac'o dyl ate
cac o phon'ic
ca coph'o ny
ca cos'mi a

ca dav'er
ca dav'er ic
ca dav'er ine
ca dav'er ous
cad'mi um
ca du'ce us
cae''ru lo plas'min
cafe' au lait
caf'er gone
caf'fe ine
caf'fe in ism
cai''no pho'bi a

cais'son
Cajal, Ramón
Cal'a bar swel'lings
ca lage'
cal'a mine
ca'la mus scrip to'ri us
cal ca'ne al
cal ca''ne o ca'vus
cal ca''ne o cu'boid
cal ca''ne o dyn'i a
cal ca''ne c na vic'u lar
cal ca''ne o val'gus
cal ca'ne us
cal'car
cal car'e ous
cal car''i u'ri a
cal ce'mi a
cal'cic
cal''ci co'sis
cal cif'er ol
cal cif'ic
cal''ci fi ca'tion
cal'ci fied
cal'ci fy
cal cig'er ous
cal'ci grade
cal cim'e ter
cal''ci na'tion
cal''ci no'sis
cal''ci pe'ni a
cal''ci to'nin
cal'ci um
cal''ci u'ri a
cal''co glob'u lin
cal''co sphe'rite
cal''cu lo gen'e sis
cal''cu lo'sis
cal'cu lous
cal'cu lus

cal''e fa'cient
calf
calf'-bone
cal'i brate
cal''i bra'tion
cal'i bra''tor
ca''li ec'ta sis
cal'i pers
cal''is then'ics
cal''li pe'di a
cal''lo ma'ni a
cal lo'sal
cal los'i tas
cal los'i ty
cal lo''so mar'gin al
cal lo'sum
cal'lous
cal'lus
cal'o mel
cal'or
cal''o ra'di ance
cal''o res'cence
ca lor'ic
cal'o rie
cal''o rif'ic
ca lor''i gen'ic
cal''o rim'e ter
ca lor''i met'ric
cal''o rim'e try
cal va'ri a
Calve, Jacques
cal vi'ti es
cal'vous
calx
ca'lyx
cam'bi um
cam'er a
cam'i sole
cam'phene

cam'phor
cam"pho ra'ceous
cam'phor ate
cam'phor ism
cam"phor o ma'ni a
cam pim'e ter
camp"to cor'mi a
camp"to dac'ty ly
camp'to spasm
ca nal'
can"a lic'u lar
can"a lic'u li
can al ic"u lo plas'ty
can"a lic'u lus
ca nal"i za'tion
can"al og'ra phy
can'cel lous
can'cer
can"cer o'gen
can"cer ol'o gist
can"cer ol'o gy
can"cer o pho'bi a
can'croid
can'crum o'ris
can"di ci'din
Can'di da al'bi cans
can"di di'as is
can"di did'
can'dle
ca nel'la
ca'nine
ca ni'nus
ca ni'ti es
can'ker
can"na bid'i ol
can'na bine
can nab'in oc
can nab'i nol
can'na bis

can'na bism
can"ni bal is'tic
can'nu la
can'nu lar
can"tha ri'a sis
can thar'i des
can thec'to my
can thi'tis
can thol'y sis
can'tho plas"ty
can thor'rha phy
can thot' o my
can'thus
ca pac'i tance
ca pac'i tate
ca pac'i tor
ca pac'i ty
cap"il lar"ec ta'si a
cap"il la rim'e ter
cap"il lar'i ty
cap"il la ros'co py
cap'il lar"y
cap"il li'ti um
cap"il lo ve'nous
ca pil'lus
cap'i tate
cap"i ta"tum
cap"i tel'lum
ca pit'u lar
ca pit'u lum
cap'ra col
cap'ric
ca pro'ic
ca pryl'ic
cap'su lar
cap'sule
cap"su lec'to my
cap"su li'tis
cap'su lo plas"ty

cap"su lor'rha phy
cap'su lo tome"
cap"su lot'o my
cap ta'tion
cap"ture
ca'put
car'a pace
car"ba mi no he"mo glo'bin
Car'bar sone
car'ba sus
carb he"me glo'bin
car'bi nol
car"bo cy'clic
car"bo hy'drase
car"bo hy'drate
car"bo hy"dra tu'ri a
car'bo late
car bol'ic
car"bo lism
car"bo lu'ri a
car bo my'cin
car'bon
car'bon ate
car'bon a"ted
car bo'nic
car bo'ni um
car"bon i za'tion
car'bon ize
car"bon om'e ter
car"bon u'ri a
car"bo run'dum
carbo'wax
car box"y he"mo glo'bin
car box'yl
car box'yl ase
car'bun cle
car bun'cu lar
car'bun"cu lo'sis
car'ci no gen

car"ci no gen'e sis
car ci"no gen'ic
car'ci noid
car"ci no'ma
car"ci nom'a toid
car"ci no"ma to'sis
car"ci no'ma tous
car"ci no sar co'ma
car'ci nous
car'di a
car'di ac
car"di al'gi a
car"di am'e ter
car"di a neu'ri a
car"di asth'ma
car"di ec'ta sis
car"di ec'to my
car"di o ac cel'er a"tor
car"di o ac'tive
car"di o an"gi ol'o gy
car"di o-a or'tic
car"di o ar te'ri al
car'di o cele
car"di o cen te'sis
car"di o cir rho'sis
car"di oc'la sis
car"di o di la'tor
car"di o di o'sis
car"di o dy nam'ics
car"di o dy"na mom'et ry
car"di o dyn'i a
car"di o e soph"a ge'al
car"di o gen'e sis
car"di o gen'ic
car'di o gram"
car'di o graph"
car"di o graph'ic
car"di og'ra phy

car"di o he pat'ic
car'di oid
car"di o in hib'i to"ry
car"di o ki net'ic
car"di o ky mog'ra phy
car"di o lip'in
car'di o lith
car"di ol'o gist
car"di ol'o gy
car"di ol'y sis
car"di o ma la'ci a
car"di o meg'a ly
car"di o mel'a no'sis
car"di o men'su ra tor
car"di o men'to pex"y
car"di om'e ter
car"di om'e try
car"di o my'o pex"y
car"di o my ot'o my
car"di o nec'tor
car"di o neph'ric
car"di o neu'ral
car"di o pal'u dism
car'di o path
car di o path'ic
car"di o pa thol'o gy
car"di op'a thy
car"di o per"i car'di o pex"y
car"dio per"i car di'tis
car"di o pho'bi a
car'di o phone
car'di o plas"ty
car"di o ple'gi a
car"di o pneu mat'ic
car"di o pneu'mo graph
car"di op to'sis
car"di o pul'mo nar y
car"di o punc'ture
car"di o py lor'ic

car"di o re'nal
car"di o re spir'a to"ry
car"di o roent'gen o gram"
car"di o roent"gen og'ra phy
car"di or'rha phy
car"di or rhex'is
car"di os'chi sis
car'di o scope"
car'di o spasm"
car"di o spec'tro gram
car"di o spec'tro graph
car"di o ste no'sis
car"di o ta chom'e ter
car"di o ther'a py
car"di ot'o my
car"di o ton'ic
car"di o tox'ic
car"di o vas'cu lar
car"di o vas'cu lar-re'nal
car"di o vec tog'ra phy
car di'tis
car"di val"vu li'tis
car"e bar'i a
ca'ri es
ca ri'na
car"i o gen'ic
car min'a tive
car'mine
car"ni fi ca'tion
car"no si ne'mi a
car'ob
car'o tene
car'o te ne'mi a
car"o te"no der'ma
ca rot'e noid
car"o te no'sis
ca rot'ic
ca rot"i co cli'noid
ca rot"i co tym pan'ic

ca rot'id
ca rot'is
car''ot o dyn'i a
car'pal
car pec'to my
car phol'o gy
car pi'tis
car''po met''a car'pal
car''po pe'dal
car''po pha lan'ge al
car'pus
car'ri er
car sick'ness
car'ti lage
car''ti la gin''i fi ca'tion
car''ti lag'in ous
car'un cle
car un'cu lar
car''y o clas'tic
car''y o phyl'lin
cas car'a
case
ca'se ase
ca'se ate
ca''se a'tion
ca'sec
ca'se in
ca''se in'o gen
ca'se ose
ca'se ous
cas''sette'
cast
cast'ing
cas'tor
cas'trate
cas tra'tion
cas''tro phre'ni a
cas'u al ty
cas''u is'tics

cat''a ba'si al
ca tab'a sis
cat a bol'ic
ca tab'o lin
ca tab'o lism
ca tab'o lite
cat''a clo'nic
cat''a clo'nus
cat''a cous'tics
cat''a crot'ic
cat ac'ro tism
cat''a gel''o pho'bi a
cat'a lase
cat'a lep''sy
cat a lep'tic
cat''a lep''to le thar'gic
ca tal'y sis
cat'a lyst
cat''a lyt'ic
cat'a ly''zer
cat''a me'ni a
cat''am ne'sis
cat''am nes'tic
cat''a mor'pho sis
cat'a pasm
cat''a pha'si a
ca taph'o ra
cat''a pho re'sis
cat''a pho'ri a
cat''a phor'ic
cat''a phy lax'is
cat''a pla'si a
cat'a plasm
cat''a plec'tic
cat'a plex''y
cat'a ract
ca tarrh'
ca tarrh'al
cat''a stal'sis

cat'a state
cat"a thy'mi a
cat"a to'ni a
cat"a ton'ic
cat"a tro'pi a
cat'e chol"am'ines
cat"e lec"trot'o nus
cat'er pil"lar
cat'gut"
ca thar'sis
ca thar'tic
ca thect'
ca thep'sin
ca ther'e sis
cath"e ret'ic
cath'e ter
cath'e ter ism
cath"e ter i za'tion
cath'e ter ize
cath'e ter o stat"
ca thex'is
cath'od al
cath'ode
ca thod'ic
cat'i"on
cat ion'ic
cat'lin
cat'a dont
ca top'trics
ca top'tro scope
cau'da
cau'dad
cau'dal
cau da'tum
cau"do ceph'al ad
caul
cau'line
cau"lo ple'gi a
cau"mes the'si a

cau sal'gi a
cause
caus'tic
cau'ter ant
cau"ter i za'tion
cau'ter ize
cau'ter y
ca'va
cav'al ry bone
cav'ern
cav"ern i'tis
cav"er no'ma
cav"er no si'tis
cav er nos'to my
cav"er no'sum
cav'er nous
cav'i tas
cav"i ta'tion
cav'i ty
ca'vus
ce"bo ce pha'li a
ce"bo ceph'a lus
ce"bo ceph'a ly
ce cec'to my
ce ci'tis
ce'ci ty
ce'co cele
ce"co co los'to my
ce"co il"e os'to my
ce'co pex"y
ce"co pli ca'tion
ce"cop to'sis
ce cor'rha phy
ce"co sig"moid os'to my
ce cos'to my
ce cot'o my
ce'cum
ce'dar
Ce"di lan'id

ce'li ac
ce"li a del'phus
ce"li ec ta'si a
ce"li o col pot'o my
ce"li o en"ter ot'o my
ce"li o gas trot'o my
ce"li o hys"ter ec'to my
ce"li o hys"ter ot'o my
ce"li o my"o mec'to my
ce"li o par"a cen te'sis
ce"li or'rha phy
ce"li os'co py
ce"li ot'o my
ce li'tis
cell
cel'la
cel loi'din
Cel'lo phane
cell'u lar
cel'lu lase
cel'lule
cel"lu lif'u gal
cel"lu li'tis
cel"lu lo'sa
cel'lu lose
ce'lo scope
ce"lo so'ma
ce"lo so'mus
ce"lo the"li o'ma
ce ment'
ce men'ti cle
ce men"ti fi ca'tion
ce men'to blast
ce men"to blas to'ma
ce men"to den'ti nal
ce men"to gen'e sis
ce"men to'ma
ce men"to per"i os-ti'tis
ce"men to'sis

ce men'tum
ce"nes the'si a
ce"nes thet'ic
ce"nes thop'a thy
ce"no gen'e sis
cen'sor ship
cen'ter
cen'ter ing
cen te'sis
cen'ti bar
cen'ti grade
cen'ti gram
cen'ti li"ter
cen'ti me"ter
cen"ti nor'mal
cen'ti pede
cen'ti poise
cen'trad
cen'trage
cen'tra phose
cen"trax o'ni al
cen"tren ce phal'ic
cen tric'i put
cen trif'u gal
cen'tri fuge
cen'tri ole
cen trip'e tal
cen'tro cyte
cen"tro des'mose
cen"tro lec'i thal
cen'tro mere
cen'tro phose
cen'tro some
cen'tro sphere"
cen'trum
ceph'al
ceph'al ad
ceph"a lal'gi a
ceph'a lal"gic

ceph"a le'a
ceph a lex'in
ceph"al'gi a
ceph"al he"ma to'ma
ceph"al hy'dro cele
ce phal'ic
ceph'a lin
ceph"a li za'tion
ceph"a lo cau'dal
ceph'a lo cele"
ceph"a lo cen te'sis
ceph'a lo chord"
ceph"a lo di pro'so pus
ceph"a lo gen'e sis
ceph"a lo gly'cin
ceph'a lo graph"
ceph"a log'ra phy
ceph"a lo gy'ric
ceph"a lo he mat'o cele"
ceph"a lo he mom'e ter
ceph'a loid
ceph a lo'ma
ceph"a lom'e lus
ceph"a lo me'ni a
ceph"a lo men"in gi'tis
ceph"a lom'e ter
ceph"a lom'e try
ceph"a lo'ni a
ceph"a lo-or'bi tal
ceph"a lop'a gus
ceph"a lop'a thy
ceph"a lo pel'vic
ceph"a lo pha ryn'ge us
ceph"a lo ple'gi a
ceph"a los'co py
ceph"a lo spo'rin
ceph"a lo spo"ri o'sis
Ceph"a lo spo'ri um
ceph"a lo tho rac'ic

ceph"a lo tho"ra cop'a gus
ceph'a lo tome
ceph"a lot'o my
ceph'a lo trac'tor
ceph'a lo tribe
ceph"a lo trid'y mus
ceph'a lo trip"sy
ceph"a lo trip'tor
ceph"a lo try pe'sis
ceph"a lox'i a
cer"a to cri'coid
cer"a to phar yn'geus
cer ca'ri a
cer ca'ri al
cer clage'
ce're a flex"i bil'i tas
cer"e bel'lar
cer"e bel lif'u gal
cer"e bel lip'e tal
cer"e bel li'tis
cer"e bel lo pon'tine
cer"e bel lo ret'i nal he"man
   gi o blas"to ma to'sis
cer"e bel"lo ru'bral
cer"e bel"lo ru"bro spi'nal
cer"e bel"lo spi'nal
cer"e bel'lum
cer'e bral
cer'e bra'tion
cer'e bric
cer'e brif'u gal
cer'e brin
cer"e brip'e tal
cer"e bri'tis
cer"e bro ma la'ci a
cer"e bro med'ul lar"y
cer"e bro phys"i ol'o gy
cer"e bro pon'tine
cer"e bro scle ro'sis

cer'e brose
cer'e bro side
cer''e bro spi'nal
cer''e bro to'ni a
cer''e bro to'nin
cer''e bro vas'cu lar
cer'e brum
ce're ous
ce'ri um
ce'roid
ce ro'sis
cer'ti fi''a ble
cer tif'i cate
ce'ru lo''plas min
ce ru'men
ce ru''mi no'sis
ce ru'min ous
cer'vi cal
cer''vi cec'to my
cer''vi ci'tis
cer''vi co ax'i al
cer''vi co brach'i al''gi a
cer''vi co buc'cal
cer''vi co buc''co ax'i al
cer''vi co dyn'i a
cer''vi co fa'cial
cer''vi co la'bi al
cer''vi co lin'gual
cer''vi co pu'bic
cer''vi co rec'tal
cer''vi co u'ter ine
cer''vi co vag'i nal
cer''vi co vag''i ni'tis
cer''vi co ves'i cal
cer'vix
Ce sar'e an sec'tion
ces to'da
ces'tode
ce''vi tam'ic ac'id

Chadwick's sign
chae to'min
cha'fing
Chagas' dis ease'
cha la'si a
cha la'za
cha la'zi a
cha la'zi on
chal co'sis
chal''i co'sis
chalk
chal'one
cha lyb'e ate
cham'ber
cham''e ceph'a lus
cham''e ceph'a ly
cham'e conch''
cham''e cra'ni al
cham''e pro sop'ic
chan'cre
chan'croid
chan croi'dal
chan'nel
chap
char'ac ter
char'coal''
Charcot's joint
Charcot-Marie-tooth dis ease'
charge
char'la tan
char'la tan ism
char'ley horse
char'tu la
chaul moo'gra oil
cheek
cheek'bone''
chees'y
chei lal'gi a
chei lec'to my

chei"lec tro'pi on
chei li'tis
chei"lo an'gi o scope"
chei log"na tho pal"a-
 tos'chi sis
chei log"na tho pros"o
 pos'chi sis
chei log"na tho u"ra nos'chi
 sis
chei'lo plas"ty
chei lor'rha phy
chei los'chi sis
chei lo'sis
chei los"to mat'o plas"ty
chei lot'o my
chei"ma pho'bi a
che'late
che'lat ing
che la'tion
chem'i cal
chem"i co cau"ter y
chem"i lu"mi nes'cence
chem"i o tax'is
chem'ist
chem'is try
che"mo bi ot'ic
chem'o cep"tor
chem"o co ag"u la'tion
chem"o dec to'ma
chem"o pro"phy lax'sis
chem'o re cep"tor
chem"o re'flex
che mo'sis
chem'o stat
chem"o sur'ger y
chem"o tax'is
chem"o ther'a py
che"mo troph'
che"mo troph'ic

che mot'ro pism
chem'ur gy
Che"no po'di um
che'o plas ty
cher"o ma'ni a
cher"o pho'bi a
cher'ry
cher'u bism
chest
Cheyne-Stokes res"pi ra'tion
Chiari's net'work
chi'asm
chi as'ma
ch as'mal
chi as'ma ta
chick'en pox"
chig'ger
chil'blain"
child
child'bed"
child'birth"
child'crow"ing
chill
chi'mer ism
chin'i o fon
chi"o na blep'si a
chi"o no pho'bi a
chi rag'ra
chi ral'gi a
chi rap'si a
chi'rap sy
chi"rar thri'tis
chi ris'mus
chi"ro kin"es thet'ic
chi rol'o gy
chi"ro meg'a ly
chi'ro plas"ty
chi rop'o dist
chi rop'o dy

chi″ro pom′pho lyx
chi″ro prac′tic
chi′ro prac tor
chi′ro scope
chi′ro spasm
chi′tin
chi′tin ous
chlam′y do spore″
chlo as′ma
chlor ac′ne
chlor bu′ta nol
chlo′ral
chlor″am phen′i col
chlo″ra ne′mi a
chlo′rate
chlor′dane
chlor hy′dri a
chlo′ric
chlo′ride
chlo″ri du′ri a
chlo′ri nat″ed
chlo″rin a′tion
chlo′rine
chlo′rite
chlo′ro form
chlo′ro form ism
chlo″ro form″i za′tion
chlo ro′ma
Chlo″ro my cet′in
chlo″ro per′cha
chlo′ro phyll
chlo′ro plast
chlo″ro plas′tin
chlo rop′si a
Chlo′ro quin
chlo ro′sis
chlo rot′ic
chlor pro′ma zine
chlor″tet ra cy′cline

chlor-tri′me ton
cho′a na
cho′a nal
choke
chol′a gogue
chol″an gi ec′ta sis
chol″an″gi o gas tros′to my
chol″an gi og′ra phy
chol an″gi o li′tis
cho lan″gi o′ma
chol″an gi os′to my
chol″an gi ot′o my
chol″an gi′tis
chol″e bil″i ru′bin
chole″e cal cif′er ol
chol″e chrom e re′sis
chol″e chro″mo poi e′sis
chol″e chry″o cy to′sis
chol″e cy′a nin
chol′e cyst
chol″e cyst′a gogue
chol″e cyst al′gi a
chol″e cyst ec ta′si a
chol″e cyst ec′to my
chol″e cyst en″ter or′rha phy
chol″e cyst en″ter os′to my
chol e cys′tic
chol″e cys ti′tis
chol″e cys″to co los′to my
chol″e cys″to du″o de′nal
chol″e cys″to e lec″tro co
  ag″u lec′to my
chol″e cys″to gas tros′to my
chol″e cys′to gram
chol″e cys tog′ra phy
chol″e cys″to il e os′to my
chol″e cys″to jej″u nos′to my
chol″e cys″to ki net′ic
chol″e cys″to ki′nin

chol''e cys''to li thi'a sis
chol''e cys''to lith ot'o my
chol''e cys'to pex''y
chol''e cys tor'rha phy
chol''e cys tos'to my
chol''e cys tot'o my
cho led'o chal
cho led''o chec ta'si a
cho led''o chec'to my
cho led''o chi'tis
cho led''o cho do chor'rha phy
cho led''o cho du''o de nos'to
   my
cho led''o cho en''ter os'to my
cho led''o cho gas tros'to my
cho led''o cho lith i'a sis
cho led''o cho li thot'o my
cho led''o cho lith'o trip''sy
cho led''o cho plas'ty
cho led''o chor'rha phy
cho led''o chos'to my
cho led''o chot'o my
cho led'o chus
chol''e glo'bin
chol''e he'ma tin
cho le'ic
chol'e lith
chol''e li thi'a sis
chol''e li thot'o my
chol''e lith'o trip''sy
cho lem'e sis
cho le'mi a
cho le'mic
chol''e poi e'sis
chol''e poi et'ic
chol''e pra'sin
chol''e pyr'rhin
chol'era
chol er a'ic

chol er e'sis
chol'er ic
chol'er i form''
chol''er i za'tion
chol'er oid
chol''er o pho'bi a
chol''er rha'gi a
cho''les cin'ti gram
cho le sta'sis
cho les''te a to'ma
cho les''te a to'ma tous
cho les''te a to'sis
chol es'ter ase
cho les''ter i nu'ri a
cho les'ter ol
cho les'ter ol ase''
cho les''ter ol er'e sis
cho les''ter ol o poi e'sis
cho les''ter o'sis
cho'lic
cho'line
cho''lin er'gic
cho''lin es'ter ase
chol'o chrome
chol'o gogue
chol'o lith
chol or rhe'a
cho lu'ri a
chon'dral
chon drec'to my
chon'dri fy
chon'dri gen
chon'drin
chon'dri o cont''
chon'dri o gene''
chon''dri o kin e'sis
chon'dri ome
chon dri'tis
chon''dro al bu'mi noid

chon'dro blast
chon''dro blas to'ma
chon''dro cal ci no'sis
chon''dro car''ci no'ma
chon dro cla'sis
chon'dro clast
chon''dro cos'tal
chon''dro cra'ni um
chon'dro cyte
chon''dro der''ma ti'tis
chon''dro dys pla'si a
chon''dro dys tro'phi a
chon''dro dys'tro phy
chon''dro ec''to der'mal
chon''dro ep''i tro chle'a ris
chon''dro fi bro'ma
chon''dro fi''bro sar co'ma
chon'dro gen
chon''dro gen'e sis
chon drog'e nous
chon''dro glos'sus
chon''dro hu mer al'is
chon'droid
chon dro'i tin
chon''dro lip''o sar co'ma
chon dro'ma
chon''dro ma la'ci a
chon''dro ma to'sis
chon dro'ma tous
chon'dro mere
chon''dro mu'coid
chon''dro myx o hem an''gi o
  end''o the''li o sar co'ma
chon''dro myx o'ma
chon''dro myx''o sar co'ma
chon''dro os''te o dys'tro phy
chon''dro-os''te o'ma
chon''dro-os''te o sar co'ma
chon drop'a thy

chon''dro pha ryn'ge us
chon'dro plast
chon'dro plas''ty
chon''dro po ro'sis
chon''dro pro'te in
chon''dro sar co'ma
chon'dro sin
chon dro'sis
chon''dro ster'nal
chon dro'tome
chon drot'o my
chor'da
chor''da blas'to pore
chor'dal
chor''da mes'o blast
chor''da mes'o derm
Chor da'ta
chor'date
chor dee'
chord''en ceph'a lon
chor di'tis
chor do'ma
chor dot'o my
cho re'a
cho're al
cho re'i form
cho''re o ath'e toid
cho''re o ath''e to'sis
cho''ri o ad''e no'ma
cho''ri o al''lan to'ic
cho''ri o al lan'to is
cho''ri o an''gi op'a gus
chor''i o blas to'sis
cho''ri o cap''il la'ris
cho''ri o car''ci no'ma
cho''ri o cele
cho''ri o ep''i the''li o'ma
cho''ri o gen'e sis
cho'ri oid

cho"ri o'ma
cho"ri o men"in gi'tis
cho'ri on
cho"ri on ep"i the"li o'ma
cho"ri o ni'tis
cho"ri o ret'i nal
cho"ri o ret"i ni'tis
cho"ri o ret"in op'a thy
chor'i sis
cho ris"to blas to'ma
cho"ri sto'ma
cho'roid
cho roi'dal
cho"roid e re'mi a
cho"roid i'tis
cho roi"do cy cli'tis
cho roi"do i ri'tis
cho roi"do ret"i ni'tis
chre"ma to pho'bi a
chro maf'fin
chro"maf fi no'ma
chro maf"fi nop'a thy
chro'ma phil
chro'ma phobe
chro ma'si a
chro'mate
chro"ma te lop'si a
chro mat'ic
chro mat'ic ness
chro'ma tid
chro'ma tin
chro"ma to der"ma to'sis
chro"ma to dys o'pi a
chro"ma tog'e nous
chro mat'o gram
chro"ma to graph'ic
chro"ma tog'ra phy
chro"ma tol'o gy
chro"ma tol'y sis

chro"ma to lyt'ic
chro mat'o mere
chro"ma tom'e ter
chro"ma tom'e try
chro"ma top'a thy
chro'ma to phil
chro"ma to pho'bi a
chro'ma to phore"
chro"ma toph'o rous
chro'ma to plasm
chro'ma to plast
chro"ma top'si a
chro"ma top tom'e try
chro"ma to'sis
chrome
chrom"hi dro'sis
chro'mic
chro'mi cize
chro mid'i um
chro'mi um
Chro"mo bac te'ri um
chro'mo blast
chro"mo blas"to my co'sis
chro'mo cen"ter
chro"mo crin'i a
chro"mo cys tos'co py
chro'mo cyte
chro"mo dac"ry or rhe'a
chro'mo gen
chro"mo gen'e sis
chro"mo gen'ic
chro'mo mere
chro"mo ne'ma
chro"mo par'ic
chro'mo phane
chro'mo phil
chro'mo phobe
chro"mo pho'bi a
chro"mo pho'bic

chro'mo phore
chro''mo phor'ic
chro'mo phose
chro''mo phy to'sis
chro'mo plasm
chro'mo plast
chro''mo pro'te in
chro mop'si a
chro''mop tom'e ter
chro mos'co py
chro''mo so'mal
chro'mo some
chro'nax ie
chron''ax im'e ter
chron'ic
chron ic'i ty
chron'o graph
chro nom'e try
chron''o pho'bi a
chron'o scope
chron''o trop'ic
chrys'a lis
chry'sene
chry si'a sis
chrys''o cy''a no'sis
Chry'sops
chry''so ther'a py
chrys''o tox'in
Chvostek's sign
chyl an''gi o'ma
chyle
chy le'mi a
chy''li dro'sis
chy'lo cele
chy''lo der'ma
chy'loid
chy''lo mi'crons
chy''lor rhe'a
chy''lo tho'rax

chy'lous
chy lu'ri a
chyme
chy'mo sin
chy''mo sin'o gen
chy''mo tryp'sin
chy''mo tryp sin'o gen
chy'mous
ci bis'o tome
ci''bo pho'bi a
cic''a tric'ial
cic'a trix
ci cat'ri zant
cic''a tri za'tion
cic'a trize
cic'er ism
cil'i a
cil''i ar'i scope
cil''i ar ot'o my
cil'i ary
cil''i ate'
cil''i at'ed
cil''i o scle'ral
cil lo'sis
cin cho'na
cin chon'ic
ci''ne an'gi o gram
cin''e flu''o rog'ra phy
ci ni're a
cin''e roent''gen og'ra phy
cin'gu late
cin''gu lec'to my
cin''gu lo trac'to my
cin'gu lum
cin nam'ic
cin'na mon
cir'ci nate
cir'cle
cir'cuit

cir'cu lar
cir"cu la'tion
cir'cu la to"ry
cir'cu lin
cir'cu lus
cir"cum a'nal
cir"cum ar tic'u lar
cir"cum ci'sion
cir"cum cor'ne al
cir"cum duc'tion
cir'cum flex
cir"cum in'su lar
cir"cum len'tal
cir"cum nu'cle ar
cir"cum o'ral
cir"cum po"lar i za'tion
cir"cum scribed'
cir"cum stan"ti al'i ty
cir"cum val'late
cir"cum vas'cu lar
cir rho'sis
cir rhot'ic
cir'rus
cir sec'to my
cir'soid
cir som'pha los
cir"soph thal'mi a
cir sot'o my
cis'sa
cis'tern
cis ter'na
cis ves'ti tism
cit'rate
cit'ric ac'id
cit'rin
cit"ron el'la oil
cit trul'line
ci"trul li ne'mi a
cit"rul lin u'ria

cit'rus
cit to'sis
clair voy'ance
clamp
cla'po
clap'ping
cla rif'i cant
clar"i fi ca'tion
clas mat'o cyte
clas"mo cy to'ma
clas'tic
clau"di ca'tion
claus"tro phil'i a
claus"tro pho'bi a
claus'trum
cla'va
clav'a cin
cla'val
cla'vate
clav"e li za'tion
clav'i cle
clav"i cot'o my
cla vic'u lar
cla vic'u late
cla vic"u lec'to my
cla'vus
claw'foot"
claw'hand"
clear'ance
cleav'age
cleft
clei'dal
clei"do cos'tal
clei"do cra'ni al
clei"do hu'mer al
clei"do hy'oid
clei'do ic
clei"do mas'toid
clei"do-oc cip'i tal

clei″do scap′u lar
clei″do ster′nal
clei dot′o my
clei″thro pho′bi a
cle′oid
cli′er
cli″ma co pho′bi a
cli mac′ter ic
cli′mate
cli″ma tol′o gy
cli″ma to ther′a py
cli′max
clin′ic
clin′i cal
cli ni′cian
clin″i co hem″a to log′ic
clin″i co pa thol′o gy
clin″i co roent″gen o log′ic
Cli′ni stix
cli″no ceph′a lus
cli″no ceph′a ly
cli″no dac′ty ly
cli′noid
cli nom′e ter
cli′no scope
clip
clis″e om′e ter
clit′i on
clit″o ral′gi a
clit″o ri daux′e
cli″to rid e′an
clit″o ri dec′to my
clit″o ri di′tis
clit″o ri dot′o my
clit′o ris
clit′o rism
clit″o ri′tis
clit″o ro ma′ni a
clit″or rha′gi a

cli′vus
clo a′ca
clo a′cal
clo fi′brate
clo′mi phene
clone
clon′ic
clo nic′i ty
clon″i co ton′ic
clon′ism
clon′o graph
clo″nor chi′a sis
Clos trid′i um
clo′sure
clot
clove
clown′ism
club′foot″
club′hand″
clump′ing
clu′ne al
clut′ter ing
Clutton's joint
cly′sis
co″a cer′vate
co″ad ap ta′tion
co ag′u la ble
co ag′u lant
co ag′u lase
co ag′u late
co ag″u la′tion
co″ag u lop′athy
co ag′u lum
co″a les′cence
coal tar
co″ap ta′tion
co arc′tate
co″arc ta′tion
co″arc tot′o my

77

co''ar tic''u la'tion
coat
co bal'a min
co'balt
Co'bra
co'bra lec'i thid
co''bra ly'sin
co'ca
co caine'
co cain'ism
co'cain ize
co cain''o ma'ni a
co''car box'yl ase
co''car cin'o gen
coc'cal
Coc cid''i oi'des
coc cid''i oi'din
coc cid''i oi''do my co'sis
coc''co ba cil'lus
coc cog'e nous
coc'coid
coc'cus
coc''cy al'gi a
coc''cy ceph'a lus
coc''cy dyn'i a
coc''cy gec'to my
coc''cy ge''o fem o ral'is
coc cyg'e us
coc''cy go dyn'i a
coc'cyx
coch''i neal'
coch'le a
coch'le ar
coch''le o ves tib'u lar
coc''to pre cip'i tin
coc''to sta'bile
co'de ine
co''ef fi'cient
coe len'ter on

coe'lom
coe lom'ic
coe'no cyte
coe nu ro'sis
co en'zyme
coeur en sab''ot'
co'fac tor
cof'fee
cof'fin
cog ni'tion
cog'wheel''
co hab''i ta'tion
co her'ence
co he'sion
co he'sive
coil
co i'tion
co''i to pho'bi a
co'i tus
co la'tion
col''a to'ri um
col'a ture
col'chi cine
co lec'to my
co''le i'tis
co'le o cele''
co''le o cys ti'tis
co''le op to'sis
co''le ot'o my
co'les
co''li bac''il le'mi a
co''li bac''il lo'sis
co''li bac''il lu'ri a
co''li ba cil'lus
col'ic
co'li ca
col'i form
col'i phage
co''li py u'ri a

co li'tis
co"li u'ri a
col'la cin
col'la gen
col'la ge nase
col"la gen'o sis
col lapse'
col'lar bone"
col lar ette'
col lat'er al
col lec'tor
Colles' frac'ture
col lic"u li'tis
col lic'u lus
col'li ma"tor
col lin'e ar
col"li qua'tion
col liq'ua tive
col li'sion
col lo'di on
col'loid
col loi'dal
col loi"do cla'sis
col loi"do pex'y
col"loid oph'a gy
col"lo ne'ma
col'lum
col"lu na'ri um
col"lu to'ri um
col lyr'i um
col'ma scope
col"o bo'ma
co"lo co los'to my
co"lo hep'a to pex"y
co'lon
col'o ny
col'o pex"y
col"o proc tos'to my
col"op to'sis

col'or
col"o rec tos'to my
col'or gus ta'tion
col"or im'e ter
col"or i met'ric
col"or im'e try
co lor'rha phy
co"lo sig"moid os'to my
co los'to my
col"os tra'tion
co los"tror rhe'a
co los'trum
co lot'o my
col pal'gi a
col"pa tre'si a
col"pec ta'si a
col pec'to my
col"pe de'ma
col"peu ryn'ter
col"peu rys'is
col pi'tis
col'po cele
col"po clei'sis
col"po hy"per pla'si a
col"po per"i ne'o plas"ty
col"po per"i ne or'rha phy
col'po pex"y
col'po plas"ty
col por'rha phy
col"por rhex'is
col'po scope
col po scop'ic
col pot'o my
col"u mel'la
col'umn
co lum'na
col'umn ing
col"um ni za'tion
co'ma

com'a tose
comb'ing
Comb's test
com'e do
com''e do-car''ci no'ma
com''e do'nes
co'mes
com'mi nute
com'mi nut ed
com''mi nu'tion
com''mis su'ra
com miss'u ral
com'mis sure
com''mis sur ot'o my
com mit'ment
com mo'ti o
com mu'ni ca ble
com mu'ni cans
com pan'ion ate
com par'a scope
com pat''i bil'i ty
com pat'i ble
com''pen sa'tion
com pen'sa to''ry
com'pe tence
com plaint'
com'ple ment
com''ple men'ta ry
com''ple men'toid
com''ple men'to phil
com'plex
com plex'ion
com''po si'tion
com po'si tus
com'pos men'tis
com'pound
com'press
com pres'sion
com pres'sor

com pul'sion
com pul'sive
co'mus
co na'tion
con'cave
con cav'i ty
con ceive'
con cen tra'tion
con cen'tric
con cep'tion
con cep'tive
con cep'tus
con'cha
con'chal
con chi'tis
con'cho tome
con com'i tant
con'cre ment
con cres'cence
con cre'tion
con cus'sion
con''den sa'tion
con dens'er
con di'tion ing
con'dom
con duct''i bil'i ty
con duc'tion
con''duc tiv'i ty
con duc'tor
con'dyle
con''dy lec'to my
con dyl'i on
con'dy loid
con''dy lo'ma
con''dy lo'ma tous
con''dy lot'o my
cone
con fab''u la'tion
con fec'tion

con fer'tus
con fine'ment
con'flict
con'flu ence
con'flu ent
con fo'cal
con"fron ta'tion
con fu'sion
con"ge la'tion
con'ge ner
con gen'i tal
con ges'tion
con ges'tive
con'gi us
con glo'bate
con glom'er ate
con glu'tin
con glu'ti nant
con glu"ti na'tion
con glu'ti nin
co nid'i um
co'ni ism
co"ni om'e ter
co"ni o'sis
co"ni o spor"i o'sis
co'ni um
con"i za'tion
con'ju gate
con"ju ga'tion
con"junc ti'va
con"junc ti'val
con junc"ti vi'tis
con junc"tiv o'ma
con"junc tiv'o plas"ty
co"no my oi'din
con"san guin'e ous
con"san guin'i ty
con'scious ness
con sen'su al

con sent'
con serv'a tive
con sist'ence
con sol'i dant
con sol"i da'tion
con sper'gent
con'stant
con"stel la'tion
con"sti pa'tion
con"sti tu'tion
con stric'tor
con sult'ant
con"sul ta'tion
con sump'tion
con sump'tive
con'tact
con tac'tant
con ta'gion
con tam'i nant
con tam'i nat ing
con tam"i na'tion
con tem'pla tive
con'tent
con tig'u ous
con'ti nence
con'ti nent
con tin'gen cy
con tor'tion
con'tour
con"tra cep'tion
con"tra cep'tive
con tract'
con trac'tile
con"trac til'i ty
con trac'tion
con trac'ture
con"tra fis su'ra
con"tra in"di ca'tion
con"tra lat'er al

con"tra stim'u lant
con"tre coup'
con"trec ta'tion
con trol'
con trude'
con tuse'
con tu'sion
co'nus
con"va les'cence
con"va les'cent
con vec'tion
con ver'gence
con ver'gent
con ver'sion
con ver'tin
con vex'
con vex'i ty
con vex'o con'cave
con vex'o con'vex
con'vo lu"ted
con"vo lu'tion
con vul'sant
con vul'sion
con vul'sive
Cooley's a ne'me i a
Coomb's test
co or"di na'tion
coot'ie
cop'per
co"pre cip"i ta'tion
cop rem'e sis
cop roc'tic
cop"ro lag'ni a
cop"ro la'li a
cop'ro lith
cop roph'a gy
cop"ro phe'mi a
cop"ro phil'i a
cop roph'i lous

cop"ro pho'bi a
cop"ro phra'si a
cop"ro por phy'ri a
cop"ro por'phy rin
cop"ro por"phy ri nu'ri a
cop"u la'tion
cor"a co a cro'mi al
cor"a co bra"chi a'lis
cor"a co cla vic'u lar
cor"a co hu'mer al
cor'a coid
cord
cor dec'to my
cor'dial
cor'di form
cor di'tis
cor'do pex"y
cor dot'o my
cor"e cli'sis
cor ec'ta sis
cor ec'tome
cor"ec to'pi a
cor"e di al'y sis
co rel'y sis
cor"e mor'pho sis
cor"en cli'sis
cor"e om'e ter
cor"on'ci on
cor'e plas"ty
cor"e ste no'ma
cor"e to me"di al'y sis
co'ri um
corn
cor'ne a
cor'ne al
cor"ne o bleph'a ron
cor"ne o scle'ra
cor'ne ous
cor'ne um

cor nic'u late
cor nic'u lum
cor"ni fi ca'tion
cor'nu
co ro'na
co'ro nar"y
co"ro na vi'rus
co ro'ne
cor'o ner
co ro'ni on
cor"o ni'tis
co ro"no bas'i lar
co ro"no fa'cial
cor'o noid
cor"o pa rel'cy sis
co roph'thi sis
co ros'co py
cor po're al
cor'po rin
cor"pro por phy rin'o gen
corpse
corps ronds
cor'pu lent
cor pul ma na'le
cor'pus
cor'pus cle
cor pus'cu lar
cor pus'cu lum
cor'pus de lec'ti"
cor rec'tion
cor rec'tive
cor"re la'tion
cor"re spond'ence
cor ro'sion
cor ro'sive
cor'ru ga"tor
cor'set
cor'tex
cor'ti cal

cor"ti co bul'bar
cor'ti coid
cor"ti co pon"to cer e bel'lar
cor"ti co spi'nal
cor"ti cos'ter oid
cor"ti cos'te rone
cor"ti co stri'ate
cor"ti co tro'phin
cor"ti co tro'pin
cor'tin
cor'ti sone
cor"us ca'tion
cor ym'bi form
Co ry"ne bac te'ri um
co ry'za
cos met'ic
cos'mo tron
cos'ta
cos'tal
cos tal'gi a
cos tal'is
cos'tate
cos tec'to my
cos"ti car'ti lage
cos'ti form
cos'tive
cos"to car'ti lage
cos"to cer"vi cal'is
cos"to chon'dral
cos"to cla vic'u lar
cos"to cor'a coid
cos"to phren'ic
cos"to scap'u lar
cos'to tome
cos tot'o my
cos"to trans verse'
cos"to trans"ver sec'to my
cos"to ver'te bral
cos"to xiph'oid

cot

cot'a zyn

cot'ton

cot''y le'don

cot'y loid

cough

cou'lomb

cou'ma rin

count

count'er

coun''ter ac'tion

coun''ter ex ten''sion

coun''ter ir'ri tant

coun'ter o''pen ing

coun'ter poi''son

coun'ter pres''sure

coun'ter punc''ture

coun'ter shock''

coun'ter stain

coun'ter stroke

coun'ter trac''tion

coun'ter trans fer'.ence

cou'ple

Courvoisier, Ludwig

co va'lence

Cowper's glands

cow''per i'tis

cow'pox''

cox al'gi a

cox''ar throc'a ce

cox'a vara

cox i'tis

Cox sack'ie vi'rus

co zy'mase

cra'dle

cramp

cra'ni ad

cra'ni al

cra''ni ec'to my

cra''ni o cele

cra''ni o cer'vi cal

cra''ni oc'la sis

cra''ni o clast

cra''ni o clei''do dys os to'sis

cra''ni o did'y mus

cra''ni o fa'cial

cra''ni o fe nes'tri a

cra'ni o graph

cra''ni og'ra phy

cra''ni o la cu'ni a

cra''ni ol'o gy

cra''ni om'e ter

cra''ni o met'ric

cra''ni om'e try

cra''ni op'a gus

cra''ni op'a thy

cra''ni o pha ryn'ge al

cra''ni o pha ryn''gi o'ma

cra'ni o plas''ty

cra''ni o rha chis'chi sis

cra''ni o sa'cral

cra''ni os'chi sis

cra''ni o spi'nal

cra'ni o stat''

cra''ni o ste no'sis

cra''ni os'to sis

cra''ni o syn''os to'sis

cra''ni o ta'bes

cra'ni o tome

cra''ni ot'o my

cra''ni o trac'tor

cra''ni o trip'so tome

cra''ni o tym pan'ic

cra'ni um

cran'ter

crap'u lent

cra''ter i za'tion

cra vat'

craw'-craw''
cream
crease
cre'a tine
cre''a ti ne'mi a
cre at'i nine
cre''a ti nu'ri a
cre''a tor rhe'a
Credé's meth'od
cre mas'ter
cre''mas ter'ic
cre ma'tion
cre'ma to''ry
crem''no pho'bi a
cre'na
cre'nate
cre na'tion
cre'o sol
cre'o sote
crep'i tant
crep''i ta'tion
crep'i tus
cres'cent
cre'sol
crest
cres'yl blue
cre'ta
cre'tin
cre'tin ism
cre'tin oid
crev'ice
crib'bing
crib'rate
crib'ri form
crib'rose
crick
cri''co ar''y te'noid
cri'coid
Crigler-Najjar syn'drome

cri''coi dec'to my
cri''co pha ryn'ge al
cri''co phar yn'ge us
cri''co thy'roid
cri cot'o my
cri''co tra'che ot'o my
crim''i nol'o gy
crimp'er
crin''o gen'ic
cri'nose
cri'sis
cris pa'tion
cris''pa tu'ra
cris'ta
crit'i cal
Crohn's dis ease'
Cro tal'i dae
crot'a line
crotch'et
cro'ton ism
cro tox'in
croup
croup'ine
Crouzon's dis ease'
crown
cru'cial
cru'ci ate
cru'ci ble
cru'ci form
cru'or
crup'per
cru'ral
cru're us
crus
crush
crust
Crus ta'ce a
crutch
cry

cry''al ge'si a
cry an''es the'si a
cry''es the'si a
cry''mo dyn'i a
cry''mo phil'ic
cry''o cau'ter y
cry'o chem
cry''o glob'u lin
cry''o glob''u li ne'mi a
cry om'e ter
cry''o pro'te in
cry'o scope
cry'o stat
cry''o ther'a py
crypt
cryp''tag glu'tin oid
crypt''an am ne'si a
cryp ti'tis
cryp''to coc co'sis
Cryp''to coc'cus
cryp'to gam
cryp''to gen'ic
cryp'to lith
cryp''to men''or rhe'a
cryp''to mer''o rha chis'chi sis
cryp''tom ne'si a
cryp''toph thal'mos
cryp top'or ous
crypt''or chid ec'to my
crypt or'chid ism
crypt''or chid'o pex y
crypt or'chism
crypt''to zo'ite
crypt toz'y gous
crys'tal
crys''tal bu'min
crys''tal fi'brin
crys'tal lin
crys''tal li za'tion

crys''tal log'ra phy
crys'tal loid
crys''tal lo mag'net ism
crys''tal lo pho'bi a
crys''tal lu'ri a
cryst i cil'lin
cry''to did'y mus
crys toid'
cu'beb
cu'beb ism
cu'bi form
cu'bi tus
cu'boid
cu boi''de o na vic'u lar
cui rass'
cul'-de-sac'
cul''do cen te'sis
cul'do scope
cul dos'co py
cul''dot'o my
Cu'lex
cu'li cide
cul'men
cult
cul''ti va'tion
cul'ture
cu'mu la''tive
cu'mu lus
cu'ne ate
cu ne'i form
cu''ne o cu'boid
cu''ne o na vic'u lar
cu''ne o scaph'oid
cu'ne us
cu nic'u lar
cu nic'u lus
cun''ni lin'guist
cun''ni lin'gus
cun'nus

cu'po la
cupped
cup'ping
cu''pram mon'ni a
cu'prex
cu'pric
cu'prous
cu'pu la
cu''pu lom'e try
cur'age
cu ra're
cu ra'ri form
cu''ra ri za'tion
cu'ra tive
curd
cure
cu ret'
cu ret'tage
cu'ric
cu'rie
cu'ri um
curled
cur'rent
cur ric'u lum
cur'va ture
curve
Cushing, Harvey
cush'ing oid''
cush'ion
cusp
cus'pid
cu ta''ne o mu co'sal
cu ta'ne ous
cu'ti cle
cu tic'u lar
cu''ti fi ca'tion
cu''ti re ac'tion
cu'tis
cu ti'tis

cu''ti za'tion
cy''an am'ide
cy'a nate
cy'a nide
cy''a no co bal'a mine
cy an'o phil
cy'a nosed
cy''a no'sis
cy''a not'ic
cy as'ma
cy''ber net'ics
cy'cla mate
cy'cle
cy clec'to my
cy''clen ceph'a lus
cy''clen ceph'a ly
cy'clic
cy''cli cot'o my
cy cli'tis
cy''clo ceph'a lus
cy''clo ceph'a ly
cy''clo cho''roid i'tis
cy''clo di al'y sis
cy''clo di'a ther my
cy clog'e ny
cy'cloid
cy''clo phor'ase
cy''clo pho'ri a
cy clo'pi a
cy''clo ple'gi a
cy''clo pro'pane
cy'clops
cy'clo scope
cy''clo thy'mic
cy clo'ti a
cy'clo tome
cy clot'o my
cy'clo tron
cy''clo tro'pi a

cy clo'tus
cy e"si ol'o gy
cy e'sis
cyl'in der
cy lin'dri form
cyl'in droid
cyl"in dro'ma
cyl"in dro'sis
cyl"in dru'ri a
cyl"lo so'ma
cyl"lo so'mus
cym"bo ceph'a ly
cy nan'thro py
cyn"i a'tri a
cyn'ic
cyn"o ceph'a lous
cyn"o don'tes
cyn"o lys'sa
cyn"o pho'bi a
cy"o pho'ri a
cy ot'ro phy
cy prid"o pho'bi a
cyr"to ceph'a lus
cyr"to cor'y phus
cyr'to graph
cyr tom'e ter
cyr"to me to'pus
cyr"to pis"tho cra'ni us
cyr to'sis
cyr"tu ran'us
cyst
cyst ad"e no car"ci no'ma
cyst"ad e no'ma
cyst"ad e no sar co'ma
cys tal'gi a
cys"ta thi"o ni nu'ri a
cyst"ec ta'si a
cys tec'to my
cys'te ine

cyst'ic
cys"ti cer'coid
cys"ti cer co'sis
cys"ti cer'cus
cys'ti form
cys'tine
cys"ti ne'mi a
cys"ti no'sis
cys"ti nu'ri a
cys ti'tis
cys tit'o my
cys"to bu bon'o cele
cys'to cele
cys"to fi bro'ma pap"il lar'e
cys"to gen'e sis
cys'to gram
cys tog'ra phy
cyst'oid
cys"to lith ec'to my
cys"to li thi'a sis
cys"to li thot'o my
cys to'ma
cys tom'e ter
cys"to met'ro gram
cys"to mor'phous
cys'to pex"y
cys"to pho tog'ra phy
cys'to plas"ty
cys"to pros ta tec'to my
cys"to py"e li'tis
cys"to py"e lo ne phri'tis
cys tor'rha phy
cys"to sar co'ma
cys'to scope
cys tos'co py
cys tos"te a to'ma
cys tos'to my
cys tot'o my
cys"to u re'thro gram

cys"to u"re throg'ra phy
cys"to u re'thro scope
cy"to ar"chi tec ton'ic
cy"to ar'chi tec"ture
cy'to blast
cy"to blas te'ma
cy"to chem'ism
cy'to chrome
cy"to chy le'ma
cy toc'la sis
cy"to crin'i a
cy'tode
cy"to dis'tal
cy to gen'ic
cy"to glob'u lin
cy to log'ic
cy tol'o gy
cy"to ly'sin
cy tol'y sis
cy"to me gal'ic
cy"to meg a"lo vi'rus
cy tom'e ter
cy"to mi'cro some
cy"to mi'tome
cy"to mor'pho sis
cy'ton

cy"to path o gen'ic
cy"to pa thol'o gy
cy top'a thy
cy toph'a gy
cy"to pe'ni a
cy'to phil
cy"to phys"i ol'o gy
cy'to plasm
cy"to plas'tin
cy"to poi e'sis
cy"to prox'i mal
cy"to re tic'u lum
cy"tos cop'ic
cy tos'co py
cy'to some
cy"to spon'gi um
cy'tost
cy'to stome
cy"to tax'is
cy toth'e sis
cy"to tox'ic
cy"to tox'in
cy"to troph'o blast
cy tot'ro phy
cy tot'ro pism
cy'to zyme

D

dac no ma'ni a
Dac'ron
dac"ry ad"e no scir'rhus
dac"ry ag"o ga tre'si a
dac'ry a gogue
dac"ry ge lo'sis
dac"ry o ad"e nal'gi a
dac"ry o ad"e nec'to my
dac"ry o ad e ni'tis
dac"ry o blen"nor rhe'a

dac'ry o cyst"
dac"ry o cys tec'to my
dac"ry o cys ti'tis
dac"ry o cys"to blen'nor rhea
dac"ry o cys'to cele
dac"ry o cys"top to'sis
dac"ry o cys"to rhi nos'to my
dac"ry o cys tos'to my
dac"ry o cys'to tome
dac"ry o cys tot'o my

dac'ry o lin
dac'ry o lith"
dac"ry o li thi'a sis
dac"ry o'ma
dac'ry on
dac'ry ops
dac"ry or rhe'a
dac"ry o so"le ni'tis
dac"ry o ste no'sis
dac"ry o syr'inx
dac'tyl
dac"ty lif'er ous
dac tyl'i on
dac"ty li'tis
dac"ty lo gram"
dac"ty lo meg'a ly
dac"ty lo sym'phy sis
dac"ty lus
dah'lin
dan'der
dan'druff
Darier's dis ease'
dar'tos
dar'trous
dau'er schlaf"
daught'er
de ac"ti va'tion
de af"fer en ta'tion
deaf'-mute"
deaf'ness
de al'bate
de al"co hol"i za'tion
de al"ler gi za'tion
de am'i dase
de am'i nase
de an"es the'si ant
de"a qua'tion
death
de bil'i tant

de bil'i ty
de bride'ment
de bris'
dec'a gram
de cal"ci fi ca'tion
de cal'ci fy
dec'a lit"er
dec'a me"ter
dec'a nor mal
de cant'
de cap'i tate
de cap"i ta'tion
de cap'i ta"tor
de cap"su la'tion
de car'bon ate
de car"bon i za'tion
de car box"y la'tion
de ca thec'tion
dec"a vi'ta min
de cay'
de cen'tered
de cer"e bel la'tion
de cer'e brate"
de cer"e bra'tion
de chlo"ri da'tion
de chlo"ru ra'tion
dec'i bel
de cid'u a
de cid'u al
de cid'u ate
de cid"u a'tion
de cid"u i'tis
de cid"u o'ma
de cid"u o'sis
de cid'u ous
dec'i gram
dec'i li"ter
dec'i me"ter
dec"i nor'mal

de cip'a ra
de clive'
De clo my'cin
de coc'tion
de''col la'tion
de'col la''tor
de col'or ant
de col'or ize
de com''pen sa'tion
de''com po si'tion
de''com pres'sion
de''con ges'tant
de''con ges'tive
de con tam'i nate
de''con tam''i na'tion
de cor''ti ca'tion
de''cu ba'tion
de cu bi'tal
de cu'bi tus
de cus'sate
de''cus sa'tion
de''den ti'tion
de''dif fer en''ti a'tion
def''e ca'tion
de fect'
de''fem i na'tion
de fense'
def'er ent
def''er en'tial
def''er en''ti o ves'i cal
def''er en ti'tis
de''fer ves'cence
de fib''ril la'tion
de fi''bri na'tion
def''i ni'tion
def''la gra'tion
de flec'tion
def''lo ra'tion
de''flo res'cence

de form'i ty
de fuse'
de gan'gli on ate
de gas'sing
de gen'er a cy
de gen'er ate
de''gen er a'tion
de''gen er a'tive
de gen''i tal'i ty
de''glu ti'tion
deg''ra da'tion
de grease'
de gree'
de''gus ta'tion
de his'cence
de hy'drate
de''hy dra'tion
de hy''dro cor''ti cos'te rone
de hy'dro gen ase
de hy'dro gen ize
de''hy dro i''so an dros'ter one
de i'on iz''er
Deiter's cells
de''ja''vu'
de jec'tion
de''lac ta'tion
de lam''i na'tion
De Lee, Joseph
de lim''i ta'tion
de lim'it ed
de lin'quen cy
de''lip i da'tion
del''i ques'cence
de liq'ui um
de lir''i fa'cient
de lir'i ous
de lir'i um
de liv'er y
de''lo mor'phous

de louse'
del'ta
del'toid
de lu'sion
de''mar ca'tion
de ment'
de ment'ed
de men'ti a
de'men tia prae'cox
De'mer ol
de meth''yl chlor''te tra cy'cline
dem''i.fac'et
dem'i lune
dem''i mon stros'i ty
de min''er al i za'tion
dem''i pen'ni form
de mog'ra phy
de''mon ol'a try
de''mon ol'ogy
de''mon o ma'nia
de''mon op'a thy
de''mon o pho'bi a
de mul'cent
de my'e lin ate
de nar'co tize
de na'tur ant
de na'tured
de na''tur i za'tion
den'drite
den''dro phil'i a
de ner'va ted
de''ner va'tion
den'gue
de ni'al
den''i da'tion
den''i gra'tion
de ni''tro gen a'tion
dens
den sim'e ter

den''sit om'e ter
den'si ty
den'so gram
den tag'ra
den'tal
den tal'gi a
den tal''o ru'bral
den tar'pa ga
den'tar y
den'tate
den ta'tum
den''te la'tion
den'tes
den'ti a pre'cox
den''ti a ski'a scope
den'ti cle
den tic'u late
den''ti fi ca'tion
den'ti form
den'ti frice
den tig'er ous
den'ti lave
den'tin
den''ti nal'gi a
den''ti no blas to'ma
den''ti no ce men'tal
den''ti no gen'e sis
den'ti noid
den''ti no'ma
den''ti nos'te oid
den tip'a rous
den'ti phone
den'tist
den'tis try
den ti'tion
den''to al ve'o lar
den''to al''ve o li'tis
den''to fa'cial
den tog'ra phy

den'toid
den''to le'gal
den ton'o my
den'ture
de nu'cle a''ted
de nude'
de ob'stru ent
de''o'dor ant
de o'dor ize
de''o ral'i ty
de or''sum duc'tion
de or''sum ver'gence
de os''si fi ca'tion
de ox''y gen a'tion
de ox''y ri bo nu cle'ic
de per''son al i za'tion
de pig''men ta'tion
dep'i late
de pil'a tory
dep'i lous
de plete'
de ple'tion
de''plu ma'tion
de po''lar i za'tion
de''po lym'er ase
de pol''y mer i za'tion
de pos'it
de'pot
de pres'sant
de pres'sion
de pres'sor
dep'side
de pu''li za'tion
der''an en''ce pha'li a
de re''al i za'tion
de're ism
der e is'tic
der''en ceph'a lus
der''en ceph'a ly

der''i va'tion
de riv'a tive
der'ma
Der''ma cen'tor
der'ma drome
der'mal
der''ma my i'a sis
der man'a plas''ty
der''ma tag'ra
der''ma tal'gi a
der''ma ta neu'ri a
der''mat he'mi a
der'ma therm
der mat'ic
der''ma ti'tis
der''ma to cel''lu li'tis
der''ma to cha la'sis
der''ma to co''ni o'sis
der''ma to cyst''
der''ma to fi bro'ma
der''ma to fi''bro sar co'ma
   pro tu'ber ans
der''ma to glyph'ics
der''ma tog'ra phy
der''ma tol'o gist
der''ma tol'o gy
der''ma tol'y sis
der'ma tome
der'ma to my'ces
der''ma to my co'sis
der''ma to my o'ma
der''ma to my''o si'tis
der''ma to neu rol'o gy
der''ma to neu ro'sis
der''ma to pa thol'o gy
der''ma to path''o pho'bi a
der''ma top'a thy
der''ma to phi li'a sis
der'ma to phyte''

der"ma toph'y tid
der"ma to phy to'sis
der'ma to plas"ty
der"ma to pol"y neu ri'tis
der"ma tor rha'gi a
der"ma tos'co py
der"ma to'sis
der'ma to some"
der"ma to stom"a ti'tis
der"ma to ther'a py
der"ma to thia'si a
der"ma tot'o my
der"ma to zo'on
der"ma to zo"on o'sis
der'mis
der mi'tis
der'mo blast
der"mo cy'ma
der"mo ep"i der'mal
der"mo graph'i a
der'moid
der"moid ec'to my
der"mo la'bi al
der mop'a thy
der"mo phle bi'tis
der"mo skel'e ton
der"mo ste no'sis
der"mos to'sis
der"mo syn"o vi'tis
der"mo syph"i lop'a thy
der"o did'y mus
de rom'e lus
der'rid
des"an i ma'ni a
de sat"u ra'tion
Descemet's mem'brane
des"ce me ti'tis
des"ce met'o cele
de scend'ens

de scen'sus
de scent'
des'e nex"
de sen"si ti za'tion
de sen'si tize
de sex"u al'i ty
de sex"u al i za'tion
des'ic cant
des"ic ca'tion
des'ic ca"tor
des'i vac
des"mi o gnath'us
des mi'tis
des"mo cra'ni um
des'mo cyte
des"mo gly'co gen
des'moid
des'mo lase
des'mone
des"mo pla'si a
des'mo some
des mot'o my
des'o gen
des sorp'tion
des ox"y cor"ti cos'te rone
des ox"y cor'ti sone
des ox"y ri"bo nu cle'ic ac'id
de spe"ci a'tion
D'Espine's sign
des'qua mate
des"qua ma'tion
de stru'do
de tach'ment
de ter'gent
de ter'mi nant
de ter"mi na'tion
de tor'sion
de tox"i ca'tion
de tox"i fi'ca tion

de tox'i fy
de tri'tion
de tri'tus
de"trun ca'tion
de tru'sion
de tru'sor
de"tu mes'cence
deu"ter a no'pi a
deu"ter a'tion
deu ter'i um
deu"ter o gen'ic
deu"ter o plasm'
deu"ter o pro'te ose
deu"ter os'to ma
deu tom'er ite
deu"to plas mol'y sis
de vel'op ment
de"vi a'tion
de"vi om'e ter
de vi'tal ize
dev"o lu'tion
dew'claw"
dew'lap"
Dex'a myl
Dex'e drine
dex'ter
dex'trad
dex'tral
dex tral'i ty
dex"tra li za'tion
Dex'tran
dex trau'ral
dex'trin
dex"tri nu'ri a
dex"tro car'di a
dex"tro car'di o gram"
dex"tro cer'e bral
dex"tro com'pound
dex"tro con'dyl ism

dex troc'u lar
dex"tro duc'tion
dex"tro man'ual
dex"tro pe'dal
dex"tro pho'bi a
dex"tro pho'ri a
dex"tro po si'tion
dex"tro ro'ta to"ry
dex'trose
dex"tro sin'is tral
dex"tro su'ri a
dex"tro tor'sion
dex"tro ver'sion
di"a bet'es
di"a bet'es in sip'i dus
di"a bet'es mel li'tus
di"a bet'ic
di"a be"to gen'ic
di"a be tog'e nous
di"a be"to pho'bi a
di ab'o lep"sy
di"a ce te'mi a
di ac"e tu'ri a
di ac"e tyl mor'phine
di ac'la sis
di'a clast
di ac"o la'tion
di"a crit'ic
di"ac tin'ic
di'ad
di'a derm
di ad"o cho ki ne'si a
di"ag nos'a ble
di"ag nose'
di"ag no'sis
di"ag nos'tic
di"ag nos ti'cian
di"a ki ne'sis
di al'y sate

di al'y sis
di'a lyze
di'a ly"zer
di"a mag net'ic
di am'e ter
di'a mine'
di"a mi nu'ri a
Di a'mox
di"a pa'son
di"a pe de'sis
di'a phane
di aph"a nom'e ter
di aph'a no scope
di aph"e met'ric
di aph'o rase
di"a pho re'sis
di"a pho ret'ic
di'a phragm
di"a phrag mat'o cele
di"a phrag mi'tis
di a phy se'al
di a phy se'al ac la'sis
di"aph y sec'to my
di aph'y sis
di ap'la sis
di"a poph'y sis
di"ar rhe'a
di ar'thric
di"ar thro'sis
di as'chi sis
di"a schis'tic
di'a scope
di"a stal'sis
di'a stase
di as'ta sis
di"a stat'ic
di"a ste'ma
di"a stem"a to my e'li a
di as'to le

di as tol'ic
di"a tax'i a
di"a ther'ma nous
di"a ther'mic
di"a ther"mo co ag"u la'tion
di"a ther mom'e ter
di'a ther"my
di ath'e sis
di"a tom'ic
di ba'sic
di cal'ci um
di ceph'a lism
di ceph'a lus
di ceph'a ly
di chei'lus
di chi'rus
di cho'ri al
di chot'o mize
di chot'o my
di chro'ic
di chro'mate
di"chro mat'ic
di chro'ma tism
di chro"ma top'si a
di'chro mism
di chro'mo phil
di"cli dot'o my
di cou'ma rin
di cou'ma rol
di crot'ic notch
di'cro tism
dic'ty o cyte
dic"ty o cy to'ma
dic"ty o ki ne'sis
dic ty'o tene
Di cum'a rol
di dac'tic
di dac'tyl ism
di del'phic

did y mi'tis
did'y mous
did'y mus
di el'drin
di''e lec trol'y sis
di em'bry o ny
di''en ceph al'ic
di''en ceph'a lon
di es'trum
di'et
di'e tar''y
di''e tet'ics
di eth''yl stil bes'trol
di''e ti'tian
dif''fer en'tial
dif''fer en''ti a'tion
dif'flu ence
dif frac'tion
dif fus'ate
dif fuse'
dif fus''i bil'i ty
dif fus''si om'e ter
dif fu'sion
di'ga len
di gas'tric
di gen'e sis
di''ge net'ic
di gen'ic
di gest'ant
di gest'er
di gest'i ble
di ges'tine
di ges'tion
dig''i fol'in
dig''i lan'id
dig'it
dig'i tal
dig''i ta'lin
dig''i tal'is

dig''i tal i za'tion
dig''i ta'tion
dig''i ti form
dig''i tox'in
dig'i tus
di glos'si a
di glos'sus
di gnath'us
di gox'in
di hy'brid
di hy''dro strep''to my'cin
di''i o'do form
di kar'y on
di lac''er a'tion
Di lan'tin
dil''a ta'tion
di la'tion
di'la tor
dil'u ent
di lute'
di lu'tion
di meg'a ly
di me'li a
di men'sion
di''mer cap'rol
di meth'yl
di me'tri a
di mor'phic
di mor'phism
dim'ple
Di o'do quin''
Di'o drast''
di'o nism
di op'ter
di''op tom'e ter
di op'tric
di op'trics
di''or tho'sis
di o'tic

di ox'ide
di pep'tide
di phal'lus
di phas'ic
di pho'ni a
diph the'ri a
diph the'ric
diph the'ri a phor
diph'the rin
diph''the ri ol'y sin
diph''the ri'tis
diph'the roid
diph thon'gi a
Diph phyl''lo both'ri um
di phy'o dont''
dip''la cu'sis
di''plas mat'ic
di ple'gi a
dip''lo al bu''mi nu'ri a
dip''lo ba cil'lus
dip''lo blas'tic
dip''lo car'di ac
dip''lo ceph'a lus
dip''lo coc'cin
Dip''lo coc'cus
dip''lo co'ri a
dip'lo e
dip''lo gen'e sis
dip'loid
dip''lo kar'y on
dip'lo mate
dip''lo mel''li tu'ri a
dip''lo my e'li a
dip''lo ne'ma
dip''lo neu'ral
di plop'a gus
di plo'pi a
di plo'sis
dip'lo some

dip''lo strep''to coc'cus
dip'lo tene
di po'lar
di'pole''
dip'pol dism
dip''ro so'pi a
di pro'so pus
dip set'ic
dip''so ma'ni a
dip''so pho'bia
dip''so ther'a py
Dip'ter a
di'pus
di py'gus
Di''py lid'i um
dir rhi'nus
di sac'char i dase
di sac'cha ride
di sac''char i du'ri a
dis ag''gre ga'tion
dis''ar tic''u la'tion
dis''as so''ci a'tion
dis charge'
dis cis'sion
disc i'tis
dis''co blas'tu la
disc'o gram
dis'coid
dis col''or a'tion
dis''com po si'tion
Dis''co my'ces
dis coph'o rous
dis''co pla cen'ta
dis crete'
dis crim''i na'tion
dis'cus
dis cu'tient
dis ease'
dis''en gage'ment

dis e″qui lib′ri um
dis″gre ga′tion
dis″in fect′ant
dis″in fec′tion
dis in″fes ta′tion
dis in″hi bi′tion
dis in′te grate
dis″in vag″i na′tion
dis joint′
disk, disc
dis″lo ca′tion
dis mem′ber
dis″mu ta′tion
dis″oc clude′
di so′ma
dis ord′**er**
dis or″gan i za′tion
dis o″ri en ta′tion
dis′pa rate
dis par′ity
dis pen′sa ry
dis pen′sa to″ry
dis pense′
dis per′sion
dis place′ment
dis″po si′tion
dis rup′tive
dis sect′
dis sec′tion
dis sec′tor
dis sem″i na′tion
dis sim″u la′tion
dis so″ci a′tion
dis″soc′i a tive
dis sog′e ny
dis″so lu′tion
dis solve′
dis′tad
dis′tance

dis tem′per
dis ten′tion
dis tich′i a
dis′til land
dis′til late
dis″til la′tion
dis″to buc′cal
dis″to buc″co oc clu′sal
dis″to oc clu′sal
dis″to clu′sion
dis″to la′bi al
dis″to lin′gual
dis″to lin″guo oc clu′sal
di sto′mi a
dis″to mi′a sis
dis″to mo′lar
di sto′mus
dis tor′tion
dis″to ver′sion
dis″tri bu′tion
dis″tri chi′a sis
dis′trix
di″u re′sis
di″u ret′ic
Di′u vil″
di″va ga′tion
di va′lent
di var″i ca′tion
di ver′gence
di″ver tic′u la
di″ver tic′u lar
di″ver tic″u lec′to my
di″ver tic″u li′tis
di″ver tic′u lo′sis
di″ver tic′u lum (a)
di vi′nyl
di vi′sion
di vul′sion
di vul′sor

di"zy got'ic
diz'zi ness
Dobell's so lu'tion
do'ca
dol"i cho ceph'a lus
dol"i cho ce phal'ic
dol"i cho ceph'a ly
dol"i cho cham"ae cra'ni al
dol"i choc ne'mic
dol"i cho co'lon
dol"i cho de'rus
dol"i cho eu"ro mes"o ceph'a lu:
dol"i cho eu"ro-o pis"tho
   ceph'a lus
dol"i cho eu"ro pro ceph'a lus
dol"i cho fa'cial
dol"i cho hi er'ic
dol"i cho ker'kic
dol"i cho lep"to ceph'a lus
dol"i cho mor'phic
dol"i cho pel'lic
dol"i cho plat'y ceph'a lus
dol'i chor rhine
dol"i cho u ran'ic
do'lor
dol"or o gen'ic
do"ma to pho'bi a
dom'in ance
dom'i nant
dom'i na tor
do"nee'
do'nor
Donovan bod'y
do'pa
dope
do"ra pho'bi a
dor'mant
dor'nase
dor'sa

dor'sad
dor'sal
dor sal'gi a
dor sa'lis
dor"si flex'ion
dor"si ven'tral
dor"so an te'ri or
dor"so ceph'al ad
dor"so ep"i tro chle a'ris
dor"so lat'er al
dor"so lum'bar
dor"so me'di an
dor"so na'sal
dor"so pos te'ri or
dor"so ra'di al
dor"so ul'nar
dor"so ven'tral
dor'sum
do'sage
do sim'e ter
do sim'e try
doub'let
douche
doug"la si'tis
dou rine'
Dover's pow'der
drachm (dram)
dra con"ti so'mus
dra cun"cu lo'sis
Dra cun'cu lus med"i nen'sis
dra gee'
Dragstedt's op"er a'tion
drain
drain'age
dram (drachm)
Dram'a mine
drap"e to ma'ni a
dread
dream

drench
drep'a no cyte
drep''a no cy the'mi a
drep''a no cy to'sis
dress'er
drib'ble
drift
driv'el ing
drom'o graph
drom''o ma'ni a
drom''o pho'bi a
drop'let
drop'si cal
drop'sy
Dro soph'i la
drug'gist
drunk'en ness
drunk om'e ter
dru'sen
du''al is'tic
duct
duct'us
du ip'a ra
dum'my
du''o crin' in
du''o de'nal
du''o de nec'ta sis
du''o de nec'to my
du''o de ni'tis
du''o de''no chlo''an gi'tis
du''o de''no chol''e cys tos'to my
du''o de''no cho led''o chot'o my
du''o de''no col'ic
du''o de''no cys tos'to my
du''o de''no en''ter os'to my
du''o de'no gram
du''o den og'raph y
du''o de''no he pat'ic
du''o de''no il''e os'to my

du''o de''no jej''u nos'to my
du''o de''no pan''cre a tec'to my
du''o de'no plas''ty
du o de''no py''lo rec'to my
du''o de nor'rha phy
du''o de nos'co py
du''o de nos'to my
du''o de not'o my
du''o de'num
du''o pa ren'tal
du'pli ca''ture
du'pli ca'tus
du plic'i tas
du plic'i ty
Dupuytren, Guillaume
du'ra
du'ra ma'ter
du'ra plas''ty
du ri'tis
du''ro ar''ach ni'tis
dwarf
dwarf'ism
dye
dy nam' e ter
dy nam'ic
dy'na mo
dy''na mo gen'e sis
dy nam'o graph
dy''na mom'e ter
dy nam'o neure
dy''na moph'a ny
dy nam'o scope
dy'na therm
dyne
dys''a cou'si a
dys ad''ap ta'tion
dys''aes the'si a
dys an''ag no'si a
dys an''ti graph'i a

dys a'phi a
dys"ap ta'tion
dys"ar te"ri ot'o ny
dys ar'thri a
dys"ar thro'sis
dys"au to no'mia
dys'bar ism
dys ba'si a
dys bu'li a
dys chi'ri a
dys chi'zi a
dys chon"dro pla'si a
dys chro"ma to der'mi a
dys"chro ma top'si a
dys chro'mi a
dys'chro nous
dys co'ri a
dys cra'si a
dys cri'nism
dys"di ad"o cho ki ne'si a
dys"e coi'a
dys em"bry o pla'si a
dys"e me'si a
dys e'mi a
dys"en doc'rin ism
dys'en ter"y
dys"er ga'si a
dys"es the'si a
dys"fi brin o"ge ne'mi a
dys func'tion
dys"ga lac'ti a
dys"gam ma glob u lin em'ia
dys gen'ic
dys"ger mi no'ma
dys geu'si a
dys glan'du lar
dys gnath'ic
dys gno'si a
dys gon'ic

dys gram'ma tism
dys graph'i a
dys hem"a to poi et'ic
dys"hi dro'sis
dys"ker a to'sis
dys"ki ne'si a
dys la'li a
dys lex'i a
dys"li po pro tein e'mi a
dys lo'gi a
dys"ma se'sis
dys"men or rhe'a
dys"mer o gen'e sis
dys me'tri a
dys mim'i a
dys mne'si a
dys mor'phi a
dys mor'phic
dys mor"pho pho'bi a
dys no'mi a
dys"o don ti'a sis
dys o'pi a
dys"o rex'i a
dys os'mi a
dys"os to'sis
dys par"a thy'roid ism
dys"pa reu'ni a
dys pep'si a
dys pep'tic
dys"per i stal'sis
dys pha'gi a
dys pha'si a
dys phe'mi a
dys pho'ni a
dys pho'ri a
dys pho'ti a
dys phra'si a
dys"pi tu'i ta rism
dys pla'si a

dysp ne'a
dys prax'i a
dys'ra phism
dys rhyth'mi a
dys se ba'ci a
dys"se cre to'sis
dys sper'ma tism
dys sta'si a
dys tax'i a
dys tec'tic

dys"tha na'si a
dys the'si a
dys thy'mi a
dys tith'i a
dys to'ci a
dys to'ni a
dys to'pi a
dys tro'phi a
dys'tro phy
dys u'ri a

E

ear
ear'ache"
ear'drum"
ear'wax"
Eaton's a'gent
Ebstein's a nom'a ly
e'bur
e"bur na'tion
ec bol'ic
ec cen'tric
ec ceph"a lo'sis
ec"chon dro'ma
ec"chy mo'sis
ec'crine
ec"cy e'sis
ec dem'ic
ec dem"o ma'ni a
ec'der on
ec'dy sis
e chid'nase
e chid'nin
e chin'e none
e chi'no coc co'sis
E chi"no coc'cus
E chi"no der'ma ta
ech"i no'sis

ech'o
ech"o a cou'si a
ech"o car di og'ra phy
ech"o graph'i a
ech"o la'li a
ech"o la'lus
ech op'a thy
ech oph'o ny
ech"o phot'o my
ech"o prax'i a
ec la'bi um
ec lamp'si a
ec lamp'sism
ec lec'ti cism
ec'ly sis
ec mne'si a
e"cog no'sis
e col'o gy
e"co ma'ni a
e'co site
e cos'tate
ec pho'ri a
e"cra"seur'
ec'sta sy
ec'tad
ec'tal

ec ta'si a
ec ten'tal
ect eth'moid
ec thy'ma
ec''to bat'ic
ec'to blast
ec''to car'di a
ec''to cho roi'de a
ec''to cor''ne a
ec''to cra'ni al
ec'to derm
ec''to der mo'sis
ec''to en'zyme
ec tog'e nous
ec tog'o ny
ec''to men'inx
ec'to mere
ec''to mes'o derm
ec'to morph
ec top'a gus
ec''to par'a site
ec'to phyte
ec to'pi a
ec top'ic
ec''to pla cen'ta
ec'to plasm
ec''to pot'o my
ec''to ret'i na
ec'to sarc
ec'to thrix
Ec''to tri choph'y ton
ec''to zo'on
ec''tro dac tyl'i a
ec trog'e ny
ec''tro me'li a
ec trom'e lus
ec tro'pi on
ec trop'o dism
ec''tro syn dac'ty ly

ec trot'ic
ec''ty lot'ic
ec'ze ma
ec zem''a ti za'tion
ec zem''a toid
ec zem''a to'sis
ec zem'a tous
e de'ma
e den'tate
e den'ti a
e den'tu lous
e''de ol'o gy
ed'i ble
ed''o ceph'al us
ef fect'
ef fec'tor
ef'fer ent
ef''fer ves'cence
ef''fer ves'cent
ef''fleu rage'
ef'.'flo res'cence
ef'flu ent
ef flu'vi um
ef fuse'
ef fu'sion
e''ga grop'i lus
e ger'sis
e ges'ta
e glan'du lar
e'go
e''go bron choph'o ny
e''go cen'tric
e'go ide'al
e''go ma ni a
e goph'o ny
Ehrlich, Paul
ei det'ic im'age
ei'do gen
ei''dop tom'e try

ein'stein

Einthoven's tri'angle

Eisenmenger's com'plex

e jac''u la'tion

e jec'ta

e jec'tion

e jec'tor

e lab''o ra'tion

el'a cin

e'lase

e las'tase

e las'tic

e las'ti ca

e las'tin

e las tom'e ter

el'bow

e lec''tric'i ty

e lec'tri fy

e lec''tri za'tion

e lec''tro af fin'i ty

e lec''tro an''es the'si a

e lec''tro bi ol'o gy

e lec''tro bi os'co py

e lec''tro cap''il lar'i ty

e lec''tro car'di o gram''

e lec''tro car'di o graph''

e lec''tro car''di og'ra phy

e lec''tro car''di o pho nog'ra phy

e lec''tro ca tal'y sis

e lec''tro cau'ter y

e lec''tro chem'is try

e lec''tro chro''ma tog'ra phy

e lec''tro co ag''u la'tion

e lec''tro co'ma

e lec''tro con''duc tiv'i ty

e lec''tro con''trac til'i ty

e lec''tro con vul'sive

e lec''tro cor ti cog'ra phy

e lec''tro cu'tion

e lec''tro cys'to scope

e lec'trode

e lec'tro dent

e lec''tro der'ma tome

e lec''tro des''ic ca'tion

e lec''tro di''ag no'sis

e lec''tro di al'y sis

e lec''tro di'a phane

e lec''tro dy nam'ics

e lec''tro dy''na mom'e ter

e lec''tro en ceph'a lo gram''

e lec''tro en ceph'a lo graph''

e lec''tro en ceph''a log'ra phy

e lec''tro fit'

e lec''tro form'

e lec''tro gas'tro graph

e lec''tro gen'e sis

e lec'tro gram''

e lec''tro he''mo sta'sis

e lec''tro hys''ter og'ra phy

e lec''tro ki net'ics

e lec''tro ky'mo graph''

e lec''tro li thot'ri ty

e lec''trol'o gy

e lec''trol'y sis

e lec'tro lyte

e lec'tro ly''zer

e lec'tro mag'net

e lec''tro mas sage'

e lec''trom'e ter

e lec''tro mo'tive

e lec''tro my'o gram

e lec''tro my og'ra phy

e lec'tron

e lec''tro nar co'sis

e lec''tro neg'a tive

e lec''tro neu rog'raphy

e lec''tro neu'ro tone

e lec''tro os mo'sis

e lec''tro pa thol'o gy
e lec''tro pho'bi a
e lec''tro pho re'sis
e lec''troph'o rus
e lec''tro pho''to ther'a py
e lec''tro phren'ic
e lec''tro phys''i ol'o gy
e lec''tro pos'i tive
e lec''tro punc'ture
e lec''tro py rex'i a
e lec''tro re sec'tion
e lec''tro ret'i no gram
e lec''tro scis'sion
e lec'tro scope
e lec''tro sec'tion
e lec'tro shock'
e lec'tro some
e lec''tro steth'o phone
e lec''tro stric'tion
e lec''tro sur'ger y
e lec''tro syn'the sis
e lec''tro tax'is
e lec''tro thal'a mo gram
e lec''tro tha na'si a
e lec''tro ther''a peu'tics
e lec''tro ther'a py
e lec'tro therm
e lec'tro tome
e lec''trot'o nus
e lec''tro tur''bi nom'e ter
e lec''tro va'go gram
e lec''tro va'lence
e lec'tu ar''y
el'e ment
el''e o'ma
el''e om'e ter
el''e o my en'chy sis
el''e phan ti'a sis
el'e va''tor

e lim'i nant
e lim''na'tion
e lin gua'tion
e lix'ir
el lip'soid
el lip'to cyte
el lip''to cy to'sis
e lon''ga'tion
el'u ate
e ma''ci a'tion
e mac''u la'tion
em''a na'tion
e man''ci pa'tion
em''a no ther'a py
e mas''cu la'tion
em balm'ing
em bed'
em''bo lec'to my
em''bo le'mi a
em bol'ic
em'bo lism
em''bo lo la'li a
em'bo lus
em'bo ly
em bra'sure
em''bro ca'tion
em''bry ec'to my
em'bry o
em'bry o blast''
em''bry oc'to ny
em'bry oid
em''bry o lem'ma
em''bry o log'ic
em''bry ol'o gist
em''bry ol'o gy
em''bry o mor'phous
em'bry o tome''
em''bry ot'o my
em''bry o tox'on

em″bry o trophe
em″bry ul′ci a
em″bry ul′cus
em′e sis
e met″a tro′phi a
e met′ic
em′e tine
em″e to ca thar′sis
em″e to ma′ni a
em″e to pho′bi a
e mic′tion
em″i gra′tion
em′i nence
em″i nen′ti a
em′is sar″y
e mis′sion
em men′a gogue
em men′i a
em men″i op′a thy
em″me nol′o gy
em″me tro′pi a
e mol′li ent
e mo″ti o met″a bol′ic
e mo″ti o mus′cu lar
e mo′tion
e mo″ti o vas′cu lar
em pasm′
em′pa thy
em′phly sis
em phrac′tic
em phrax′is
em″phy se′ma
em″phy se′ma tous
em pir′ic
Em′pir in
em plas′trum
em″pros thot′o nos
em″pros tho zy go′sis
em″py e′ma

em″py e′sis
em″py reu mat′ic
e mul′si fi″er
e mul′si fy″
e mul′sion
e munc′to ry
en am′el
en am″e lo blas′ma
en am″el o′ma
en″an the′ma
en an″ti o la′li a
en an′ti o morph″
en″ar thro′sis
en can′this
en cap″su la′tion
en cap′suled
en ceph″a lal′gi a
en ceph″a lat′ro phy
en ceph″a lit′ic
en ceph″a lit′ic
en ceph″a li′tis
en ceph″a li to gen′ic
en ceph′a lo cele″
en ceph″a lo dys pla′si a
en ceph′a lo gram″
en ceph″a log′ra phy
en ceph′a loid
en ceph′a lo lith″
en ceph″a lol′o gy
en ceph″a lo′ma
en ceph″a lo ma la′ci a
en ceph″a lo men″in gi′tis
en ceph″a lo me nin′go cele
en ceph″a lo men″in gop′a thy
en ceph′a lo mere″
en ceph″a lom′e ter
en ceph″a lo my″e li′tis
en ceph″a lo my″e lo
    neu rop′a thy

107

en ceph"a lo my"e lop'a thy
en ceph"a lo my"e lo
   ra dic"u li'tis
en ceph"a lo my"e lo
   ra dic"u lop'a thy
en ceph"a lo my el o'sis
en ceph"a lo my"o car di'tis
en ceph'a lon
en ceph"a lo nar co'sis
en ceph"a lop'a thy
en ceph"a lo punc'ture
en ceph"a lo py o'sis
en ceph"a lo ra chid'i an
en ceph"a lor rha'gi a
en ceph'a lo scope
en ceph"a lo sep'sis
en ceph"a lo'sis
en ceph'a lo tome
en ceph"a lot'o my
en ceph"a lo tri gem'i nal
en"chon dro'ma
en chon"dro ma to'sis
en chon"dro sar co'ma
en"chon dro'sis
en"chy le'ma
en clit'ic
en"co pre'sis
en cra'ni us
en"cy e'sis
en"cys ta'tion
en cyst'ed
en cyst'ment
en"da del'phus
En"da moe'ba
en"dan gi i'tis
en"da or ti'tis
end'-ar"bor i za'tion
en"dar ter ec'to my
en"dar te'ri al

en"dar te ri'tis
end au'ral
end"ax o neu'ron
end'-bulb"
en dem'ic
end ep"i der'mis
end"er gon'ic
en der'mic
en"der mo'sis
en"do ab dom'i nal
en"do an"eu rys mor'rha phy
en"do an"gi i'tis
en"do a"or ti'tis
en"do bi ot'ic
en"do bron'chi al
en"do car di'al
en"do car di'tis
en"do car'di um
en"do car'do fi bro'sis
en"do ce'li ac
en"do cer"vi ci'tis
en"do cer'vix
en"do chol'e doch al
en"do chon'dral
en"do col pi'tis
en"do cra'ni al
en"do cra ni'tis
en"do cra'ni um
en'do crine
en"do cri nol'o gy
en"do cri nop'a thy
en"do crin"o ther'a py
en'do cy'ma
en'do cyst
en'do derm
en"do der"ma to zo"o no'sis
en"do don'tics

en"do don'tist
en"do en'zyme
en dog'a my
en dog'e nous
en"do gna'thi on
en"do la ryn'ge al
en'do lymph
en'do lym phat'ic
en"do lym phan'gi al
en"do me trec'to my
en"do me"tri o'ma
en"do me"tri o'sis
en"do me tri'tis
en"do me'tri um
en dom'e try
en"do mi to'sis
en'do morph
en'do mor"phy
En"do my'ces
en"do my o car'di al
en"do my"o car di'tis
en"do mys'i um
en"do na'sal
en"do neu'ral
en"do neu'ri um
en"do nu cle'o lus
en"do par'a site
en"do pep'ti dase
en"do per"i car di'tis
en"do per"i my"o car di'tis
en"do phle bi'tis
en doph"thal mi'tis
en'do plasm
en'do scope
en"do scop'ic
en"do skel'e ton

en"dos mom'e ter
en"dos mo'sis
en'do sperm
en'do spore
en dos"te o'ma
en dos'te um
en"dos ti'tis
en"dos to'sis
en"do sub til'y sin
en"do ten din'e um
en"do the'li al
en"do the"li o an"gi i'tis
en"do the"li o cho'ri al
en"do the'li oid
en"do the"li o ly'sin
en"do the"li o'ma
en"do the"li o ma to'sis
en"do the"li o'sis
en"do the'li um
en"do ther'mic
en'do thrix
en"do tox"i co'sis
en"do tox'in
en"do tra'che al
en'e ma
en"er get'ics
en"er gom'e ter
en'er gy
en"er va'tion
en gage'ment
en gas'tri us
en globe'ment
en gorge'ment
en'gram
en hem'a to spore
en large'ment

109

en"oph thal'mos
en"o si ma'ni a
en"os to'sis
en'si form
en som'pha lus
en'stro phe
en"ta cous'tic
en'tad
en'tal
En"ta moe'ba
en ta'si a
en tel'e chy
en'ter al
en"ter al'gi a
en"ter ec'ta sis
en"ter ec'to my
en"ter e pip'lo cele
en ter'ic
en ter'i coid
en"ter i'tis
en"ter o a nas"to mo'sis
en'ter o bac"ter i a'ceae
en"ter o bi'a sis
En"ter o'bi us
en'ter o cele"
en"ter o cen te'sis
en"ter o'cin
en"ter oc'ly sis
en"ter o coc'cus
en'ter o coele"
en"ter o co lec'to my
en"ter o co li'tis
en"ter o co los'to my
en'ter o cyst"
en"ter o cys'to cele
en"ter o cys to plas'ty

en"ter o cys tos'che o cele
en"ter o en ter'ic
en"ter o en"ter os'to my
en"ter o gas'tro cele
en"ter o gas'trone
en"ter og'e nous
en'ter o graph"
en"ter o ki'nase
en'ter o lith
en"ter o li thi'a sis
en'ter ol'o gist
en"ter ol'y sis
en"ter o me'ro cele
en"ter o my co'sis
en"ter o my'ia sis
en 'ter on
en"ter op'a thy
en"ter o pex'y
en'ter o plas"ty
en"ter o ple'gi a
en"ter o proc'ti a
en"ter op to'sis
en"ter or rha'gi a
en"ter or'rha phy
en"ter or rhex'is
en'ter o scope
en"ter o sep'sis
en'ter o spasm
en"ter o sta'sis
en"ter o ste no'sis
en"ter os'to my
en'ter o tome
en"ter ot'o my
en"ter o tox'in
en"ter o vi'rus
en"ter o zo'on

en''the o ma'ni a
en'the sis
en thet'ic
en ti'ris
en'to blast
en'to cele
en''to cho roid'e a
en'to cone
en''to co'nid
en'to derm
en''to derm'al
en'to mere
en to'mi on
en to mog'e nous
en''to mol'o gist
en''to mol'o gy
en''to mo pho'bi a
ent''oph thal'mi a
ent op'tic
ent''op tos'co py
en''to ret'i na
ent''os to'sis
ent o'tic
en''to zo'on
en train'ment
en tro'pi on
en'tro py
en'ty py
e nu'cle ate
en''u re'sis
en vi'ron ment
en''zy mat'ic
en'zyme
en''zy mol'o gy
en''zy mol'y sis
e'on ism
e'o sin
e''o sin''o pe'ni a

e''o sin'o phil
e''o sin''o phil'i a
e''o sin''o phil'ic
e pac'tal
ep''ar te'ri al
ep ax'i al
ep en'dy ma
ep en''dy mi'tis
ep en''dy mo blas to'ma
ep en'dy mo cyte
e''pen dy mo'ma
ep en''dy mop'a thy
eph''e bo gen'e sis
e phed'rine
eph e'lis
e phem'er al
eph''i dro'sis
ep''i a gnath'us
ep'i blast
ep''i bleph'a ron
e pib'o ly
ep''i bulb'ar
ep''i can'thus
ep''i car'di um
ep''i chor'dal
ep''i cho'ri al
ep''i cho'ri on
ep''i col'ic
ep''i co'mus
ep''i con''dyl al'gi a
ep''i con'dy lar
ep''i con'dyle
ep''i con''dy li'tis
ep''i cra'ni o tem''po ral'is
ep''i cra'ni um
ep''i cra'ni us
ep''i cri'sis
ep''i crit'ic
ep''i cys ti'tis

ep"i cys tot'o my
ep'i cyte
ep"i dem'ic
ep"i de"mi ol'o gist
ep"i de"mi ol'o gy
ep"i der'mal
ep"i der"ma to plas'ty
ep"i der"ma to'zo"on o sis
ep"i der'mic
ep"i-der"mi dal i za'tion
ep"i der'mis
ep"i der mi'tis
ep"i der"mi za'tion
ep"i der"mo dys pla'si a
    ver ru"ci for'mis
ep"i der'moid
ep"i der mol'y sis
ep"i der"mo my co'sis
ep"i der moph'y tid
Ep"i der moph'y ton
ep"i der"mo phy to'sis
ep"i der mo'sis
ep"i did"y mec'to my
ep"i did'y mis
ep"i did"y mi'tis
ep"i did'y mo-or chi'tis
ep"i did"y mot'o my
ep"i did"y mo vas os'to my
ep"i du'ral
ep"i fas'ci al
ep"i fol lic"u li'tis
ep"i gas tral'gi a
ep"i gas'tric
ep"i gas'tri o cele"
ep"i gas'tri um
ep"i gas'tri us
ep"i gas'tro cele
ep"i gen'e sis
ep"i glot'tic

ep"i glot"ti dec'to my
ep"i glot'tis
ep"i glot ti'tis
e pig'na thus
ep"i hy'oid
ep"i.la mel'lar
ep"i la'tion
ep"i lem'ma
ep'i lep"sy
ep"i lep'tic
ep"i lep"to gen'ic
ep"i lep'toid
ep"i loi'a
ep'mere
ep"i my"o car'di um
ep"i mys'i um
ep"i neph'rine
ep"i ne phri'tis
ep"i neu'ral
ep"i neu'ri um
ep"i ot'ic
ep"i pal'a tum
ep"i pas'tic
ep"i phar'ynx
ep"i phe nom'e non
e piph'o ra
ep"i phy lax'is
ep"i phys"e o ne cro'sis
ep"i phys"e op'a thy
ep"i phys"i o de'sis
ep"i phys"i ol'is the'sis
ep"i phys"i ol'y sis
e piph'y sis
e piph"y si'tis
ep"i pi'al
ep"i pleu'ral
e pip'lo cele
ep"i plo ec'to my
e pip"lo en'ter o cele"

e pi plo'ic
e pip''lom phal'o cele''
e pip'lo on
e pip'lo pex''y
ep''i plor'rha phy
ep''ip ter'ic
ep''i py'gus
ep''i scle'ra
ep''i scle'ral
ep''i scle ri'tis
e pi''si o cli'si a
e pi''si o el''y tror'rha phy
e pi''si o per''i ne'o plas''ty
e pi''si o per''i ne or'rha phy
e pi'si o plas''ty
e pi''si or rha'gi a
epi''si or'rha phy
e pi''si o ste no'sis
e pi''si ot'o my
ep'i sode
ep''i spa'di as
ep''i spas'tic
ep''i sphe'noid
ep''i spi'nal
ep''i sta'sis
ep''i stat'ic
ep''i stax'is
ep''i stern'um
ep''i stro'phe us
ep''i sym'pus
ep''i ten din'e um
ep''i thal'a mus
ep''i tha lax'i a
ep''i the'li a
ep''i the''li o cho'ri al
ep''i the''li o ge net'ic
ep''i the'li oid
ep''i the''li o'ma
ep''i the li'tis

ep''i the'li um
ep''i the''li za'tion
ep'i them
ep''i to'nos
ep''i trich'i um
ep''i troch'le ar
ep''i troch''le ar'is
ep''i troch'le o-ol''e cra no'nis
ep''i tu ber''cu lo'sis
ep''i tym pan'ic
ep''i tym'pa num
ep''i zo'ic
ep''i zo ot'ic
ep''o nych'i um
ep'o nym
ep'o oph'o ron
ep ox'y
Ep'som salt
ep u'lis
ep'u loid
ep''u lo fi bro'ma
e qua'tion
e qua'tor
e''qui ax'i al
e''qui li bra'tion
e''qui lib'ri um
eq'uine
eq''ui no ca'vus
eq''ui no va'rus
e qui'nus
eq''ui se to'sis
e quiv'a lent
e ra'sion
Erb's pal'sy
e rec'tile
e rec'tion
e rec'tor
er''e mi o pho'bi a
e rep'sin

er'e thism
er''e this'tic
erg
er ga'si a
er ga'si a try
er ga''si o ma'ni a
er ga''si o pho'bi a
er''gas'the'ni a
er gas'to plasm
er'go graph
er gom'e ter
er''go no'vine
er''go pho'bi a
er'go phore
er gos'ter ol
er'got
er got'a mine
er''go ther'a py
er'got ism
Er''go trate'
er'i gens
Erlenmeyer flask
e rog'e nous
eros
e rose'
e ro'si o in''ter dig''i ta'lis
   blas''to my ce'ti ca
e ro'sion
e rot'ic
e rot'i ca
er'o ti cism
er'o tism
er''o to gen'ic
er''o to ma'ni a
er''o top'a thy
er''o to pho'bi a
e''ruc ta'tion
e ru'ga to''ry
e rup'tion

e rup'tive
er''y sip'e las
er''y sip''e lo coc'cus
er''y sip'e loid
e rys'i phake
er''y the'ma
er''y the'moid
er''y thras'ma
e ryth''re de ma pol''y
   neu rop'a thy
er''y thre'mi a
er''yth re'mic
e ryth'ro blast
e ryth''ro blas to'ma
e ryth''ro blas''to pe'ni a
e ryth''ro blas to'sis foe tal'is
e ryth''ro chlo ro'pi a
E ryth'ro cin
e ryth''ro cy''a no'sis
e ryth'ro cyte
e ryth''ro cy the'mi a
e ryth''ro cyt'ic
e ryth''ro cy''to ly'sin
e ryth''ro cy tol'y sis
e ryth''ro cy tom'e ter
e ryth''ro cy'to-op'so nin
e ryth'' cy''to poi e'sis
e ryth''ro cy''tor rhex'is
e rythro cy tos'chi sis
e ryth''ro cy to'sis
e ryth''ro de gen'er a tive
e ryth''ro der'ma
e ryth''ro dont'i a
e ryth'ro gen'e sis
er''yth ro gen'in
e ryth'ro gone
er'y throid
e ryth''ro leu''ko blas to'sis
e ryth''ro leu ko'sis

er''y throl'y sin
er''y throl'y sis
e ryth''ro me lal'gi a
e ryth''ro me'li a
er''y throm'e ter
e ryth''ro my'cin
e ryth''ro my''e lo'sis
er'y thron
e ryth''ro ne''o cy to'sis
e ryth''ro no cla'si a
er''y thro pe'ni a
e ryth'ro phage
e ryth''ro pha''go cy to'sis
e ryth'ro phil
e ryth''ro phle'um
e ryth''ro pho'bi a
e ryth'ro phose
e ryth'ro pla'si a
e ryth''ro poi e'sis
e''ryth ro poi e'tic
e ryth''ro sar co'ma
e ryth ro'sis
e ryth''ro sta'sis
er''y thru'ri a
Esbach's re a'gent
es cape'
es'char
es''cha rot'ic
Esch''er ich'i a co'li
es cutch'eon
es'er ine
e soph''a gal'gi a
e soph''a ge'al
e soph''a gec ta'si a
e soph''a gec'to my
e soph''a gec'to py
e soph''a gi'tis
e soph''a go du''o de nos'to my
e soph''a go en''ter os'to my

e soph''a go e soph''a gos'to my
e soph''a go gas trec'to my
e soph''a go gas'tro plas''ty
e soph''a go gas'tro scope''
e soph''a go gas tros'to my
e soph''a go je''ju nos'to my
e soph''a gom'e ter
e soph''a go my'o to my
e soph''a gop'a thy
e soph'a go plas''ty
e soph'a gop to'sis
e soph'a go scope''
e soph'a gos'copy
e soph'a go spasm''
e soph''a go ste no'sis
e soph''a gos'to ma
e soph''a gos''to mi'a sis
e soph''a gos'to my
e''so phag'o tome
e soph''a got'o my
e soph'a gus
e soph''o gram
es''o pho'ri a
es''o tro'pi a
es'sence
es sen'tial
es'ter
es'ter ase
es ter''i fi ca'tion
es the'si a
es the''si ol'o gy
es the''si om'e ter
es the''si o phys''i ol'o gy
es thet'ic
es''thi om'e ne
es'ti val
es''ti va'tion
es tra di'ol
est'ri ol

es'tro gen
es tro gen'ic
es'trus
es''tu a ri'um
eth'ane
eth'a nol
eth'e noid
e'ther
eth''mo ceph'a lus
eth''mo fron'tal
eth'moid
eth moi'dal
eth''moid ec'to my
eth''moid i'tis
eth''moid ot'o my
eth''mo lac'ri mal
eth''mo max'il lar''y
eth''mo na'sal
eth''mo tur'bi nal
eth'nic
eth nol'o gy
eth'yl
eth'yl ene
eth'y nyl
e''ti o la'tion
e''ti o log'ic
e''ti ol'o gy
e''ti o path''o gen'e sis
eu''ca lyp'tus
eu chol'i a
eu chro'ma tin
eu chro''ma top'si a
eu''di om'e ter
eu''es the'si a
eu gen'ics
eu gnath'ic
eu gon'ic
eu''ki ne'si a
eu mor'phic
eu noi'a
eu'nuch

eu'nuch oid
eu'nuch oid ism
eu pho'ni a
eu pho'ri a
eu phys''i o log'ic
eu prax'i a
eu''ro don'ti a
eu''ro pis''o ceph'a lus
eu''ro pro ceph'a lus
eu''ry ce phal'ic
eu''ry chas'mus
eu''ry gnath'ism
eu''ry mer'ic
eu'ry on
eu''ry ther'mal
eu'scope
eu sta'chi an
eu sys'to le
eu''tha na'si a
eu then'ics
Eu the'ri a
eu thy'roid ism
eu to'ci a
e vac'u ant
e vac''u a'tion
e vac'u a tor''
e vag''i na'tion
ev''a nes'cent
e''ven tra'tion
e ver'sion
ev'i dence
ev''i ra'tion
e vis''cer a'tion
e vis''cer o neu rot'o my
ev''o ca'tion
ev''o lu'tion
e vul'sion
ex ac''er ba'tion
ex''al ta'tion
ex am''i na'tion
ex an'them
ex''an the'ma

ex ar''te ri'tis
ex''ca va'tion
ex'ca va''tor
ex''ce men to'sis
ex cer''e bra'tion
ex cip'i ent
ex ci'sion
ex cit''a bil'i ty
ex ci'tant
ex''ci ta'tion
ex clu'sion
ex''coch le a'tion
ex co'ri ate
ex co''ri a'tion
ex'cre ment
ex cres'cence
ex cre'ta
ex'cre tin
ex cre'tion
ex'cre to ry
ex cur'sion
ex cur'va ture
ex cy''clo pho'ri a
ex cy''clo tro'pi a
ex''cys ta'tion
ex'e dens
ex''en ce pha'li a
ex en''ter a'tion
ex'er cise
ex er'e sis
ex''fe ta'tion
ex fo''li a'tion
ex fo''li a'tive
ex''ha la'tion
ex haust'er
ex haus'tion
ex''hi bi'tion
ex''hi bi'tion ism
ex''hi bi'tion ist
ex hil'a rant
ex''hu ma'tion
ex''is ten'tia lism

ex'i tus
Exner's area
ex''o car'di a
ex''o car'di ac
ex''o cat''a pho ri a
ex''o ce lom'ic
ex''oc cip'i tal
ex''o cho'ri on
ex''o coe'lom
ex'o crine
ex''o don'ti a
ex''o don'tist
ex og'a my
ex''o gas'tru la
ex og'e nous
ex''o hys'ter o pex''y
ex om'pha los
ex''o pho'ri a
ex''oph thal mom'e ter
ex''oph thal mom'e try
ex''oph thal'mos
ex''o skel'e ton
ex''os''to sec'to my
ex''os to'sis
ex''o ther'mic
ex''o tox'in
ex''o tro'pi a
ex pan'sive
ex pec'to rant
ex pec'to rate
ex pec''to ra'tion
ex pel'
ex per'i ment
ex''pi ra'tion
ex pi'ra tory
ex pire'
ex''plan ta'tion
ex''plo ra'tion
ex po'sure
ex pres'sion
ex pul'sion
ex san'gui nate

ex san"gui na'tion
ex sic'cant
ex"sic ca'tion
ex'stro phy
ex"suf fla'tion
ex ten'sion
ex ten'sor
ex te"ri or i za'tion
ex'tern
ex ter'nal ize
ex'ter o cep"tor
ex"ter o fec'tive
ex tinc'tion
ex"tir pa'tion
ex tor'sion
ex"tra ar tic'u lar
ex"tra buc'cal
ex"tra bulb'ar
ex"tra cap'su lar
ex"tra car'pal
ex"tra cel'lu lar
ex"tra cer'e bral
ex"tra cor po're al
ex"tra cor pus'cu lar
ex"tra cra'ni al
ex'tract
ex trac'tion
ex"tra cyst'ic
ex"tra du'ral
ex"tra em"bry on'ic
ex"tra ep"i phys'e al
ex"tra e"so phag'e al
ex"tra gen'i tal

ex"tra he pat'ic
ex"tra lig"a men'tous
ex"tra med'ul lar"y
ex"tra mu'ral
ex"tra nu'cle ar
ex"tra oc'u lar
ex"tra pa ren'chy mal
ex"tra pel'vic
ex"tra per"i ne'al
ex"tra per"i to ne'al
ex"tra pla cen'tal
ex"tra pros tat'ic
ex"tra py ram'i dal
ex"tra sen'sor y
ex"tra sys'to le
ex"tra tu'bal
ex"tra u'ter ine
ex"tra vag'i nal
ex trav"a sa'tion
ex"tra vas'cu lar
ex"tra ven tric'u lar
ex"tra vis'u al
ex trem'i ty
ex trin'sic
ex'tro phy
ex'tro vert
ex tru'sion
ex"tu ba'tion
ex'u date
ex"u da'tion
ex u"vi a'tion
eye
eye'lash"

F

fa bel'la
fab"ri ca'tion
face
fac'et
fa'cial

fa'ci es
fa cil"i ta'tion
fac"i o scap"u lo hu'mer al
fac ti'tious
fac'tor

fac'ul ta"tive
fag"o py'rism
Fahrenheit
fail'ure
faint
fal'ci form
fal'cu la
fal'cu lar
fal lo'pi an
Fallot, tetral'o gy of
false
falx
fa'mes
fa mil'ial
fa nat'i cism
Fanconi, Guido
fang
fan"go ther'a py
fan'ta sy
far'ad
Faraday, Michael
fa rad'ic
far"a dim'e ter
fa rad"i punc'ture
far'a dism
far"a di za'tion
far"a do con"trac til'i ty
far"a do mus'cu lar
far"i na'ceous
fas'ci a
fas'ci cle
fas cic'u la"ted
fas cic"u la'tion
fas cic'u lar
fas cic'u lus
fas"ci ec'to my
fas ci'num
fas"ci od'e sis
fas ci'o la ci ne're a
Fas"ci o loi'des
fas'ci o plas"ty
fas"ci or'rha phy

fas"ci o scap"u lo hu'mer al
fas"ci ot'o my
fas ci'tis
fas tig'i um
fa tigue'
fau'ces
fau'na
fa vag'i nous
fa ve'o lus
fa'vi des
fa'vism
fa'vus
fear
fea'ture
feb'ri cant
fe brif'ic
feb'ri fuge
fe'brile
feb"ri pho'bi a
fe'cal
fe'ca lith
fe'cal oid
fe'ces
fec'u lent
fe"cun da'tion
fe cun'di ty
feed'ing
Fehling's re a'gent
fe'line
fel la'ti o
fel"la tor'
fel"la trice'
fel'on
Felty's syn'drome
fe'male
fem'i nism
fem"i ni za'tion
fem'i niz ing
fem'o ral

119

fem"o ro tib'i al
fe'mur
fe nes'tra
fen"es tra'tion
Fe'o sol
fer'ment
fer"men ta'tion
fer'ra ted
fer'ric
fer"ri he"mo glo'bin
fer'rous
fer'tile
fer"ti li za'tion
fer'ti li zin
fes'ter
fes'ti na"ting
fes"ti na'tion
fes toon'
fe'tal ism
fe ta'tion
fe'ti cide
fet'id
fe'tish
fe'tish ism
fet'lock
fe tom'e try
fe"to pel'vic
fe'tor
fe'tus
fe'ver
fi'ber
fi'bril
fi'bril lat ed
fi"bril la'tion
fi bril"lo gen'e sis
fi'brin
fi brin'o gen
fi brin"o gen"o pe'ni a
fi"brin o glob'u lin

fi'bri noid
fi"bri no ly'sin
fi"brin ol'y sis
fi"brin o ly'tic
fi'brin ous
fi"bro ad"e no'ma
fi"bro ad'i pose
fi"bro an"gi o'ma
fi"bro a re'o lar
fi'bro blast
fi"bro blas'tic
fi"bro blas to'ma
fi"bro bron chi'tis
fi"bro cal car'e ous
fi"bro car"ci no'ma
fi"bro car'ti lage
fi"bro cel'lu lar
fi"bro chon dro'ma
fi"bro chon dro-os"te o'ma
fi"bro cys'tic
fi"bro cys to'ma
fi'bro cyte
fi"bro dys pla'si a
fi"bro e las'tic
fi"bro e las to'sis
fi"bro en"chon dro'ma
fi'bro gen
fi"bro gli o'ma
fi'broid
fi"broid ec'to my
fi"bro lam'i nar
fi"bro lei"o my o'ma
fi"bro li po'ma
fi"bro li po sar co'ma
fi"bro ly'sin
fi bro'ma
fi bro'ma toid
fi bro"ma to'sis
fi"bro mus'cu lar

fi"bro my o'ma
fi"bro my"o mec'to my
fi"bro my"o si'tis
fi"bro myx"o en do the"li o'ma
fi"bro myx"o li po'ma
fi"bro myx o'ma
fi"bro myx"o sar co'ma
fi"bro neu ro'ma
fi"bro-os"te o chon dro'ma
fi"bro-os te o' ma
fi"bro-os"te o sar co'ma
fi"bro pla'si a
fi"bro plas'tic
fi'bro plate"
fi"bro psam mo'ma
fi"bro pu'ru lent
fi"bro sar co'ma
fi"bro se'rous
fi bro'sis
fi"bro si'tis
fi brot'ic
fi'brous
fib'u la
fib"u lo cal ca'ne al
Fielder's my"o car di'tis
fig'ure
' fi la'ceous
fil'a ment
fil"a men ta'tion
fi la'ri a
fi lar'i al
fil"a ri sis
fi lar'i cide
fi lar'i form"
fil'i form"
fil'i punc"ture
fil'let
fil'ter
fil'tra ble

fil'trate
fil tra'tion
fil'trum
fi'lum
fim'bri a
fim'bri al
fin'ger
fis'sion
fis sip'a rous
fis'su la
fis'sure
fis'sure-in-a'no
fis'tu la
fis'tu lar
fis"tu lec'to my
fis"tu li za'tion
fis"tu lo en"ter os'to my
fis"tu lot'o my
fix a'tion
fix'a tive
flac'cid
flag'el late
flag"el la'tion
fla gel'li form"
fla gel'lum
flail
flap
flare
flat'u lence
flat'u lent
fla'tus
fla'vin
fla"vo bac ter'i a
flex"i bil'i tas
flex'i ble
flex im'e ter
flex'ion
Flexner's ba cil'lus
flex'or

121

flex'u ous
flex'ure
flick'er
floc''cu la'tion
floc'cu lent
floc'cu lus
flor'id
flo ta'tion
flow'me''ter
flu'id
fluke
flu'mi na pi lor'um
flu''o res'ce in
flu''o res'cence
flu''o ri da'tion
flu'o ride
flu''o ri na'tion
flu'o rine
flu'o rite
flu''o ro pho tom'e try
flu'o ro scope''
flu or os'co py
flu''o ro'sis
flut'ter
flux
foam
fo'cal
fo'cus
foil
fold
Foley cath'e ter
fo'lic ac'id
fo lie'a''deux
fo lin'ic
fo'li um
fol'li cle
fol lic'u lar
fol lic''u li'tis
fol lic''u lo'ma

fo''men ta'tion
fo'mes
fo'mi tes
fon''ta nel'
fo ra'men
fo ra'mi na
for''a min'u lum
for'ceps
Forcheimer's sign
Fordyce's dis ease'
fore'arm''
fore'brain''
fore'fin''ger
fore'foot''
fore'gut''
fore'head
for'eign
fo ren'sic
fore'pleas''ure
fore'skin''
fore'wa''ters
form al'de hyde
For'ma lin
for ma'tion
form'a tive
for'ma zan
for'mic
for''mi ca'tion
for'mu la
for'mu lar''y
for'ni cate
for''ni ca'tion
for'nix
Foshay's se'rum
fos'sa
fos sette'
fos'su la
found'ling
four chette'

fo've a
fo ve'o la
frac''tion a'tion
fract'ure
fra gil'tas
fra gil'i ty
frag''men ta'tion
fram be'si a
free'mar''tin
Frei test
frem'i tus
fre'nal
fre not'o my
fren'u lum
fre'num
fren'zy
fre'quen cy
Freud, Sigmund
fri'a ble
fric'tion
Friedlander ba cil'li
Friedman test
Friedreich's a tax'i a
fri gid'i ty
Froehlich's syn'drome
frole''ment'
fron'tal
fron ta'lis
fron''to ma'lar
fron''to max'il lar
fron''to men'tal
fron''to na'sal
fron''to-oc cip'i tal
fron''to-tem''po ra'le
frost'bite''
frot''tage'
frot''teur'
fruc'tose
frus tra'tion

Fu a'din
fuch'sin
fu'gi tive
fugue
ful'gu ra''ting
ful''gu ra'tion
fu lig'i nous
ful'mi nant
ful'mi na''ting
fu'ma rase
fu''mi ga'tion
fu'ming
func tion
func'tion al
fun'da ment
fun'di form
fun'dus
fun'du scope
fun''du sec'to my
fun'gate
fun'gi
fun''gi ci'dal
fun'gi cide
fun'gi form
fun''gi stat'ic
Fun gi'zone
fun'goid
fun'gus
fu'ni cle
fu nic'u lar
fu nic''u li'tis
fu nic'u lus
fu'nis
fun'nel
Fu'ra cin
Fu''ra dan tin
fur'cu la
fur'fur
fur'fur yl

fu'ror
fu ro'se mide
fur'row
fu'run cle
fu''run'cu lar
fu run''cu lo'sis
fus'cin

fu'sel oil
fu'si ble
fu'si form
fu'sion
fu''so cel'lu lar
fu''so spi''ro che'tal
fu''so spi''ro che to'sis

G

gait
ga lac''ta cra'si a
ga lac'ta gogue
ga lac'tase
gal''ac te'mi a
ga lact''hi dro'sis
ga lac'tic
gal''ac tis'chi a
ga lac'to cele
ga lac'to gen
ga lac'toid
gal''ac tom'e ter
gal''ac toph'a gous
gal''ac toph'ly sis
ga lac'to phore
gal''ac toph''o ri'tis
gal''ac toph'y gous
ga lac''to poi et'ic
ga lac''tor rhe'a
gal''ac tos'che sis
ga lac'to scope
ga lac'tose
gal ac''to se'mi a
gal''ac to'sis
gal''ac tos'ta sis
ga lac''to su'ri a
ga lac''to ther'a py
ga lac''to tox'in

gal''ac tot'ro phy
gal''ac tu'ri a
ga'le a
gal''e o phil'i a
gal''e o pho'bi a
gal''e ro'pi a
gall'blad''der
gal'lop
gall'stone
gal van'ic
gal'va nism
gal'van ize
gal''va no con''trac til'i ty
gal''va no far''a di za'tion
gal''va nom'eter
gal''va no mus'cu lar
gal'va no scope''
gal''va no sur'ger y
gal''va no ther'a py
gal'va no ther''my
gam'bi an
gam'ete
ga me'to cyte
gam''e to gen'e sis
ga me'to phyte
gam'ma
gam'ma cism
gam''o ma'ni a

gam"o pho'bi a
gan'gli a"ted
gan'gli o blast"
gan"gli o blas to'ma
gan'gli o cyte"
gan"gli o gli o'ma
gan'gli oid
gan'gli on
gan"gli on ec'to my
gan"gli o neu ro'ma
gan"gli on'ic
gan"gli o ni'tis
gan'gli o side
gan"glio si do'sis
gan"gli o sym path"i co
    blas to'ma
gan go'sa
gan'grene
gan'gre nous
gan'o blast
Gan ta'nol
Gan'tri sin
gar'get
gar'gle
gar'goyl
gar'goyl ism
gar'lic
gar rot'ing
Gartner's cyst
gasp
Gasserian gan'gli on
Gas"ter oph'i lus
gas tral'gi a
gas"tral go ke no'sis
gas"tras the'ni a
gas"tra tro'phi a
gas trec'ta sis
gas trec'to my
gas'tric

gas'trin
gas tri'tis
gas"tro a ceph'a lus
gas"tro a mor'phus
gas"tro an as"to mo'sis
gas'tro cele
gas"troc ne'mi us
gas"tro col'ic
gas"tro co lot'o my
gas"tro col pot'o my
gas"tro di'a phane
gas"tro di aph"a nos'co py
gas"tro did'y mus
gas"tro du"o de'nal
gas"tro du"o de ni'tis
gas"tro du"o de nos'to my
gas"tro en'ter ic
gas"tro en"ter i'tis
gas"tro en"ter o a nas"to mo'sis
gas"tro en"ter ol'o gist
gas"tro en"ter ol'o gy
gas"tro en"ter op to'sis
gas"tro en"ter os'to my
gas"tro ep"i plo'ic
gas"tro e'soph a ge"al
gas"tro e soph"a gi'tis
gas"tro gas tros'to my
gas"tro ga"vage'
gas'tro graph
gas"tro he pat'ic
gas"tro hy"per ton'ic
gas"tro hys"ter ot'o my
gas"tro in tes'ti nal
gas"tro je ju'nal
gas"tro je"ju ni'tis
gas"tro je"ju no col'ic
gas"tro je"ju nos'to my
gas"tro lav'age
gas'tro lith

gas"tro li thi'a sis
gas trol'o gy
gas trol'y sis
gas"tro ma la'ci a
gas"tro meg'a ly
gas trom'e lus
gas"tro my co'sis
gas"tro mu ot'o my
gas trop'a thy
gas'tro pex"y
gas"tro pho'tor
gas"tro phren'ic
gas"tro plas'ty
gas"tro pli ca'tion
gas"trop to'sis
gas"tro ph"lo rec'to my
gas"tror rha'gi a
gas tror'rha phy
gas"tror rhe'a
gas tros'chi sis
gas'tro scope
gas tros'co py
gas'tro spasm
gas"tro splen'ic
gas"tro stax'is
gas tros'to my
gas"tro tho ra cop'a gus
gas trot'o my
gas"tro tym'pa ni'tes
gas'tru la
gat"o phil'i a
gat"o pho'bi a
Gaucher's dis ease'
gauze
ga'vage
gaze
gel so'ma
ge las'mus
ge lat"i fi ca'tion

gel'a tin
ge lat"i no lyt'ic
ge lat'i nous
geld
geld'ing
Gel'foam
ge lot'o lep"sy
ge mel'lus
gem'i nate
gem"i na'tion
gem'ma
gem'mule
Gem'o nil
gene
ge ner'ic
ge ne"si ol'o gy
gen'e sis
ge net'ic
ge net'i cist
ge net'ics
ge net"o troph'ic
ge'ni al
ge nic'u lar
ge nic'u late
ge nic'u lum
ge"ni o glos'sus
ge"ni o hy'oid
ge'ni on
ge"ni o pha ryn'ge us
ge'ni o plas"ty
gen'i tal
gen"i ta'li a
gen'i ta loid
gen"i to cru'ral
gen"i to fem'o ral
gen"i to u'ri nar"y
gen'i us
Gennari's lay'er
gen'o cide

gen'o copy
gen"o der ma to'sis
ge'nome
gen"o pho'bi a
gen ta mi'cin
gen'o type
gen'tian
gen'u clast
gen"u cu'bi tal
gen"u fa'cial
gen"u pec'tor al
ge'nus
gen"y chei'lo plas"ty
gen'y plas"ty
ge"o pha'gi a
ge oph'a gy
Ge ot'ri chum
ge phy"ro pho'bi a
ge rat'ic
ger"a tol'o gy
ger"i a tri'ci an
ger"i at'rics
ger"i o psy cho'sis
ger ma'ni um
ger mi ci'dal
ger'mi cide
ger"mi na'tion
ger mi no'ma
ger"o der'ma
ger"o don'ti a
ger"o don'tics
ger"o ma ras'mus
ger"o mor'phism
ge ron'tic
ger"on tol'o gy
ge ron"to phil'ia
ge ron"to pho'bi a
ge ron'to ther'a py
ger"on tox'on

Gerstmann's syn'drome
Gesell, Arnold
ges ta'tion
Ghon tu'ber cle
Gi ar'di a
Gi ar'di a Lam'blia
gi"ar di'a sis
gib bos'i ty
gib'bous
gib'bus
gid'di ness
Giemsa stain
gi gan'tism
gi gan'to blast
gi gan'to cyte
Gigli's saw
gin'gi va
gin'gi val
gin"gi val'gi a
gin"gi vec'to my
gin"gi vi'tis
gin"gi vo glos si'tis
gin"gi vo'sis
gin"gi vo sto"ma ti'tis
gin'gly mus
gi"o tri cho'sis
gir'dle
git'o nin
gi tox'in
giz'zard
gla bel'la
gla'brous
gla'cial
glad"i o'lus
glair'y
gland
glan'ders
gland'u lar
glans

glass'y
Glauber's salt
glau co'ma
gleet
gle"no hu'mer al
gle'noid
gli'a
gli'al
gli'a cyte
gli'a din
gli"o bac te'ri a
gli"o blas to'ma mul"ti for'me
gli"o coc'cus
gli"o fi"bro'sar co'ma
gli o'ma
gli"o ma to'sis
gli o'ma tous
gli"o sar co'ma
gli o'sis
gli'o some
globe
glo'bin
glob'ule
glob'u li cide"
glob u lin
glob"u li nu'ri a
glo'bus
gloe'a
glome
glom'er ate
glo mer'u lar
glo mer"u lo ne phri'tis
glo mer"u lo scle ro'sis
glo mer'u lus
glo'mus
glos'sa
glos'sal
glos sal'gi a
glos san'thrax

glos sec'to my
glos si'tis
glos'so cele
glos"so dy"na mom'e ter
glos"so dyn'i a
glos"so ep"i glot'tic
glos'so graph
glos"so hy'al
glos"so kin"es thet'ic
glos"so la'bi al
glos"so la'li a
glos sol'o gy
glos"so man'ti a
glos"so pal'a tine
glos"so pal a ti'nus
glos sop'a thy
glos"so pha ryn'ge al
glos"so pha ryn'ge us
glos'so plas"ty
glos"so ple'gi a
gloss"op to'sis
glos"so py ro'sis
glos sor'rha phy
glos sos'co py
glos'so spasm"
glos sot'o my
glos"so trich'i a
glot'tic
glot'tis
glu'ca gon
glu"co cor'ti coid
glu"co ki'nase
glu"co ne"o gen'e sis
Glu"cos'a mine
glu'cose
glu'co side
glu"co su'ri a
glu"co syl cer"bro
  sid o'sis

glu″cu ron′ic ac′id
glu tam′ic ac′id
glu″ta thi′one
glu′ten
glu te′us
glu′tin
glut′ton y
gly ce′mi a
glyc′er ide
glyc′er in
glyc′er ol
glyc′er yl
gly′cine
gly′co gen
gly′co ge nase″
gly″co gen′e sis
gly″co gen′ic
gly″co ge nol′y sis
gly″co ge no′sis
gly′col
gly col′ic
gly col′y sis
gly″co me tab′o lism
gly″co ne″o gen′e sis
gly″co phil′i a
gly″co pty′a lism
gly″cor rha′chi a
gly″cor rhe′a
gly″co si al′i a
gly′co side
gly″co su′ri a
gly″co su′ric
glyc″u re′sis
Gmelin′s test
gnat
gnath al′gi a
gnath′ic
gna′thi on
gnath i′tis

gnath″o ceph′a lus
gnath″o̧ dy″na mom′e ter
gnath″o dyn′i a
gnath′o plas″ty
gnath os′chi sis
Gnath os′to ma
gno′sis
gnos′tic
Goetsch′s test
goi′ter
goi″tro gen′ic
Goldblatt clamp
Goldthwait′s op″e ra′tion
Golgi net′work″
gom phi′a sis
gom pho′sis
gon″a cra′ti a
gon′ad
gon′ad arch″e
gon″a dec′to my
gon″a do cen′tric
gon″a do ther′a py
gon″a do tro′pic
gon″a do tro′pin
gon′a duct
go nag′ra
go nal′gi a
gon″an gi ec′to my
gon″ar thri′tis
gon″ar throc′a ce
gon″a throt′o my
go nat′o cele
gon′e cyst
gon″e cys ti′tis
gon″e cys′to lith
gon″e cys″to py o′sis
gon″e poi e′sis
gon′ic
go″ni o chei los′chi sis

go"ni o cra"ni om'e try
go"ni om'e ter
go'ni on
go"ni o punc'ture
go'ni o scope
go ni ot'o my
go ni'tis
go'ni um
gon'o blast
gon"o coc'cal
gon"o coc ce'mi a
gon"o coc'ci
gon"o coc'cide
gon"o coc'cin
gon"o coc'cus
gon'o cyte
go nom'er y
gon"or rhe'a
gon"y ba'ti a
gon"y camp'sis
gon"y on'cus
gor'get
Gottschalk's op"e ra'tion
gouge
goun'dou
gout
Graafian fol'li cle
grac'i lis
Gradenigo's syn'drome
gra'di ent
grad'u ate
graft
grain'age
gram"i ci'din
gran'di ose
grand" mal'
gran'u lar
gran'u la"ted
gran"u la'tion

gran'ule
gran'i li form"
gran'u lo blast"
gran'u lo cyte"
gran"u lo cy"to pe'ni a
gran"u lo cy"to poi e'sis
gran"u lo'ma
gran"u lo"ma to'sis
gran"u lo'ma tous
gran"u lo plas'tic
gran"u lo poi e'sis
gran"u lo'sa
gran"u lo'sis ru'bra na'si
graph
graph"e the'si a
graph'ite
graph ol'o gy
graph"o ma'ni a
graph"o mo'tor
graph"o pho'bi a
graph"or rhe'a
grat tage'
grav'el
grav'id
gra'vi da
grav"i do car'di ac
gra vim'e ter
grav"i stat'ic
grav"i ta'tion
grav'i ty
Grawitz's tu'mor
gref'fo tome
gre ga'ri ous ness
grip, grippe
gris'e o ful vin
Grocco's sign
groin
Gruber's test
Grübler stain

gry po'sis
guai'ac
guan'i dine
Guarnieri's bod'ies
gu"ber nac'u lum
Guillain-Barre syn'drome
guil'lo tine
gul'let
gum'boil"
gum'ma
gum'ma tous
gus ta'tion
gus'ta to"ry
Guthrie test
gut'ta
gut'ta-per'cha
gym nas'tics
gym"no pho'bi a
gy nan'der
gy nan"dro blas to'ma
gy nan'dro morph
gy nan"dro mor'phism
gy nan'dro mor"phy
gy nan'drous

gy nan'dry
gyn"a tre'si a
gy ne'cic
gyn"e co gen'ic
gyn"e cog'ra phy
gyn'e coid
gyn"e co log'ic
gyn"e co log'i cal
gyn"e col'o gist
gyn"e col'o gy
gyn"e co ma'ni a
gyn"e co mas'ti a
gyn"e cop'a thy
gyn"e pho'bi a
gyn"e phor'ic
Gy'ner gen
gyn"i at'rics
gyn'o plas ty
gyp'sum
gy ra'tion
gy rec'to my
gyr"en ceph'a late
gy'ro mele
gy'rus

H

ha ben'u la
hab'it
hab'i tat
ha bit"u a'tion
hab'i tus
hack'ing
ha"de pho'bi a
haem"a to ther'mal
hae"mo coe'lom
Hagedorn nee'dle
Hageman fac'tor
hair

hal'a kone
ha la'tion
ha'la zone
hal'ite
hal"i to'sis
hal lu"ci na'tion
hal lu'ci"no gen
hal lu"ci no gen'ic
hal lu"ci no'sis
hal'lux
hal'o gen
hal'o thane

Halsted's op''e ra'tion
ham ar''to blas to'ma
ham''ar to'ma
ham''ar to pho'bi a
ham'ate
ha ma'tum
ham'ster
ham'u lus
hand'ed ness
hang'nail''
Hansen's dis ease'
haph''al ge'si a
haph''e pho'bi a
hap'lo dont
ha plo'pi a
hap'lo scope
hap'ten
hap''te pho'bi a
hap'tics
hap''to dys pho'ri a
hap''to glo'bin
hard'ness
hare'lip''
har''pax o pho'bi a
Hashimoto's stru'ma
hash'ish
Hassall's cor'pus cle
haunch
haus'trum
Haverhill fe'ver
ha ver'sian sys'tem
head'ache''
heal'ing
hear'ing
heart
he''be phre'ni a
Heberden's nodes
he bet'ic
heb'e tude

hec''a ter o mer'ic
hec'tic
hec'to gram
hec'to li''ter
hec'to me''ter
he do'ni a
he'don ism
he''do no pho'bi a
Hegar's sign
he gem'o ny
Heinz bod'ies
hel'i cine
hel'i cis
hel'i coid
hel'i co pod
hel''i co tre'ma
he''li en ceph''a li'tis
he''li o phobe''
he''li o pho'bi a
he'li o stat''
he''li o tax'is
he''li o ther'a py
he'li um
he'lix
Heller's test
Helmholtz's the'o ry
hel'minth
hel''min them'e sis
hel''min thi'a sis
hel''min thol'o gist
hel''min tho'ma
hel min''tho pho'bi a
he lo'ma
he lot'o my
he'ma chrome
he''ma dy''na mom'e ter
he''mag glu''ti na'tion
he''mag glu'ti nin
he'mal

he man''gi ec'ta sis
he man''gi o blas to'ma
he man''gi o en''do the''li o'ma
he man''gi o'ma
he man''gi o per i cy to'ma
he man''gi o sar co'ma
he''ma poph'y sis
he''mar thro'sis
he''ma te'in
he''ma tem'e sis
he''mat hi dro'sis
he mat'ic
hem'a tin
hem''a ti ne'mi a
hem''a tin'ic
hem''a to aer om'e ter
hem'a to blast''
hem'a to cele''
hem''a to chy'lo cele
hem''a to chy lu'ri a
hem''a to col'pus
hem'a to crit''
hem'a to cyst''
hem''a to cy tol'y sis
hem''a to dys cra'si a
hem''a to gen'e sis
he'ma toi'din
he''ma tol'o gist
he''ma tol'o gy
hem''a to lym''phan gi o'oma
hem''a to lym phu'ri a
he''ma tol'y sis
he''ma to'ma
hem''a to me''di a sti'num
he''ma tom'e ter
hem''a to me'tra
hem''a to my e'li a
hem''a to my''e li'tis
hem''a to pa thol'o gy

he''ma top'a thy
hem''a toph'a gus
hem''a to plas'tic
hem''a to poi e'sis
hem''a to poi et'ic
hem''a to por'phy rin
hem''a to por''phy ri ne'mi a
hem''a to por''phy ri nu'ri a
hem''a to pre cip'i tin
hem''a tor rha'chis
hem''a tor rhe'a
hem''a to sal'pinx
hem'a to scope
hem'a tose
hem''a to si phon i'a sis
he''ma to'sis
hem''a to spec'tro scope
hem''a to sper'ma to cele''
hem''a to sper'mi a
hem''a to tym'pa num
he''ma tox'y lin
hem''a tu'ri a
heme
hem''er a lo'pi a
hem''er a pho'ni a
hem'i a car'di us
hem''i a ceph'a lus
hem''i a geu'si a
hem''i an''a cu'si a
hem''i an''al ge'si a
hem''i an''es the'si a
hem''i an op'si a
hem''i a tax'i a
hem''i ath''e to'sis
hem''i at'ro phy
hem''i bal lis'mus
he'mic
hem''i car'di a
hem''i cel'lu lose

hem"i ceph'a lus
hem"i ceph'a ly
hem"i cho re'a
hem"i co lec'to my
hem"i cra'ni a
hem"i cra"ni o'sis
hem"i de cor"ti ca'tion
hem"i di'a phragm
hem'i dys"es the'si a
hem"i fa'cial
hem"i glos sec'to my
hem"i glos"so ple'gi a
hem"i gna'thi a
hem"i hy"pal ge'si a
hem"i hy"per es the'si a
hem"i hy"per hi dro'sis
hem"i hy"per to'ni a
hem"i hy"per'tro phy
hem"i hy"pes the'si a
hem"i hy"po to'ni a
hem"i lab"y rin thec'to my
hem"i lam"i nec'to my
hem"i lar"yn gec'to my
hem"i man"di bu lec'to my
hem"i me'li a
hem"i me'lus
hem"i me tab'o lous
he'min
hem"i ne phrec'to my
he mip'a gus
hem"i pal"a to la ryn"go ple'gi a
hem"i pa re'sis
hem"i pel vect'o my
hem"i ple'gi a
hem"i ra chis'chi sis
hem"i scler o der'ma al'ter nans
hem"i sco to'sis
hem"i sec'tion
hem"i so'mus

hem'i spasm
hem'i sphere
hem"i spher ec'to my
hem"i syn er'gi a
hem"i sys'to le
hem"i thy"roid ec' to my
hem"i ver'te bra
hem"i zy'gote
he"mo al"ka lim'e ter
he"mo bil'i a
he"mo bil"i ru'bin
he'mo blast
he"mo cho'ri al
he"mo chro"ma to'sis
he"mo chro'mo gen
he"mo chro mom'e ter
he"mo cla'si a
he"mo con"cen tra'tion
he"mo co'ni a
he"mo cry os'co py
he"mo cy'a nin
he'mo cyte
he"mo cy'to blast
he"mo cy"to gen'e sis
he"mo cy tol'y sis
he"mo cy tom'e ter
he mo'di a
he"mo di"ag no'sis
he"mo di al'y sis
he"mo di lu'tion
he"mo dy nam'ics
he"mo en"do the'li al
he"mo glo'bin
he"mo glo"bi ne'mi a
he"mo glo"bin if'er ous
he"mo glo"bi nom'e ter
he"mo glo"bin o'path ies
he"mo glo"bi nu'ri a
he'mo gram

he″mo his′ti o blast
he″mo hy per ox′i a
he″mo hy pox′i a
he′mo lith
he′mo lymph
he mol′y sin
he mol′y sis
he mo lyt′ic
he mol″y to poi et′ic
he′mo lyze
he″mo ma nom′e ter
he mom′e ter
he″mo pa thol′o gy
he mop′a thy
he″mo per″i car′di um
he″mo per″i to ne′um
he′mo phage
he′mo phil
he″mo phil′i a
he″mo phil′i ac
he″mo phil′ic
He moph′i lus
he″mo pho′bi a
he″moph thal′mi a
he″moph thi′sis
he″mo pneu″mo tho′rax
he mop′ty sis
hem′or rhage
hem″or rhag′ic
hem″or rhoi′dal
hem″or rhoid ec′to my
hem′or rhoids
he″mo sid′er in
he″mo sid″er i nu′ri a
he″mo sid″er o′sis
he″mo sta′sis
he′mo stat
he″mo stat′ic
he″mo ta chom′e ter

he″mo ther′a py
he″mo tho′rax
he″mo tox′ic
he″mo tox′in
he′mo trophe
he″mo troph′ic
he″mo tym′pa num
he″mo vil′lous
hen′bane
Henoch's pur′pu ra
he′par
hep′a rin
hep′a rin e′mia
hep′a rin ize
hep a′rin ized
hep″a rin′o cyte
hep″a tal′gi a
hep″a tec′to my
he pat′ic
he pat″i co du″o de nos′to my
he pat″i co en″ter os′to my
he pat″i co gas tros′to my
he pat″i co li thot′o my
he pat″i co pan″cre at′ic
he pat″i cos′to my
he pat″i cot′o my
hep″a tit′i des
hep″a ti′tis
he″pat o bil′i ary
hep″a to cell′u lar
he″pat o ce re′bral
hep″a to cho lan″gi o du″o de nos′to my
hep″a to cho lan″gi o en″ter os′to my
hep″a to cho lan″gi o gas tros′to my
hep″a to cho lan″gi o je″ju nos′to my

hep"a to col'ic
hep"a to cyst'ic
hep"a to du"o de'nal
hep"a to du"o de nos'to my
hep"a to gen'ic
hep'a to gram
hep"a tog'ra phy
hep"a to len tic'lar
hep"a to li e'nal
hep"a to li"en og'ra phy
hep'a to lith
hep"a to lith ec'to my
hep"a to li thi'a sis
he pat"o ly'sin
hep"a to'ma
hep"a to meg'a ly
hep'a to pex"y
he"pat o phos"phor'y lase
he"pat o por'tal
hep"a top to'sis
hep"a to re'nal
hep"a tor'rha phy
hep"a tor rhex'is
hep"a tos'co py
hep"a to'sis
hep"a to sple"no meg'a ly
hep"a to sple"nop'a thy
hep"a to ther'a py
hep"a tot'o my
hep"a to tox'ic
hep"a to tox'in
Hep'ta chlor
hep to su'ri a
herb
her ba'ceous
her biv'o rous
he red'i ty
her"e do ak"i ne'si a
her"e do fa mil'i al

her"e do path'i a
her'it age
her maph'ro dite
her maph'ro dit ism
her"mar thro'sis
her met'ic
her'nia
her'ni ate
her'ni at"ed
her"ni a'tion
her'ni o plas"ty
her"ni or'rha phy
her'ni o tome
her"ni ot'o my
her'o in
her pan'gin a
her'pes
her pet'ic
her pet'i form
her"pe tol'o gy
Herxheimer's re ac'tion
Hesselback's tri'an"gle
het"er a de'ni a
het"er a'li us
het"er es the'si a
het"er o ag glu'ti nin
het"er o aux'one
het"er o blas'tic
het"er o cel'lu lar
het"er o ceph'a lus
het"er o chro'ma tin
het"er o chro'mi a
het'er o dont"
het"er o dro'mi a
het"er o er'o tism
het"er o fer men'ta tive
het"er o ga met'ic
het"er og'a my
het"er o ge'ne ous

het"er og'o ny
het'er o graft"
het"er o hyp no'sis
het"er o ki ne'si a
het"er o ki ne'sis
het"er ol'o gy
het"er o mer'ic
het"er o met"a pla'si a
het"er o me tro'pi a
het"er o mor'phic
het"er on'y mous
het"er o os'te o plas"ty
het"er op'a thy
het'er o phe"my
het'er o phil
het'er o pho'ni a
het'er o pho'ri a
het'er o pla'si a
het'er o plas"ty
het'er o ploid
het"er op'si a
Het"er op'ter a
het"er op'tics
het'er o scope"
het"er o sex"u al'i ty
het"er o sug ges'tion
het"er o tax'is
het"er o to'ni a
het"er o to'pi a
het"er o trans plan ta'tion
het"er o tro'pi a
het"er o ty'pus
het"er o zy'gote
het"er o zy'gous
hex"a chro'mic
hex'ad
hex"a dac'ty lism
hex"a gen'ic
hex'ane

hex"o bar'bi tal
hex"o ki'nase
hex'ose
hex"yl res or'cin ol
hi a'tal
hi a'tus
hi"ber na'tion
hi"ber no'ma
hic'cough
hic'cup
hid rad"e ni'tis
hid rad"e car"ci no'ma
hid rad'e no cyte
hid rad"e no'ma
hid ro'a
hid"ro cys to'ma
hid"ro poi e'sis
hid"ror rhe'a
hi"dros ad"e ni'tis
hid ros'che sis
hi dro'sis
hi drot'ic
hid"ro to path'ic
hi"er o pho'bi a
hi'lar
hi'lum
hi'lus
hip pan'thro py
hip"po cam'pus
Hippocrates
hip'po lith
hip"po myx o'ma
hip pu'ri a
hip pu'ric ac'id
hip'pus
Hirschsprung's dis ease'
hir'sute
hir su'ti es
hir'sut ism

hir′u din
his′ta mine
his″ta min′ic
his′ti dine
his″ti di ne′mi a
his′ti o cyte
his″ti o cy to′ma
his″ti o cy″to sar co′ma
his″ti o cy to′sis
his′to blast
his″to chem′is try
his″to di al′y sis
his″to flu″o res′cence
his″to gen′e sis
his′toid
his to log′ic
his tol′o gist
his tol′o gy
his tol′y sis
his″to lyt′ic
his to′ma
his″to met″a plas′tic
his″to mor phol′o gy
his″to pa thol′o gy
his″to phys″i ol′o gy
His″to plas′ma
his″to plas′min
his″to plas mo′sis
his″to spec tros′co py
his″to ther′a py
his″to throm′bin
his′to tome
his tot′o my
his″to tox′ic
his′to trophe
his″tri on′ic
hives
hoarse
hoar′y

hob′ble
Hodgkin's dis ease′
ho″do pho′bi a
Hofmeister-Finsterer
  op″e ra′tion
hol″er ga′si a
hol″o a car′di us
hol″o blas′tic
hol″o ce phal′ic
hol″o cra′ni a
hol′o crine
hol″o di″as tol′ic
hol″o gas tros′chi sis
hol″o gyn′ic
hol″o met″a bol′ic
hol″o ra chis′chi sis
hol″o so mat′ic
hol″o sys tol′ic
hom″a lo ceph′a lus
hom″a lo cor′y phus
hom″a lo me′to′pus
hom″a lo pis″tho cra′ni us
hom″a lu ra′nus
hom at′ro pine
hom ax′i al
ho′me o chrome″
ho″me o ki ne′sis
ho″me o mor′phous
ho″me o path′ic
ho″me op′a thy
ho″me o pla′si a
ho″me o′sis
ho″me os′ta sis
ho″me o ther′mal
ho″mi chol pho′bi a
hom′i cide
ho″mo cen′tric
ho′mo chrome
ho″mo chro″mo i som′er ism

ho"mo clad'ic
ho"mo cys'tin e mia
ho"mo cys tin u'ria
ho'mo dont
ho'mo dy'na my
ho"mo er'o tism
ho"mo ga met'ic
ho"mo ge'ne ous
ho"mo gen'ic
ho"mo ge"ni za'tion
ho mog'e nous
ho"mo gen tis'ic ac'id
ho'mo graft
ho"mo i other'mic
ho"mo lac'tic
ho mol'o gous
ho mon'o mous
ho"mo mor'phic
ho mon'y mous
ho'mo plas"ty
ho'mo sex"u al'i ty
ho"mo ther'mic
ho"mo trans"plan ta'tion
ho'mo type
ho"mo zy'gote
ho"mo zy'gous
ho mun'cu lus
hor de'o lum
hor"me pho'bi a
hor'mi on
Hor"mo den'drum
hor mo'nal
hor'mone
hor mo"no poi e'sis
hor'mo zone
Horner's syn'drome
horn"i fi ca'tion
ho rop'ter
hos'pi tal

hos"pit al i za'tion
hot flash'es
Houssay, Bernardo Alberto
Hoyne's sigh
hu man'o scope
Hu'ma tin
hu mec'tant
hu'mer al
hu"mer o ra'di al
hu"mer o scap'u lar
hu"mer o ul'nar
hu'mer us
hu mid"i fi ca'tion
hu mid'i ty
hu'min
hu'mor
hu'mor al
hu'mu lus
hu'mus
Hurler's dis ease'
hy'a lin
hy'a line
hy"a lin i za'tion
hy"a lin o'sis
hy"a li nu'ri a
hy"a li'tis
hy"a lo cap"su li'tis
hy al'o gen
hy'a loid
hy'a lo mere
hy"a lo mu'coid
hy"a lo nyx'is
hy"a lo pho'bi a
hy'a lo plasm
hy"a lo se"ro si'tis
hy"a lu ron'i dase
hy'brid
hy"brid i za'tion
hy dan'to in

139

hy dat'id
hy da tid'i form"
hy"da tid'o cele
hy dat"i do'sis
hy'dra gogue
hy dral'a zine
hy dram'ni os.
hy"drar gyr'i a
hy"drar gyr"o pho'bi a
hy"drar gyr"oph thal'mi a
hy"drar thro'sis
hy'drase
hy'drate
hy dra'tion
hy drau'lics
hy'dra zine
hy"dre lat'ic
hy dre'mi a
hy"dren ceph'a lo cele
hy"dren ceph"a lo me nin'go cele
hy dri od'ic ac'id
hy dro'a
hy"dro bil"i ru'bin
hy"dro bro'mic
hy"dro ca'lix
hy"dro car'bon
hy'dro cele
hy"dro ce lec'to my
hy"dro ce phal'ic
hy"dro ceph'a lus
hy"dro ceph'a ly
hy"dro chin"o nu'ri a
hy"dro chlo'ric ac'id
hy"dro chlo'ride
hy"dro col'loid
hy"dro col'pos
hy"dro co'ni on
hy"dro cor'ti sone
hy"dro dip"so ma'ni a

hy"dro dy nam'ics
hy'dro gen
hy"dro gen'a tion
hy"dro gen ly'ase
hy"dro glos'sa
hy"dro gym nas'tics
hy"dro hem"a to ne phro'sis
hy"dro ki net'ic
hy"dro lac tom'e ter
hy'dro lase
hy drol'o gy
hy drol'y sis
hy drol'y zate
hy"dro ma'ni a
hy"dro mas sage'
hy'dro mel
hy"dro me nin'go cele
hy drom'e ter
hy"dro me"tro col'pos
hy"dro mi"cro ceph'a ly
hy"dro my e'li a
hy"dro my'e lo cele"
hy"dro my'rinx
hy"dro ne phro'sis
hy drop'a thy
hy"dro per"i car di'tis
hy"dro per"i car'di um
hy"dro per'i on
hy"dro per"i to ne'um
Hy droph'i dae
hy'dro phil
hy"dro phil'ic
hy'dro phobe
hy"dro pho'bi a
hy'dro phone
hy"droph thal'mos
hy drop'ic
hy'dro plasm
hy"dro pneu"ma to'sis

hy"dro pneu"mo per"i car'di um
hy"dro pneu"mo per"i to ne'um
hy"dro pneu"mo tho'rax
hy'drops
hy"dro py"o ne phro'sis
hy"dror rhe'a
hy"dro sal'pinx
hy"dro sat'ur nism
hy"dro sol'u ble
hy"dro sper'ma to cyst"
hy"dro spi rom'e ter
hy'dro stat
hy"dro sy rin"go my e'li a
hy"dro tax'is
hy"dro ther"a peu'tics
hy"dro ther'a py
hy"dro ther'mal
hy"dro thi"o nu'ri a
hy"dro tho'rax
hy dro'tis
hy drot'ro pism
hy"dro tym'pa num
hy"dro-u re'ter
hy drox'ide
hy drox'yl
hy dru'ri a
hy"e tom'e try
Hygeia
hy'giene
hy'gi en ist
hy"gre che'ma
hy"gro ble phar'ic
hy gro'ma
hy grom'e ter
hy"gro pho'bi a
hy'gro scope
hy"gro scop'ic
hy"gro sto'mi a
Hy'ki none

hy"lo pho'bi a
hy"lo trop'ic
hy"lo zo'ism
hy'men
hy"me nec'to my
hy"me ni'tis
Hy"me nol'e pis
hy"me nol'o gy
Hy"me nop'ter a
hy"me nor'rha phy
hy men'o tome
hy"me not'o my
hy"o ep"i glot'tic
hy"o glos'sal
hy"o glos'sus
hy'oid
hy"o man dib'u lar
hy o'cine
hy"os cy'a mine
hy"o sta pe'di al
hy"o ver"te brot'o my
hyp"a cu'si a
hyp"al bu"min o'sis
hyp"al ge'si a
hyp am'ni o૬
hy pan"i sog'na thism
hy"par te'ri al
hy"pas the'ni a
hy pax'i al
hy pen"gy o pho'bi a
hy"per ab duc'tion
hy"per a cid'i ty
hy"per a cu'i ty
hy"per a cu'si a
hy"per a cu'sis
hy"per ad"e no'sis
hy"er ad re'nal ism
hy"per ad re'ni a
hy"per ad re"no cor'ti cism

hy"per a"er a'tion
hy"per al dos'ter on ism
hy"per al ge'si a
hy"per al"i men ta'tion
hy"per al"i men to'sis
hy"per am mon e'mi a
hy"per an"a ki ne'si a
hy"per a'phi a
hy"per bar'ic
hy"per bar'ism
hy"per bil"i ru"bi ne'mi a
hy"per brach"y ceph'a ly
hy"per bu'li a
hy"per cal ce'mi a
hy"per cal ci nu'ri a
hy"per cap'ni a
hy"per car"o te ne'mi a
hy"per ca thar'sis
hy"per ca thex'is
hy"per ce"men to'sis
hy"per ce"nes the'si a
hy"per cham'aer rhine
hy"per chlo re'mi a
hy"per chlor hy'dri a
hy"per cho les"ter e'mi a
hy"per cho'li a
hy"per chro mat'ic
hy"per chro'ma tism
hy"per chro"ma to'sis
hy"per chy'li a
hy"per chy"lo mi cro ne'mi a
hy"per cor'ti cism
hy"per cry"al ge'si a
hy"per di crot'ic
hy"per dis ten'tion
hy"per dy nam'ic
hy"per e che'ma
hy"per e"las to'sis
hy"per em'e sis

hy"per e'mi a
hy"per en ceph'a lus
hy"per ep"i thy'mi a
hy"per e"qui lib'ri um
hy"per er'gi a
hy'per er gy
hy"per es"o pho'ri a
hy"per es the'si a
hy"per es'trin ism
hy"per es"tro ge ne'mi a
hy"per ex"o pho'ri a
hy"per ex ten'sion
hy"per flex'ion
hy"per func'tion
hy"per gam"ma glob u li ne'mi a
hy"per gen'e sis
hy"per geu'si a
hy"per gi gan"to so'ma
hy"per glob'u li ne'mi a
hy"per gly ce'mi a
hy"per gly ce'mic
hy"per gly cer e'mi a
hy"per gly ci ne'mi a
hy"per gly"co ge nol'y sis
hy"per gly"cor rha'chi a
hy"per gly"co su'ri a
hy"per gon'ad ism
hy"per go'ni a
hy"per he do'ni a
hy"per hi dro'sis
hy"per his"ta mi ne'mi a
hy"per hor mo'nal
hy"per in"o se'mi a
hy"per i no'sis
hy"per in'su lin ism
hy"per in"vo lu'tion
hy"per ka le'mi a
hy"per ker"a to'sis
hy"per ker"a tot'ic

hy"per ke"to nu'ri a
hy"per ki ne'mi a
hy"per ki ne'si a
hy"per ki net'ic
hy"per lac ta'tion
hy"per lep'tor rhine
hy"per ley'dig ism
hy"per li pe'mi a
hy"per li"po pro tein e'mi a
hy"per li sin e'mi a
hy"per li thu'ri a
hy"per lo'gi a
hy"per mac"ro glob u lin e'mi a
hy"per ma'ni a
hy"per ma'nic
hy"per mas'ti a
hy"per ma ture'
hy"per mel an o'sis
hy"per men"or rhe'a
hy"per me tro'pi a
hy"per mi"cro so'ma
hy"per mim'i a
hy"perm ne'si a
hy"per mo til'i ty
hy"per na tre'mi a
hy"per neph'roid
hy"per ne phro'ma
hy"per noi'a
hy"per nu tri'trion
hy"per on cho'ma
hy"per on'to morph
hy"per o nych'i a
hy"per o'pi a
hy"per o rex'i a
hy"per or'tho gna"thy
hy"per os'mi a
hy"per os"mo lar'i ty
hy"per os"te og'e ny
hy"per os to'sis

hy"per ox a lu'ri a
hy"per ox e'mi a
hy"per ox"y gen a'tion
hy"per par'a site
hy"per par"a thy'roid ism
hy"per path'i a
hy"per pep sin'i a
hy"per per"i stal'sis
hy"per pha'gi a
hy"per pha lan'gism
hy"per pho ne'sis
hy"per pho'ni a
hy"per phos pha tas'i a
hy"per phos"pho li pi de'mi a
hy"per phos pha te'mi a
hy"per pi e'si a
hy"per pig"men ta'tion
hy"per pi tu'i ta rism
hy"per pla'si a
hy"per plas mi ne'mi a
hy"per plas'tic
hy"per plat"y mer'ic
hy"perp ne'a
hy"per po ro'sis
hy"per pot"as se'mi a
hy"per pra'gi a
hy"per prax'i a
hy"per pres"by o'pi a
hy"per pro"cho re'sis
hy"per pro ges"ter o ne'mia
hy"per pro lin e'mi a
hy"per pro sex'i a
hy"per pro"te in e'mi a
hy"per psy cho'sis
hy"per py rex'i a
hy"per re flex'i a
hy"per res'o nance
hy"per sal"i va'tion
hy"per sar co si ne'mi a

hy"per se cre'tion
hy"per sen"si tiv'i ty
hy"per som'ni a
hy"per sple'nism
hy"per ster"e o roent"gen
  og'ra phy
hy"per sthe'ni a
hy"per sthen'ic
hy"per sus cep"ti bil'i ty
hy"per syn'chro ny
hy"per tel'or ism
hy"per ten'sin
hy"per ten'sin ase
hy"per ten sin'o gen
hy"per ten'sion
hy"per the'li a
hy'per therm"
hy"per ther"mal ge'si a
hy"per ther'mi a
hy"per ther'my
hy"per thy"mi za'tion
hy"per thy'roid ism
hy"per to'ni a
hy"per ton'ic
hy"per tri cho'sis
hy per tro'phi a
hy"per troph'ic
hy per'tro phy
hy"per tro'pi a
hy"per u"ri ce'mi a
hy"per val in e'mi a
hy"per vas'cu lar
hy"per veg'e ta"tive
hy"per ven"ti la'tion
hy"per vi"ta min o'sis
hy"per vo le'mi a
hyp"es the'si a
hy'pha
hyp"he do'ni a

hy phe'ma
hyp"hi dro'sis
hyp"i no'sis
hyp"na gog'ic
hyp'na gogue
hyp nal'gi a
hyp'nic
hyp"no a nal'y sis
hyp"no gen'ic
hyp"no go'gic
hyp'noid
hyp"no lep"sy
hyp nol'o gy
hyp"no nar co'sis
hyp"no pho'bi a
hyp"no phre no'sis
hyp"no pom'pic
hyp"no si gen'e sis
hyp no'sis
hyp"no ther'a py
hyp not'ic
hyp'no tism
hyp'no tist
hyp'no tize
hyp'no toid
hyp"no tox'in
hy'po
hy"po a cid'i ty
hy"po ac tiv'i ty
hy"po ad ren"i ne'mi a
hy"po ad re'nal ism
hy"po ad re'ni a
hy"po ag'na thus
hy"po al dos'ter on ism
hy"po al"bu min e'mi a
hy"po al ler gen'ic
hy"po az"o tu'ri a
hy"po bar'ic
hy"po bar'ism·

hy''po ba rop'a thy
hy''po be ta li''po pro tein e'mi a
hy''po bran'chi al
hy''po bu'li a
hy''po cal ce'mi a
hy''po cal''ci fi ca'tion
hy''po cap'ni a
hy''po ca thex'is
hy''po chlo re'mi a
hy''po chlor hy'dri a
hy''po chlo'rite
hy''po chlor u'ri a
hy''po cho les''ter e'mi a
hy''po chon'dri a
hy''po chon'dri ac
hy''po chon dri'a sis
hy''po chon'dri um
hy''po chor'dal
hy''po chro mat'ic
hy''po chro'mic
hy''po chy'li a
hy''po coe'lom
hy'po cone
hy''po con'id
hy''po con'ule
hy''po con'u lid
hy''po cy clo'sis
hy''po cy the'mi a
hy''po der mi'a sis
hy''po der'mic
hy''po der'mis
hy''po der moc'ly sis
hy''po don'ti a
hy''po er'gy
hy''po es''o pho'ri a
hy''po es'trin ism
hy''po ex''o pho'ri a
hy''po fer re'mi a
hy''po func'tion

hy''po gal ac'ti a
hy''po gam ma glob''u lin e'mi a
hy''po gas'tric
hy''po gas'tri um
hy''po gas trop'a gus
hy''po gas tros'chi sis
hy''po gen'i tal ism
hy''po geu'si a
hy''po glos'sal
hy''po glos si'tis
hy''po glos'sus
hy''po gly ce'mi a
hy''po gly''co ge nol'y sis
hy''po gnath'ous
hy''po gon'ad ism
hy''po gran''u lo cy to'sis
hy''po in'su lin ism
hy''po kal i e'mi a
hy''po ki ne'si a
hy''po lem'mal
hy''po lep''si o ma'ni a
hy''po ley'dig ism
hy''po li po pro''tein e'mi a
hy''po lo'gi a
hy''po mag''ne se'mi a
hy''po ma'ni a
hy''po ma'nic
hy''po mas'ti a
hy''po men''or rhe'a
hy'po mere
hy''po me tab'o lism
hy''po me tro'pi a
hy''po mi''cro gnath'us
hy''po mi'cron
hy''po mi''cro so'ma
hy''pom ne'si a
hy''po mo til'i ty
hy''po nan''o so'ma
hy''po nat re'mi a

hy″po no′ic
hy″po nych′i um
hy″po os to′sis
hy″po par″a thy′roid ism
hy″po per″me a bil′i ty
hy″po pha lan′gism
hy″po phar″yn gos′co py
hy″po phar′ynx
hy″po pho′ni a
hy″po pho′ri a
hy″po phos″pha ta′sia
hy″po phos″pha te′mi a
hy″po phre′ni a
hy poph″y sec′to my
hy poph′y sis
hy″po pi e′si a
hy″po pin′e al ism
hy″po pi tu′i ta rism
hy″po pla′si a
hy pop′nea
hy″po pot″as se′mi a
hy″po prax′i a
hy″po pro sex′i a
hy″po pro″te i ne′mi a
hy″po pro throm″bi ne′mi a
hy″po psel″a phe′si a
hy″po psy cho′sis
hy″po′py on
hy″po sal″i va′tion
hy″po scle′ral
hy″po se cre′tion
hy″po sen″si tiv′i ty
hy pos′mi a
hy″po som′ni a
hy″po spa′di ac
hy″po spa′di as
hy″po sper″ma to gen′e sis
hy″pos phre′si a
hy′po spray

hy pos′ta sis
hy″po stat′ic
hy″pos the′ni a
hy pos″the nu′ri a
hy″po sto′mi a
hy″po syn er′gi a
hy″po tax′i a
hy″po tax′is
hy″po tel′or ism
hy″po ten′sion
hy″po ten′sive
hy″po ten′sor
hy″po thal′a mus
hy″po the′nar
hy″po therm″es the′sia
hy″po ther′mal
hy″po ther′mi a
hy″poth′e sis
hy″po thy′mi a
hy″po thy′roid ism
hy″po thy ro′sis
hy″po to′ni a
hy″po ton′ic
hy″po tri cho′sis
hy″po tro′pi a
hy″po tym′pan um
hy″po veg′e ta″tive
hy po ven′ti la″tion
hy″po vi″ta min o′sis
hy″po vo le′mi a
hy″pox e′mi a
hy pox′i a
hyp″sar rhyth′mia
hyp″si brach″y ce phal′ic
hyp″si ceph′a ly
hyp′si conch″
hyp″si sta phyl′i a
hyp so chro′mic
hyp″so pho′bi a

hys'sop
hys"ter al'gi a
hys"ter ec'to my
hys"ter e'sis
hys"ter eu ryn'ter
hys te'ri a
hys ter'i cism
hys ter'i cal
hys ter'ics
hys ter'i form
hys"ter o bu bon'o cele
hys'ter o cele"
hys"ter o clei'sis
hys"ter o de"mon op'a thy
hys"ter o dyn'i a
hys"ter o ep'i lep"sy
hys"ter o fren'ic
hys"ter og'e ny
hys"ter og'ra phy
hys'ter oid
hys"ter o lap"a rot'o my
hys'ter o lith
hys"ter o li thi'a sis
hys"ter ol'o gy
hys"ter ol'y sis
hys"ter o ma'ni a
hys"ter om'e ter
hys"ter o my o'ma

hys"ter o my"o mec'to my
hys"ter o my ot'o my
hys"ter o-o"pho rec'to my
hys"ter op'a thy
hys'ter a pex"y
hys"ter o phil'i a
hys"ter o plas'ty
hys"ter op to'sis
hys"ter or'rha phy
hys"ter or rhex'is
hys"ter o sal"pin gec'to my
hys"ter o sal"pin gog'ra phy
hys"ter o sal pin"go
 o"o pho rec'to my
hys"ter o sal pin"go
 o"o the cec'to my
hys"ter o sal"pin gos'to my
hys'ter o scope"
hys"ter os to ma 'tomy
hys'ter o tome"
hys"ter ot'o my
hys"ter o tra"che lec'to my
hys"ter o tra'che lo plas"ty
hys"ter o tra"che lor'rha phy
hys"ter o tra"che lot'o my
hys"ter o trau'ma tism
hy'ther

I

i am"a tol'o gy
i at"ro chem'is try
i at"ro gen'ic
i at"ro phys'ics
ich'no gram
i'chor
i"chor rhe'a
i"chor rhe'mi a

ich'tham mol
ich"thy is'mus
ich"thy o col'la
ich'thy oid
ich"thy ol'o gy
ich"thy oph'a gous
ich"thy o pho'bi a
ich"thy o'sis

ich"thy o tox'i con
ich"thy o tox is'mus
i'con
i"co nog'ra phy
i con"o lag'ny
i con"o ma'ni a
ic'tal
ic ter'ic
ic"ter o gen'ic
ic'ter oid
ic'ter us
ic'tus
id
i de'a
i de"al i za'tion
i"de a'tion
id"e o ge net'ic
id"e o glan'du lar
id"e ol'o gy
id"e o me tab'o lism
id"e o mo'tor
id"e o mus'cu lar
id"e o pho'bi a
id'e o plas"ty
id"e o syn chy'si a
id"e o vas'cu lar
id"i o chro'mo some
id"i oc'ra sy
id"i oc to'ni a
id'io cy
id"i og'a mist
id"i o gen'e sis
id"i o glos'si a
id"i o hyp'no tism
id"i ol'o gism
id"i o me tri'tis
id"i o mus'cu lar
id"i o path'ic
id"i op'a thy

id'i o phone
id'i o plasm
id"i o psy chol'o gy
id"i o re'flex
id"i o ret'i nal
id'i o some"
id'i o syn'cra sy
id"i o syn crat'ic
id'i ot
id"i o ven tric'u lar
i dol"o ma'ni a
i dro'sis
ig'ni punc"ture
ig ni'tion
il'e ac
il"e ec'to my
il"e i'tis
il"e o ce cos'to my
il"e o ce'cal
il"e o ce'cum
il"e o col'ic
il"e o co li'tis
il"e o co los'to my
il"e o il"e os'to my
il"e or'rha phy
il"e o sig"moid os'to my
il"e os'to my
il"e ot'o my
il'e um
il'e us
il'i a
il'i ac
i li'a cus
il"i o cap"su lar'is
il"i o cap" su lo tro"chan ter'i cu
il"i o coc cyg'e al
il"i o coc cyg'e us
il"i o cos tal'is
il"i o cos"to cer"vi cal'is

il″i o fem′o ral
il″i o hy″po gas′tric
il″i o in′gui nal
il″i op′a gus
il″i o par″a si′tus
il″i o pec tin′e al
il″i o pso′as
il″i o sac ral′is
il″i o tho″ra cop′a gus
il″i o xi phop′a gus
il′i um
il laq″ue a′tion
il″le git′i mate
il″li ni′tion
il lin′i um
ill′ness
il lu′mi nance
il lu″mi na′tion
il lu′mi nism
il lu′sion
I lo ty′cin
i′ma
im′age
im ag″i na′tion
i ma′go
im bal′ance
im′be cile
im″be cil′i ty
im″bi bi′tion
im′bri ca″ted
Imhotep
im″i ta′tion
im″ma ture′
im med′i ca ble
im mer′sion
im mis′ci ble
im mo″bi li za′tion
im″mor tal′i ty
im mune′

im mu′ni ty
im″mu ni za′tion
im′mu nize
im mu′no blasts
im mu″no chem′is try
im mu′no cytes
im mu″no gen′ic
im″mu no glob′u lin
im mu′no-he″ma tol′o gy
im mu″no log′ic
im″mu nol′o gist
im″mu nol′o gy
im mu″no trans fu′sion
im pac′tion
im pal′pa ble
im′par
im par″i dig′i tate
im passe′
im pe′dance
im per′a tive
im″per cep′tion
im per′fo rate
im per′me a ble
im per′vi ous
im″pe tig″i ni za′tion
im″pe ti′go
im pin′ger
im″plan ta′tion
im′plants
im pon′der a ble
im′po tence
im′po tent
im preg′nate
im pres′sion
im pro′cre ant
im pu′ber al
im′pulse
im pul′sion
im pu″ta bil′i ty

in''a cid'i ty
in ac'ti vate
in ad'e qua cy
in al''i men'tal
in an'i mate
in''a ni'tion
in ap'pe tence
in''ar tic'u late
in ar tic'u lo mor'tis
in''as sim'i la ble
in'born''
in'breed''ing
in car''cer a'tion
in ca'ri al
in car'nant
in'cest
in'ci dence
in'ci dent
in cin''er a'tion
in cip i ent
in ci'sal
in cised'
in ci'sion
in ci'sive
in ci si'vis la'bi i in''fer i or'is
in ci si'vis la'bi i su''per i or'is
in ci'sor
in''ci su'ra
in''ci sur'ae he'li cis
in ci'sure
in''cli na'tion
in''cli nom'e ter
in clu'sion
in''co ag'u la ble
in''co her'ence
in''co her'ent
in''com bus'ti ble
in''com pat'i ble
in''com pen sa'tion

in com'pe tence
in con'gru ence
in''con gru'i ty
in con'ti nence
in con'ti nent
in con tin en'ti a pig men'ti
in''co or''di na'tion
in cor''po ra'tion
in'cre ment
in cre'tion
in''crus ta'tion
in''cu ba'tion
in'cu ba''tor
in'cu bus
in''cu dec'to my
in''cu do mal'le al
in''cu do sta pe'di al
in cur'a ble
in'cus
in cy''clo pho'ri a
in cly''clo tro'pi a
i de'cent
in''de ci'sion
in''den ta'tion
in'dex
in'di can
in'di cant
in''di ca nu'ri a
in''di ca'tion
in'di ca''tor
in'di ces
in dig'e nous
in''di ges'tion
in dig''i ta'tion
in'di go
in'dole
in'do lent
in duc tion
in''duc to'ri um

in duc'to ther"my
in'du rat"ed
in"du ra'tion
in e'bri ant
in e"bri a'tion
in"e bri'e ty
in ef'fi ca cy
in"e nu'cle a ble
in er'ti a
in'fant
in fan'ti cide
in'fantile
in fan'ti lism
in farct'
in farct'ion
in fec'tion
in fec'tious
in fec'tious ness
in"fe cun'di ty
in fe'ri or
in fe"ri or'i ty
in"fer til'i ty
in"fes ta'tion
in fib u la'tion
in fil'trate
in"fil tra'tion
in fin'i ty
in firm'
in fir'ma ry
in fir'mi ty
in"flam ma'tion
in fla'tion
in flec'tion
in"flo res'cence
in"flu en'za
in"fra car'di ac
in"fra cla vic'u lar
in"fra cla vic u lar'is
in"fra con'dyl ism

in"fra cos'tal
in frac'tion
in"fra di"a phrag mat'ic
in"fra glenoid'
in"fra glot'tic
in"fra hy'oid
in"fra oc clu'sion
in"fra or'bit al
in"fra pa tel'lar
in"fra phys"i o log'ic
in"fra red'
in"fra scap'u lar
in"fra spi na'tus
in"fra spi'nous
in"fra ster'nal
in"fra tem"po ra'le
in"fra ten to'ri al
in"fra troch'le ar
in fric'tion
in"fun dib'u li form"
in"fun dib u lo'ma
in"fun dib'u lo pel'vic
in"fun dib'u lar
in"fun dib'u lum
in fu'sion
in"fu so'ri a
in ges'ta
in ges'tion
in"gra ves'cent
in gre'di ent
in'grow"ing
in'guen
in'gui nal
in"gui no dyn'i a
in"gui no fem'o ral
in"gui no scro'tal
in ha'lant
in"ha la'tion
in'ha la"tor

in ha′ler
in her′ent
in her′it ance
in her′it ed
in hib′in
in″hi bi′tion
in hib′i tor
in″i en ceph′a lus
in″i od′y mus
in′i on
in″i op′a gus
in′i ops
in ject′
in jec′tion
in′ju ry
in′lay″
in′let
in′nate
in″ner va′tion
in′no cent
in noc′u ous
in nom′nate
in nox′ious
in″oc ci pit′i a
in″o chon dri′tis
in oc″u la′tion
in oc′u la″tor
in oc′u lum
in′o gen
in op′er a ble
in″or gan′ic
in os′cu late
in os″cu la′tion
in″o se′mi a
in′o sine
in o′si tol
in″stil la′tion
in″o trop′ic
in′quest

in″qui si′tion
in sal″i va′tion
in″sa lu′bri ous
in″sa lu′bri ty
in san′i tar″y
in san″i ta′tion
in san′i ty
in scrip′tion
in scrip″ti o′nes
in′sect
in sec′ti cide
in sec′ti fuge
in″se cu′ri ty
in sem″i na′tion
in sen′si ble
in sheathed′
in sid′i ous
in′sight″
in sip′id
in si′tu
in″so la′tion
in sol′u ble
in som′ni a
in spec′tion
in″spi ra′tion
in spi′ra to″ry
in″spi rom′e ter
in spis′sant
in spis′sate
in″spis sat′ed
in″sta bil′i ty
in′step
in″stil la′tion
in′stil la″tor
in′stinct
in stinc′tive
in′stru ment
in″stru men ta′tion
in″suf fi′cien cy

in″suf fla′tion
in′suf fla″tor
in′su la
in′su lin
in″su lin e′mi a
in″su lin o′ma
ın″sus cep″ti bil′i ty
in″te gra′tion
in″teg′u ment
in′tel lect
in tel′li gence
in tel′li gent
in tem′per ance
in″ten″si fi ca′tion
in″ten sim′e ter
in ten′si ty
in ten′tion
in″ter ac ces′so ry
in″ter ac′i nous
in″ter al ve′o lar
in″ter ar″y te noid′e us
in″ter a′tri al
in ter′ca la″ted
in″ter cap′il lar″y glo
    mer″u lo scle ro′sis
in″ter car′pal
in″ter cav′ern ous
in″ter cel′lu lar
in″ter chon′dral
in″ter cli′noid
in″ter co lum′nar
in″ter con′dy lar
in″ter cos′tal
in″ter cos″to bra′chi al
in″ter coup′ler
in′ter course
in″ter cri″co thy rot′o my
in″ter cris′tal
in″ter cru′ral

in″ter cur′rent
in″ter cusp′ing
in″ter den′tal
in″ter den′ti um
in″ter dic′tion
in″ter dig′i tal
in″ter dig″i ta′tion
in′ter face
in″ter fere′
in″ter fer′ence
in″ter fer om′e ter
in″ter fer om′e try
in″ter fer′on
in″ter fi′bril lar
in″ter fol lic′u lar
in″ter glob′u lar
in″ter go′ni al
in te′ri or
in″ter kin e′sis
in″ter la′bi al
in″ter la mel′lar
in″ter lam′i nar
in″ter lin′gua
in″ter lo′bar
in″ter lob′u lar
in″ter mar′riage
in″ter max′il lar″y
in″ter me′din
in″ter me″di o lat′er al
in″ter mem′bra nous
in″ter me nin′ge al
in″ter men′stru al
in ter′ment
in″ter mes″o blas′tic
in″ter met″a mer′ic
in″ter mi cel′lar
in″ter mi tot′ic
in″ter mit′tent
in″ter mu′ral

in"ter mus'cu lar
in ter'nal
in"ter na'ri al
in"ter neu'ron
in"ter neu'ro nal
in ter'nist
in'ter node"
in"ter nun'ci al
in"ter o cep'tor
in"ter o fec'tive
in"ter ol'i var"y
in"ter os'se us
in"ter pal'pe bral
in"ter pa ri'e tal
in"ter pe dun'cu lar
in"ter pha lan'ge al
in"ter prox'i mal
in"ter prox'i mate
in"ter pu'pil la"ry
in'ter sex"
in"ter spi nal'es
in"ter spi'nous
in ter'sti ces
in"ter sti'tial
in"ter tar'sal
in"ter trans"ver sa'ri i
in"ter trans verse'
in"ter tri'go
in"ter tro"chan ter'ic
in"ter tu'bu lar
in"ter vas'cu lar
in"ter ven tric'u lar
in"ter ver'te bral
in"ter vil'lous
in"ter zo'nal
in tes'tin al
in tes'tine
in'ti ma
in tol'er ance

in tort'er
in tox'i cant
in tox"i ca'tion
in"tra ab dom'i nal
in"tra ac'i nar
in"tra ar tic'u lar
in"tra a'tri al
in"tra cap'su lar
in"tra car"ti lag'i nous
in"tra cav'i ta ry
in"tra cel'lu lar
in"tra cer e'bral
in"tra cra'ni al
in tract'able
in"tra cu ta'ne ous
in"tra cys'tic
in"tra der'mal
in"tra du'ral
in"tra e soph'a geal
in"tra fu'sal
in"tra gem'mal
in"tra he pat'ic
in"tra lig"a men'tous
in"tra lo'bar
in"tra lob'u lar
in"tra lu'mi nal
in"tra med'ul lar y
in"tra mem'bra nous
in"tra mu'ral
in"tra mus'cu lar
in"tra na'sal
in"tra nu'cle ar
in"tra oc'u lar
in"tra o'ral
in"tra or'bit al
in"tra pa ri'e tal
in"tra pel'vic
in"tra per i to ne'al
in"tra pleu'ral

in''tra scro'tal
in''tra spi'nal
in''tra stro'mal
in''tra the'cal
in''tra tra'che al
in''tra tu'bal
in''tra u re'thral
in''tra u'ter ine
in''tra vas'cu lar
in''tra ve'nous
in''tra ven tric'u lar
in''tra ves'i cal
in''tra vi'tal
in trin'sic
in''tro ces'sion
in''tro flex'ion
in tro'i tus
in''tro jec'tion
in''tro mis'sion
in''tro mit'tent
in''tro spec'tion
in''tro ver'sion
in'tro vert''
in''tu ba'tion
in''tu mes'cence
in''tus sus cep'tion
in''tus sus cep'tum
in''tus sus cip'i ens
in'u lin
in unc'tion
in u'te ro
in vac'u o
in vag'i nate
in vag''i na'tion
in'valid
in va'sion
in ver'sion
in vert'
in ver'tase

in ver'te bral
in ver''te bra'ta
in ver'te brate
in vest'ment
in vet'er ate
in''vi ril'i ty
in''vis ca'tion
in vit'ro
in vi'vo
in''vo lu'crum
in vol'un tar''y
in'vo lute
in''vo lu'tion
i'o dide
i'o dine
i''o din'o phil
i'o dism
i'o dized
i o''do der'ma
i o'do form
i''o dom'e try
i o''do phil'i a
i''o dop'sin
i o''do ther'a py
i''o do thy''ro glob'u lin
i om'e ter
i'on
i o'ni um
i''on i za'tion
i''on om'e ter
i on''to pho re'sis
i''o pho'bi a
ip'e cac
ip''si lat'er al
i ras''ci bil'i ty
ir''i dad''e no'sis
i'ri dal
ir''i dal'gi a
ir''i daux e'sis

ir″i da vul′sion
ir″i dec′tome
ir″i dec′to mize
ir″i dec′to my
ir″i dec tro′pi um
ir″i de′mi a
ir″i den clei′sis
ir″i den tro′pi um
i rid″e re′mi a
ir′i des
ir″i des′cence
i rid′ic
i rid′i um
ir″i di za′tion
ir″i do a vul′sion
ir″i do cap″su li′tis
ir″i do cap″su lot′o my
i rid′o cele
ir″i do cho″roid i′tis
ir″i do col″o bo′ma
ir″i do cy clec′to my
ir″i do cy cli′tis
ir″i do cy″clo cho″roid i′tis
ir″i do cys tec′to my
ir′i do cyte″
ir′i do di″ag no′sis
ir″i do di al′y sis
ir″i do di la′tor
ir″i do do ne′sis
ir″i do ki ne′si a
ir″i do lep tyn′sis
ir″i do ma la′ci a
ir″i do mo′tor
ir″i don co′sis
ir″i don′cus
ir″i do pa ral′y sis
ir″i do pa rel′ky sis
ir″i do pa re′sis

ir″i do per″i pha ki′tis
ir″i do ple′gi a
ir″i dop to′sis
ir″i do pu′pil lar″y
ir″i do rhex′is
ir″i dos′chi sis
ir″i do scle rot′o my
ir″i dot′a sis
ir′i do tome
ir″i dot′o my
ir″i dot ro mos
i′ris
i rit′ic
i ri′tis
ir″i to ec′to my
i′ron
ir ra′di ate
ir ra″di a′tion
ir ra′tion al
ir″re du′ci ble
ir reg″u lar′i ty
ir″re sus′ci ta ble
ir″re ver′si ble
ir″ri ga′tion
ir″ri ta bil′i ty
ir′ri ta ble
ir′ri tant
ir″ri ta′tion
i″sa del′phi a
is che′mi a
is che′sis
is″chi al′gi a
is″chi a ti′tis
is″chi dro′sis
is″chi o bul bo′sus
is″chi o cap′su lar
is″chi o cav″er no′nous
is″chi o coc cyg′e al

is″chi o coc cyg′e us
is″chi o did′y mus
is″chi o fe mo ra′lis
is chi om′e lus
is″chi o my″e li′tis
is″chi o neu ral′gi a
is chi op′a gus
is″chi o pu′bi cus
is″chi o pu″bi ot′o my
is″chi o pu′bis
is″chi o rec′tal
is′chi um
isch″no pho′ni a
is″cho ga lac′ti a
is″cho gy′ri a
is″cho me′ni a
is chu′ri a
Ishihara (color vision test)
is′let
i″so ag glu′ti nin
i″so an′ti bod″ies
i″so an′ti gen
i″so bar
i″so bar′ic
i″so cel″lo bi′ose
i″so cel′lu lar
i″so chro mat′ic
i soch′ro nal
i″so chro′ni a
i″so co′ri a
i″so cor′tex
i″so cy tol′y sin
i″so dac′ty lism
i″so di″ag no′sis
i′so dont
i″so do′ses
i″so dy nam″ic

i″so e lec′tric
i″so gam′ete
i sog′a mous
i″so gen′e sis
i″sog′na thous
i′so graft
i″so he″mag glu′ti nin
i″so he mol′y sin
i″so he mol′y sis
i″so i co′ni a
i″so im″mu ni za′tion
i″so la′tion
i′so mer
i som′er ism
i″so met′ric
i″so me tro′pi a
i′so morph
i″so mor′phic
i″so ni′a zid
i″so os mot′ic
i sop′a thy
i″so pho′ri a
i so′pi a
i″so plas′tic
i″so pro′pyl
i sop′ters
i′so therm
i′so tope
i″so trop′ic
isth mec′to my
isth′mus
i su′ri a
itch′ing
i′ter
ix″od′i dac
ix″od′ic
ix″y o my″e li′tis

157

J

Jacksonian at tack'
jac"ti ta'tion
jar'gon
jaun'dice
je ju'nal
jej"u nec'to my
jej"u ni'tis
jej"u no ce cos'to my
jej"u no co los'to my
jej"u no il"e i'tis
jej"u no il"e os'to my
jej"u no il'e um
jej"u no jej"u nos'to my
jej"u nor'rha phy
jej"u nos'to my
jej"u not'o my

je ju'num
Jimson weed
joint
jug'u lar
ju jit'su
ju men'tous
junc'tion
junc tu'ra
ju"ris pru'dence
jus'to ma'jor
ju've nile
jux"ta-ar tic'u lar
jux"to glo mer'u lar
jux"ta po si'tion
jux"ta py lor'ic

K

Kahn test
kai"no pho'bi a
kak"or raph"i o pho'bi a
ka'la-a zar'
kal"li kre'in
ka le'mi a
ka"na my'cin
ka' o lin
ka"o li no'sis
Ka o pec'tate
Kaposi's dis ease'
Kartagener's syn'drome
ka"ry en'chy ma
ka'ry o blast"
ka'ry o chrome"
ka'ry og'a my
ka"ry o ki ne'sis
ka"ry o lo'bic

ka"ry ol'y sis
ka'ry o mere
ka"ry o mi"cro so'ma
ka"ry o mi'tome
ka"ry o mi to'sis
ka'ry o phage"
ka'ry o plasm
ka"ry or rhex'is
ka'ry o some"
ka"ry os'ta sis
kar"y o the'ca
kar"y o type'
kath"i so pho'bi a
Kef'lin
ke'loid
kelp
ken"o pho'bi a
ken"o tox'in

ker"a phyl'lo cele
ker"a phyl'lous
ker'a sin
ker"a tal'gi a
ker"a tec ta'si a
ker"a tec'to my
ke rat'ic
ker'a tin
ker"a tin i za'tion
ker"a tin'o cytes
ke rat'i nous
ker"a ti'tis
ker"a to ac"an tho'ma
ker'a to cele"
ker"a to cen te'sis
ker"a to chro"ma to'sis
ker"a to con junc"ti vi'tis
ker"a to co'nus
ker"a to der'ma
ker"a to gen'e sis
ker"a to glo'bus
ker"a to hel co'sis
ker"a to hy'a lin
ker'a toid
ker"a to ir'i do scope
ker"a to i ri'tis
ker"a to leu ko'ma
ker"a tol'y sis
ker"a to lyt'ic
ker"a to me la'ci a
ker'a tome
ker"a tom'e ter
ker"a to my co'sis
ker"a to nyx'is
ker'a to plas"ty
ker"a tor rhex'is
ker"a to scle ri'tis
ker'a to scope
ker"a tos'co py

ker'a tose
ker"a to'sis
ker a tot'o my
ke rau"no pho'bi a
ke'ri on
ker nic'ter us
Kernig's sign
ker'o cele
ke"to ac i do'sis
ke"to gen'i sis
ke'tone
ke"to ne'mi a
ke"to nu'ri a
ke'tose
ke to'sis
ke"to ster'oid
kid'ney
Kiesselbach's tri'angle
kil'o cal"o rie
kil'o gram
kil'o me"ter
Kimmelstiel-Wilson syn'drome
ki'nase
kin"e mat'o graph
kin'e plas"ty
kin"e ra"di o ther'a py
kin'e scope
ki ne'si a
ki ne"si at'rics
ki ne"si es the"si om'e ter
kin"e sim'e ter
ki ne"si ol'o gy
ki ne'sis
ki ne"so pho'bi a
kin"es the'si a
ki net'ic
ki ne'tism
kin"e to car'di o gram
ki ne'to chore

ki"no cen'trum
ki'o tome
Klebs-Loeffler ba cil'lus
Kleb si el'la
klep"to lag'ni a
klep"to ma'ni a
klep"to pho'bi a
Kline test
Kline-Felter's syn'drome
Klippel-Feil syn'drome
knee
knee'cap"
knit'ting
knob
knock'-knee"
knuck'le
knuck'ling
Koch, Robert
koi"lo nych'i a
Kolmer's test
ko"ly phre'ni a

ko'ni me"ter
ko"ni o cor'tex
Koplik's spots
kop"o pho'bi a
Ko rot'koff
kra tom'e ter
krau ro'sis
Krukenberg tu'mor
Kupffer cells
Kussmaul's re"spi ra'tion
kwash i or'kor
ky es'te in
ky'mo gram
ky'mo graph
Ky'nex
ky"pho ra chi'tis
ky"pho sco"li o ra chi'tis
ky"pho sco"li o'sis
ky pho'sis
ky phot'ic

L

la'bi a
la'bi al ism
la'bile
la bil'i ty
la"bi o al ve'o lar
la"bi o cer'vi cal
la"bi o den'tal
la"bi o gin'gi val
la"bi o glos"so la ryn'ge al
la"bi o gres'sion
la"bi o men'tal
la"bi o pal'a tine
la'bi o plas"ty
la'bi um
la'bor

lab'o ra to"ry
la'brum
lab'y rinth
lab"y rin thec'to my
lab"y rin thi'tis
lab"y rin thot'o my
lac'er at"ed
lac"er a'tion
la cer'tus
la cin'i ate
lac'ri mal
lac"ri ma'le
lac"ri ma'tion
lac'ri ma"tor
lac'ri mo tome"

lac''ri mot'o my
lac tac''i du'ri a
lac''tal bu'min
lac'tant
lac'tase
lac'tate
lac ta'tion
lac'te al
lac'tic
lac tif'er ous
lac'ti fuge
Lac'ti gen
lac tig'e nous
lac''ti su'gi um
lac tiv'o rous
Lac''to ba cil'lus
lac'to cele
lac'to crit
lac'to gen
lac''to gen'ic
lac''to glob'u lin
lac tom'e ter
lac'tose
la cu'na
la cu'nu la
la'dre rie''
Laennec's cir rho'sis
Lafora bo'dies
lag''neu o ma'ni a
lag''oph thal'mos
la'i ty
lal''o pho'bi a
lal la'tion
la lop'a thy
lal''o pho mi'a trist
lal''o ple'gi a
lamb'da cism
lamb'doid
lam bli'a sis

la mel'la
la mel'lar
lame'ness
lam'i na
lam''i na'tion
lam''i nec'to my
lam''i ni'tis
lam''i nog'ra phy
lam''i not'o my
lam'pas
lamp'black''
lam proph'o ny
lan'a to side''
Lancefield group'ing
lan'cet
lan'ci na''ting
Langerhan's is'lets
lan'o lin
Lansing po'lio vi'rus
lan'to cide-C
la nu'go
lan'u lous
lap''a ror'rha phy
lap''a rot'o mist
lap''a rot'o my
lap''a ro tra''che lot'o my
la pros'co py
lap'sus
lar da'ceous
lar'va
lar'val
lar'vate
lar'vi cide
lar''yn gal'gi a
lar''yn ge'al
lar''yn gec'to my
lar''yn gem phrax'is
lar''yn gis'mus
lar''yn gi'tis

161

la ryn'go cele
la ryn''go cen te'sis
la ryn''go fis'sure
la ryn'go graph
lar''yn gol'o gist
lar''yn gol'o gy
lar''yn go ma la'ci a
lar''yn gom'e try
la ryn''go pa ral'y sis
lar''yn gop'a thy
la ryn''go phan'tom
la ryn''go pha ryn'ge al
la ryn''go phar''yn gec'to my
la ryn''go pha ryn'ge us
la ryn''go phar''yn gi'tis
la ryn''go phar'ynx
lar''yn goph'o ny
la ryn'go plas''ty
la ryn''go ple'gi a
la ryn''gc pto'sis
la ryn''go rhi nol'o gy
la ryn''gor rha' gi a
lar''yn gor'rha phy
la ryn''gor rhe'a
la ryn''go scle ro'ma
la ryn'go scope
lar''yn go scop'ic
lar''yn gos'co pist
lar''yn gos'co py
la ryn'go spasm''
lar''yn gos'ta sis
lar''yn go ste no'sis
lar''yn gos'to my
la''ryn''go stro'bo scope
la ryn''go syr'inx
la ryn'go tome
lar''yn got'o my
la ryn''go tra'che al
la ryn''go tra''che i'tis

la ryn''go tra''che o bron chi'tis
la ryn''go tra''che ot'o my
la ryn''go xe ro'sis
lar'ynx
las civ'i a
las civ'i ous
Lasegue's sign
Lassar's paste
las'si tude
la'tent
lat'er ad
lat'er al
lat''er o ab dom'i nal
lat''er o duc'tion
lat''er o flex'ion
lat''er o mar'gin al
lat''er o pul'sion
lat''er o tor'sion
lat''er o ver'sion
la'tex
la tis''si mo con''dy lar'is
la tis'si mus
la trine'
Lat''ro dec'tus mac'tans
la'tus
laud'a ble
lau'da num
laugh
laugh'ter
la vage'
la va'tion
lax'a tive
lax'i ty
lay'er
lay ette'
lay'man
leach'ing
lead
lec''a no so''ma top'a gus

162

lec'i thal
lec'i thin
leech
Leiner's dis ease'
lei''o der'ma tous
lei''o der'mi a
lei''o my''o fi bro'ma
lei''o my o'ma
lei''o my''o sar co'ma
lei ot'ri chous
lei''po me'ri a
Leishman-Donovan bod'ies
Leish ma'ni a
leish''man i'a sis
leish'man oid
lem'mo cyte
lem nis'cus
lem'no blast
le''mo ste no'sis
len'i ceps
len'i tive
lens om'e ter
Len'te in'su lin
len''ti co'nus
len tic'u lar
len tic'u late
len tic''u lo stri'ate
len tic''u lo tha lam'ic
len'ti form''
len''ti glo'bus
len ti'go
le''on ti'a sis
lep'er
lep''i do'ma
Lep''i dop'ter a
lep'o thrix
lep'ro lin
lep rol'o gist
lep rol'o gy

lep ro'ma
lep'ro min
lep''ro pho'bi a
lep''ro sar'i um
lep'ro sin
lep'ro sy
lep'rous
lep''to ce pha'li a
lep''to ceph'a lus
lep''to chro mat'ic
lep''to cy'tic
lep''to cy to'sis
lep''to dac'ty lous
lep''to don'tous
lep''to me nin'ges
lep''to me nin''gi o'ma
lep''to men''in gi'tis
lep''to men''in gop'a thy
lep''to me'ninx
lep''to mi''cro gnath'i a
lep''to pel'lic
lep''to pho'ni a
lep''to pro so'pi a
lep'tor rhine''
lep'to scope''
Lep''to spi'ra
Lep''to spi'ra ic''ter
    o hae mor rha'gi ae
lep''to spi ro'sis
lep'to tene
Lep'to thrix
le re'sis
Les'bi an
le'sion
le'thal
leth'ar gy
le'the
Letterer-Siwe syn'drome
leu cae'thi op

leu'cine
leu"ci no'sis
leu"ci nu'ri a
leu"ka ne'mi a
leu ke'mi a
leu kem'id
leu ke'moid
leu'kin
leu'ko blast"
leu"ko blas to'sis
leu ko'ci din
leu'ko cyte"
leu"ko cy'to blast"
leu"ko cy'to ly'sin
leu"ko cy tol'y sis
leu"ko cy to'ma
leu"ko cy tom'e ter
leu"ko cy to'sis
leu"ko der'ma
leu"ko dys'tro phy
leu"ko en ceph a lop'athy
leu ko'ma
leu"ko nych'i a
leu kop'a thy
leu"ko pe de'sis
leu"ko pe'ni a
leu"ko pe'nic
leu"ko phleg ma'si a
leu"koph thal'mous
leu"ko pla'ki a
leu kop'sin
leu"kor rha'gi a
leu"kor rhe'a
leu"ko sar co'ma
leu"ko sar co"ma to'sis
leu'ko scope"
leu'ko tome"
leu"ko tox'ic
leu"ko tox'in

leu"ko trich'i a
leu"ko u"ro bil'in
leu'kous
lev"ar ter'en ol
le va'tor
le'ver
lev"i ga'tion
lev"i ta'tion
le vo car'di a
le"vo car'di o gram"
le"vo con'dyl ism
le"vo duc'tion
le"vo gy'rous
le"vo pho'bi a
le"vo pho'ri a
le"vo ro ta'tion
le"vo ro'ta to"ry
lev'u lose
lew'is ite
Leydig cell
lib"er a'tion
li bi'do
Li'bri um
li'cense
li cen'ti ate
li'chen
li"chen if i ca'tion
li"chen i za'tion
lic'o rice
li"e ni'tis
li e'no cele
li"en og'ra phy
li e"no ma la'ci a
li"e nop'a thy
li e"no re'nal
li e"no tox'in
li'en ter"y
li"en un'cu lus
lig'a ment

lig"a men'to pex"y
lig"a men'tum
li'gate
li ga'tion
lig'a ture
lig'ne ous
lig"ni fi ca'tion
lig'num
limb
lim'bic
lim'bus
li'men
li'mes
lim'i na
lim'i nal
lim"i troph'ic
lim nol'o gy
li moph'thi sis
lin'dane
lin'e a
lin'e ar
lin'gua
lin'gual
lin'gu la
lin'gu lar
lin"guo dis'tal
lin"guo gin'gi val
lin'i ment
lin"o le'ic
lin"o le'nic
lin"o no pho'bi a
lin'seed
li'pa
lip"a ro trich'i a
lip'a rous
li'pase
lip ec'to my
li pe'mi a
lip"id

li pi'o dol
lip"o blas to'sis
lip"o cal"ci no gran"u
   lo ma to'sis
lip"o chon"dro dys'tro phy
lip"o chon dro'ma
lip"o chrome"
lip'o cyte"
lip"o dys'tro phy
lip"o fi"bro myx o'ma
lip"o fi"bro sar co'ma
lip"o gen'e sis
li pog'e nous
lip"o gran"u lo'ma
lip"o gran u lo ma to'sis
lip"o he"mar thro'sis
lip'oid
lip"oi do'sis
li pol'y sis
li po'ma
lip o'ma toid
li po"ma to'sis
lip"o me tab'o lism
li pom'pha lus
lip"o my o hem an"gi o'ma
lip"o my o'ma
lip"o my o sar co'ma
lip"o pe'ni a
lip"o pha'gic
lip'o phil
lip"o phre'ni a
lip"o pro'te in
lip"o sar co'ma
li po'sis
lip"o sol'u ble
li pos'to my
lip"o tro'pic
lip"o vac'cine
lip"pi tu'do

li pu′ri a
liq″ue fac′tion
liq′uid
liq′uor
lisp
lis″sen ce pha′li a
lis″sen ceph′a lous
Lis te′ri a
li′ter
lith′a gogue
lith′arge
lith ec′to my
li the′mi a
li thi′a sis
lith″i co′sis
lith′i um
lith″o di al′y sis
lith″o gen′e sis
lith′oid
lith″o kel″y pho pe′di on
lith′o labe
li thol′a pax″y
lith″o ne phri′tis
lith″o ne phrot′o my
lith″o pe′di on
lith′o phone″
lith′o scope″
li tho′sis
li thot′o mist
li thot′o my
lith′o trip″sy
lith′o trite
lith′ous
lith″u re′sis
li thu′ri a
lit′mus
Litten′s sign
lit′ter
Littré, glands of

liv′er
liv′id
lo″a i′a sis
lo′bar
lobe
lo bec′to my
lo be′li a
lo bot′o my
lob′u lar
lob′u le
lob′u lus
lo′bus
lo″cal i za′tion
lo′cal ized
lo′chia
lo″chi o col′pos
lo′chi o cyte
lo″chi o me′tra
lo″chi o me tri′tis
lo″chi or rha′gi a
lo″chi or rhe′a
lo″chi os′che sis
lo″cho me tri′tis
lo″cho per″i to ni′tis
lo′ci
lock′jaw″
lo″co mo′tion
loc″u la′tion
loc′u li
loc′u lus
lo′cum te′nens
lo′cus
Loeffler′s syn′drome
log″a dec′to my
log″a di′tis
log″a do blen″nor rhe′a
log″ag no′si a
log″a graph′i a
log″am ne′si a

log"a pha'si a
log"o ko pho'sis
log"o ma'ni a
log"o neu ro'sis
log op'a thy
log"o pe'dics
log"o pha'si a
log"o ple'gi a
log'o spasm
lo i'a sis
loin
lon gev'i ty
lon"gi lin'e al
lon"gi ma'nous
lon"gi ped'ate
lon gis'si mus
lon"gi tu'di nal
lon"gi tu"di na'lis
lon"gi typ'i cal
lon'gus
lo'pho dont
lo quac'i ty
lor do'sis
lor dot'ic
lo'ti o
lo'tion
loupe
louse
lous'y
lu cid'i ty
lu cif'u gal
lu'dic
lu'es
lu e'tic
Lugol's so lu'tion
lum ba'go
lum'bar
lum"bo co los'to my
lum"bo co lot'o my

lum"bo cos'tal
lum"bo dor'sal
lum"bo in'gui nal
lum"bo is'chi al
lum"bo sa'cral
lum'bri cal
lu'men
lu'mi nal
lu'mi nance
lu"mi nes'cence
lu"mi nif'er ous
lu"mi nos'i ty
lu'na cy
lu'nar
lu'nate
lu'na tic
lung
lu'nu la
lu po'ma
lu'pus
lu'pus er"y thy ma to'sis
lu'sus na tu'rae
lu'te al
lu'te in
lu"te in iz'ing
lu"te o'ma
lux a'tion
lux u'ri ant
lux'us
ly'cine
ly"co rex'i a
ly"go phil'i a
ly"ing-in'
lymph
lym phad"e nec'to my
lym phad"e ni'tis
lym phad"e no'ma
lym phad"e no ma to'sis
lym phad"e nop'a thy

167

lym phad"e no'sis
lym phad"e not'o my
lym'pha gogue
lym"phan gi ec tas'i a
lym phan"gi ec'ta sis
lym phan"gi ec'to my
lym phan"gi o en"do the"
   li o'ma
lym phan"gi og'ra phy
lym phan"gi o'ma
lym phan'gi o plas"ty
lym phan"gi o sar co'ma
lym phan"gi ot'o my
lym"phan gi'tis
lym phat'ic
lym phat"i cos'to my
lym"phe de'ma
lym'pho blast
lym"pho blas to'ma
lym"pho car'ci no ma
lym'pho cyte
lym"pho cy'tic
lym"pho cy to'ma
lym"pho cy"to pe'ni a
lym"pho cyto poi e'sis
lym"pho cy to'sis
lym"pho der'mi a
lym"pho ep'i the"li o'ma
lym phog'en ous
lym"pho go'ni a
lym"pho gran"u lo'ma
lym"pho gran"u lo ma to'sis

lym'phoid
lym pho'ma
lym"pho ma to'sis
lym"pho path'i a ve ne're um
lym"pho pe'ni a
lym"pho poi e'sis
lym"pho re tic"u lo'ma
lym"pho re tic"u lo'sis
lym'phor rhage
lym'phor rhe'a
Lym"pho sar co'ma
lym"pho sar"co ma to'sis
lym phu'ri a
ly'o phile
ly"o phil i za'tion
ly'o phobe
ly'o sol
ly"o sorp'tion
ly'o trope
lyse
ly ser'gic ac'id
   di"eth yl am'ide
ly sim'e ter
ly'sine
ly'sis
ly"so ceph'a lin
Ly'sol
ly'so zyme
lys'sic
lys"so dex'is
lys'soid
lys"so pho'bi a

M

McBurney's in ci'sion
mac'er ate
mac'er a"ter
Macewen, William

mac"ra cu'si a
mac"ren ce phal'ic
mac"ren ceph'a ly
mac"ro bac te'ri um

mac''ro ble phar'i a
mac''ro bra'chi a
mac''ro car'di us
mac''ro ce pha'li a
mac''ro ceph'a lus
mac''ro chei'li a
mac''ro chei'ri a
mac''ro cyte
mac'ro cyt'ic
mac''ro cy to'sis
mac''ro dac tyl'i a
mac''ro don'ti a
mac''ro en ceph'a ly
mac''ro gam'ete
mac''ro glob''u lin e'mi a
mac''ro glos'si a
mac''ro gnath'ic
mac''ro gy'ri a
mac''ro lymph'o cyte
mac''ro mas'ti a
mac''ro me'li a
ma crom'e lus
mac''ro mo lec'u lar
mac''ro mon'o cyte
mac''ro my'e lo blast
mac''ro nor'mo blast
mac''ro nu'cle us
mac''ro nych'i a
mac'ro phage
mac''ro po'di a
mac''ro pol'y cytes
mac''ro pro so'pi a
mac''ro pro'so pus
ma crop'si a
mac''ro scop'ic
mac''ros mat'ic
mac''ro so'mi a
mac'ro spore''
mac''ro sto'mi a

ma cro'ti a
mac'u la
mac'u lar
mac'ule
mac''u lo pap'u lar
mad''a ro'sis
mad'i dans
ma du'ra foot
ma''du ro my co'sis
Maffucci's syn'drome
ma'gen bla se
mag'en stras''se
ma gen'ta
mag'got
mag'is tral
mag'ma
mag ne'si a
mag ne'si um
mag'net
mag'net ism
mag''net i za'tion
mag ne''to ɛ lec''tric'i ty
mag ne'to graph
mag ne'to in duc'tion
mag''ne tom'e ter
mag ne''to-op'tic
mag ne''to ther'a py
mag'ne tron
mag''ni fi ca'tion
mag'num
maid'en head''
ma ieu''si o ma'ni a
ma ieu''si o pho'bi a
ma ieu'tic
maim
mal
mal''ab sorp'tion
ma la'ci a
mal''a co pla'ki a

mal''ad just'ment
mal'a dy
ma laise'
mal'an ders
ma'lar
ma lar'i a
ma lar''i ol'o gist
mal''as sim''i la'tion
mal''di ges'tion
mal''for ma'tion
ma lig'nant
ma lin'ger er
mal''in''ter dig i ta'tion
mal'le a ble
mal''le a'tion
mal''le o in'cu dal
mal le'o lus
mal''le ot'o my
mal'let
mal'le us
mal''nu tri'tion
mal''oc clu'sion
mal''po si'tion
mal pos'ture
mal''prac'tice
mal''pres''en ta'tion
mal''re duc'tion
malt'ase
mal turned'
ma'lum
mal un'ion
mam'e lon
mam'ma
mam'mal
mam mal'gi a
Mam ma'li a
mam'ma plas''ty
mam'ma ry
mam mec'to my

mam'mi form
mam mil'la
mam'mil lar''y
mam'mil la''ted
mam''mil la'tion
mam mil'li form''
mam mil'li plas''ty
mam''mil li'tis
mam''mil lo tha lam'ic
mam mog'ra phy
mam'mose
mam mot'o my
man del'ic ac'id
man'di ble
man dib''u lo glos'sus
man dib''u lo mar''gin al'is
man'drin
man''du ca'tion
man'ga nese
mange
ma'ni a
ma'nic
man'i kin
ma nip''u la'tion
man'ni tol
ma nom'e ter
man om'e try
man'tle
Mantoux test
ma nu'bri um
man''u duc'tion
ma'nus
man''u stu pra'tion
ma ran'tic
ma ras'mus
mar''ble i za'tion
mar che'-a-pet it-pas
Marfan's syn'drome
mar'gin

mar"gi na'tion
mar'gi no plas"ty
Marie-Strumpell dis ease'
ma"ri hua'na
mar'lex
mar'row
mar su"pi al i za'tion
mas'cu line
mas"cu lin i za'tion
mask'ing
mas'o chism"
mas sage'
mas se'ter
mas seur'
mas seuse'
mas"so ther'a py
mast"ad e ni'tis
mast"ad e no'ma
mas tal'gi a
mast"a tro'phi a
mas tec"chy mo'sis
mas tec'to my
mast"hel co'sis
mas'tic
mas"ti ca'tion
mas"ti ca'tor
mas'ti ca to"ry
mas ti'tis
mas"to car"ci no'ma
mas"to de al'gi a
mas"to dyn'i a
mas'toid
mas"toid ec'to my
mas"toid i'tis
mas"toid ot'o my
mas ton'cus
mas top'a thy
mas'to pex"y
mas"to pla'si a

mas'to plas"ty
mas"tor rha'gi a
mas"to scir'rhus
mas to'sis
mas tos'to my
mas'tous
mas"tur ba'tion
ma ter'nal
ma ter'ni ty
ma'trix
mat'ter
mat'u rate
mat"u ra'tion
ma tu'ri ty
ma tu'ti nel
max ill'la
max'ill ary
max il"lo fa'cial
max il"lo-fron ta'le
max'i mal
max'i mum
may'hem
ma zal'gi a
ma'zic
maz"o mor'ro
ma zop'a thy
ma'zo pex"y
mea'sles
meas'ly
me"a ti'tis
me"a tot'o my
me a'tus
mech'a nism
mech"a no ther'a py
me'cism
Meckel's di'ver tic"u lum
me com'e ter
me"co nal'gi a
mec'on ate

171

mec″o neu″ro path′i a
mec″o ni or rhe′a
me co′ni um
me cys′ta sis
MEDEX
me′di a
me′di ad
me′di al
me′di an
me″di as ti′nal
me″di as″ti ni′tis
me′di as ti″no per″i car di′tis
me″di as″ti not′o my
me″di as ti′num
me′di ate
med′i ca ble
me dic′a ment
med″i ca men to′sus
med′i ca″ted
med″i ca′tion
med′i ca″tor
me dic′i nal
med″i co eth′i cal
med″i co le′gal
med″i co psy chol′o gy
me″di o car′pal
me″di o dor′sal
me″di o fron′tal
me″di o ne cro′sis
me″di o tar′sal
Med″i ter ra′ne an a ne′mi a
me′di um
me′di us
me dul′la
med′ul la″ry
med′ul la″ted
med″ul la′tion
med″ul li za′tion
med′ul lo blast″

med″ul lo blas to′ma
meg″a car′di a
meg″a ce′cum
meg″a coc′cus
meg″a co′lon
meg′a dont
meg″a du″o de′num
meg′a dyne
meg″a e soph′a gus
meg″a gna′thus
meg″a kar′y o blast
meg″a kar′y o cyte
meg″a kar″y oph′thi sis
me gal′gi a
meg′a lo blast
meg″a lo car′di a
meg″a lo ce phal′ic
meg″a lo ceph′a ly
meg″a loc′er us
meg″a lo chei′rous
meg″a lo cor′ne a
meg′a lo cyte
meg″a lo cy to′sis
meg″a lo en′ter on
meg″a lo gas′tri a
meg″a lo he pat′i a
meg″a lo ma′ni a
meg″a lo me′li a
meg″a lo ny cho′sis
meg″a lo pe′nis
meg″a loph thal′mus
meg″a lo po′di a
meg″a lo splanch′nic
meg′a lo spore″
meg″a lo u re′ter
meg′a phone
meg″a pros′o pous
meg″a rec′tum
meg″a sig′moid

meg'a volt''
meg'ohm''
mei o'sis
me la'gra
me lal'gi a
mel''an cho'li a
mel''an chol'ic
mel''a ne'mi a
mel''an id ro'sis
mel''a nif'er ous
mel'a nin
mel'a nism
mel''a no am''e lo blas to'ma
mel'a no blast''
mel'a no cyte''
mel''a no der'ma
mel''a no der''ma ti'tis tox'i ca
mel''a no der''ma to'sis
me lan'o gen
mel''a no gen'e sis
mel''a no glos'si a
mel'a noid
mel''a no'ma
mel''a no ma to'sis
mel''a no nych'i a
mel'a no phage''
mel'a no phore''
mel''a no pla'ki a
mel''a nor rhe'a
mel''a no'sis
me lan'o some
mel''a not'ri chous
mel''a nu'ri a
me las'ma
me le'na
me''li oi do'sis
me lis''so pho'bi a
me li'tis
mel''i tu'ri a

mel''o di dy'mi a
mel''o did'y mus
mel''o ma'ni a
me lom'e lus
mel''o rhe''os to'sis
me los'chi sis
me lo'tus
mem'brane
mem''bra no cra'ni um
mem'brum
mem'o ry
me nac'me
men ad'i one
me nar'che
Mendel, Gregor
Ménière's syn'drome
me nin'ge al
me nin''ge or'rha oht
me nin''gi o'ma
me nin''gi o''ma to'sis
me nin''gi o sar co'ma
me nin''gi o the''li o'ma
me nin'gism
men''in gis'mus
men''in git'i des
men''in gi'tis
men''in git''o pho'bi a
me nin''go ar''te ri'tis
me nin'go cele
me nin''go coc'cal
me nin''go coc ce'mi a
me nin''go coc'cic
me nin''go coc'cus
me nin''go cor'ti cal
me nin'go cyte
me nin''go-en ceph''a li'tis
me nin''go-en ceph'a lo cele
me nin''go-en ceph''a lo my''
   e li'tis

me nin"go-en ceph"a lop'a thy
me nin"go my"e li'tis
me nin"go my'e lo cele
men"in gop'a thy
me nin"go ra dic'u lar
me nin"go rha chid'i an
me nin"gor rha'gi a
men"in go'sis
me nin"go vas'cu lar
men"in gu'ri a
me'ninx
men"is cec'to my
men"is ci'tis
me nis'co cyte
me nis'cus
men"o ce'lis
men"o lip'sis
men'o pause
men"o pha'ni a
men"o pla'ni a
men"or rha'gi a
men"or rhal'gi a
men"or rhe'a
me nos'che sis
men"o sta'si a
men"o stax'is
men"o xe'ni a
mens
men'sa
men'ses
men'stru al
men'stru ant
men'stru ate
men"stru a'tion
men'stru um
men'su al
men"su ra'tion
men'tal
men ta'lis

men tal'i ty
men ta'tion
men'thol
men"to hy'oid
men"tu lo ma'ni a
me per'i dine
me phit'ic
me ral'gi a
me ra lo'pi a
mer"a mau ro'sis
mer cap'tan
Mer cre'sin
Mer"cu hy'drin
mer cu'ri al
mer cu'ri al ism
mer cu"ri al i za'tion
mer cu'ric
Mer"cur o'chrome
mer cu'rous
mer'cu ry
mer"er ga'si a
me rid'i an
mer"in tho pho'bi a
mer'i spore
me ris'tic
mer"o a cra'ni a
mer"o gen'e sis
mer"o mi"cro so'mia
me ro'pi a
mer"o ra chis'chi sis
me ros'mi a
mer"o som'a tous
mer'o some
me rot'o my
Mer thio'late
Mes an'to in
mes"a or ti'tis
mes ar"te ri'tis
mes"a ti pel'lic

mes cal'
mes ec'to derm
mes en''ce phal'ic
mes''en ceph''al i'tis
mes''en ceph'a lon
mes''en ceph a lot'o my
me sen'chy ma
mes'en chyme
mes''en chy''mo blas to'ma
mes''en chy mo'ma
mes''en ter ec'to my
mes''en ter'ic
mes''en ter''i co mes''o col'ic
mes''en ter''i o'lum
mes''en ter''i or'rha phy
mes''en ter''i pli ca'tion
mes''en ter'ri um
mes'en ter''y
me sen'to derm
mes''en tor rha phy
me'si al
me''si o buc'cal
me''si o buc''co oc clu'sal
me''si o clu'sion
me''si o dis'tal
me''si o gres'sion
me''si o in ci'sal
me''si o la'bi al
me'si o lin'gual
me''si o lin''guo oc clu'sal
me''si o oc clu'sal
mes'mer ism
mes''o ap pen'dix
mes''o bil''i ru'bin
mes'o blast
mes''o blas te ma
mes''o blas tem'ic
me so car'di a
mes''o car'di um

mes'o carp
mes''o ce'cum
mes''o ce phal'ic
mes''oc ne'mic
mes''o co'lon
mes'o conch
mes'o derm
mes''o du''o de'num
mes''o e soph'a gus
mes''o gas'ter
mes''o gle'a
mes''o gnath'ic
mes'o gna'thi on
mes'o mere
mes''o me'tri um
mes'o morph
mes'o mor''phy
mes'on
mes''o ne phro'ma
mes''o neph'ros
mes'o pex''y
mes''o phle bi'tis
mes o'pic
mes''o pul'mo num
me sor'chi um
mes''o rec'tum
mes''o rop'ter
mes or'rha phy
mes'or rhine
mes''o sal'pinx
mes''o sig'moid
mes''o ten'don
mes''o the''li o'ma
mes''o the'li um
me sot'o my
mes'o tron
mes''o var'i um
met''a bi o'sis
met''a bol'ic fail'ure

met″a bo lim′e ter
me tab′o lism
me tab′o lite
me tab′o lize
met″a bol′o gy
met″a car′pal
met″a car pec′to my
met″a car″po pha lan′ge al
met″a car′pus
met″a chro ma′si a
met″a chro′sis
met′a coele
met′a cone
met″a con′id
met′a con′ule
met″a dra′sis
met″a kar′y o cyte
met′al
me tal′lic
met′al loid
met″al lo pho′bi a
met al′o phil
met′a mere
met″a mor′phic
met″a mor phop′si a
met″a mor′pho sis
met″a mor′phous
met″a my′e lo cyte
met″a neph″ro gen′ic
met″a neph′ros
met′a phase
me taph′y sis
met″a phys i′tis
met″a pla′si a
met′a plasm
met″a pneu mon′ic
met″ar te′ri ole
met′a sta ble
me tas′ta sis

me tas′ta size
met a stat′ic
met″a tar sal′gi a
met″a tar sec′to my
met″a tar″so pha lan′ge al
met″a tar′sus
met″a thal′a mus
met″a troph′ic
Met″a zo′a
me″te or′ic
me′te or o graph″
me″te or ol′o gy
me″te or o path″o log′ic
me′ter
me tes′trus
meth′a done
meth′a nol
met he″mo glo′bin
met he″mo glo″bi ne′mi a
met he″mo glo″bi nu′ri a
meth i′o nine
meth′yl
meth′yl ene blue
meth″yl ep′si a
Me ti cort′e lone″
Me ti cort′en
met″my o glo′bin
met″o don ti′a sis
me top′a gus
met″o pan tral′gi a
me top′ic
me to′pi on
met″ra pec′tïc
met″ra to′ni a
met″ra tro′phi a
Met′ra zol
me′trec
met″rec ta′si a
met″rec to′pi a

me tre′mi a

met″reu ryn′ter

met reu′ry sis

me′tri a

met′ric

met″ri o ce phal′ic

me tri′tis

me′tro cele

me′tro clyst

me″tro col′po cele

me″tro cys to′sis

me′tro cyte

me″tro dy″na mom′e ter

me″tro dyn′i a

me″tro ec ta′si a

me″tro en″do me tri′tis

met rog′ra phy

me trol′o gy

me″tro lym″phan′gi tis

me″tro ma la′ci a

met′ro nome

me″tro pa ral′y sis

me″tro path′i a

me trop′a thy

me″tro per″i to ni′tis

me″tro phle bi′tis

me″trop to′sis

me″tror rha′gi a

me″tror rhe′a

me″tror rhex′is

me″tro sal″pin gi′tis

me″tro sal″pin gog′ra phy

me′tro scope

me″tro stax′is

me′tro tome

me try″per ci ne′sis

me try″per es the′si a

me try″per tro′phi a

Met′y caine Hy″dro chlo′ride

Meulengracht di′et

mi′ca

mi ca′ce ous

mi celle′

mi″cra cous′tic

mi″cren ceph′a lon

mi″cren ceph′a lous

mi″cren ceph′a ly

mi″cro ab′scess

mi″cro a″er o phil′ic

mi″cro au′di phone

Mi″cro bac te′ri um

mi′crobe

mi cro′bi cide

mi″cro bin ert′ness

mi″cro bi ol′o gist

mi″cro bi ol′o gy

mi″cro bi″o pho′bi a

mi″cro bi ot′ic

mi′cro bism

mi′cro blast″

mi″cro bleph′a ron

mi″cro bra′chi a

mi″cro brach″y ce pha′li a

mi″cro bu ret′

mi″cro cal′o rie

mi″cro car′di a

mi″cro cen′trum

mi″cro ceph′a lus

mi″cro ceph′a ly

mi″cro chei′li a

mi″cro chem′is try

mi″cro chi′ri a

mi″cro coc′cin

Mi″cro coc′cus

mi″cro co′lon

mi″cro co nid′i um

mi″cro cou′lomb

mi″cro cu′rie

mi′cro cyst
mi′cro cyte
mi″cro cy the′mi a
mi″cro cy to′sis
mi″cro dac tyl′i a
mi″cro de ter″min na′tion
mi″cro dis sec′tion
mi′cro dont
mi″cro don′ti a
mi″cro drep′a no cyt ic
   dis ease′
mi″cro e elec″tro pho ret′ic
mi″cro e ryth′ro cyte
mi″cro far′ad
mi″cro fi lar′i a
mi″cro frac′ture
mi″cro gam′ete
mi″cro ga me′to cyte
mi crog′a my
mi″cro gas′tri a
mi″cro gen′e sis
mi″cro ge′ni a
mi″cro gen′i tal ism
mi″cro glos′si a
mi″cro gna′thi a
mi″cro go′ni o scope
mi′cro gram
mi′cro graph
mi crog′ra phy
mi″cro gy′ri a
mi′crohm
mi″cro in cin″er a′tion
mi″cro in jec′tion
mi″cro len′ti a
mi″cro leu′ko blast
mi′cro li″ter
mi′cro lith
mi″cro li thi′a sis
mi″cro ma′ni a

mi″cro ma nip′u la″tor
mi″cro mas′ti a
mi″cro ma′zi a
mi″cro me′li a
mi crom′e lus
mi crom′e ter disk
mi″cro mi′cron
mi″cro mil′li me″ter
mi″cro mon″o spo′rin
mi″cro mo′to scope
mi″cro my e′li a
mi″cro my′e lo blast
mi″cro my″e lo lym′pho cyte
mi′cron
mi′cro nee″dles
mi cron′e mous
mi″cro nu′cle us
mi″cro nu′tri ents
mi″cro nych′i a
mi″cro or′chism
mi″cro or′gan ism
mi″cro par′a site
mi″cro pe′nis
mi′cro phage
mi″cro pha′ki a
mi″cro phal′lus
mi″cro pho′bi a
mi′cro phone
mi″cro pho′ni a
mi″cro pho′no graph
mi″cro pho′no scope
mi″cro pho′to graph
mi″cro pho tom′e ter
mi″croph thal′mus
mi″cro phys′ics
mi″cro pi pet′
mi″cro ple thys mog′ra phy
mi″cro po′di a
mi″cro po lar′i scope

mi″cro pro jec′tion
mi″cro pro so′pi a
mi″cro pro′so pus
mi crop′si a
mi″cro psy′chi a
mi′cro pus
mi″cro pyk″nom′e ter
mi′cro pyle
mi″cro ra″di og′ra phy
mi″cro res′pi ra″tor
mi″cro rrhi′ni a
mi″cro scel′ous
mi′cro scope
mi″cro scop′ic
mi cros′co pist
mi cros′co py
mi″cros mat′ic
mi′cro some
mi″cro so′mi a
mi″cro spec trog′ra phy
mi″cro spec″tro pho tom′e try
mi″cro spec′tro scope
mi″cro spher′o cyte
mi″cro sphyg′my
mi″cro sphyx′i a
Mi″cro spo′ron
mi″cro spo ro′sis
Mi″cro spo′rum au″dou i′ni
mi″cro steth′o phone
mi″cro steth′o scope
mi″cro sto′mi a
mi″cro sur′ger y
mi″cro the′li a
mi′cro therm
mi cro′ti a
mi′cro tome
mi crot′o my
mi″cro trau′ma
mi″cro u′nit

mi′cro volt
mi cro wave
mi crox′y cyte
mi″cro zo o sper′mi a
mic′tu rate
mic″tu ri′tion
mid″ax il′la
mid′bod″y
mid′brain″
mid″fron′tal
midge
midg′et
mid′gut
mid′pain″
mid′riff
mid′wife″
mid′wife″ry
mi′graf
mi′graine
mi′grate
mi gra′tion
Mikulicz's dis ease′
mil′dew
mil′i a
mil″i a ri′a
mil′i ar″y
Mi′li bis
mi lieu′
mil′i um
mil″li am′me″ter
mil″li am′pere
mil″li am′pere me″ter
mil′li bar
mil″li cu″rie
mil″li e quiv′a lent
mil′li gram
mil″li li″ter
mil′li me″ter
mil″li mi′cron

mil'li mol
mil"li nor'mal
mil"li os'mol
mil"li ruth'er ford
mil'li volt
mil pho'sis
Mil'town
mi me'sis
mim ma'tion
min"a mo'ta
min'er al
min"e ral o cor'ti coids
min'im
min'i mal
min'i mum
mi nom'e ter
mi"o car'di a
mi"o did'y mus
mi o'pus
mi o'sis
mi ot'ic
mire
mir'ror
mis an'thro py
mis car'riage
mis car'ry
mis'ce
mis"ce ge na'tion
mis'ci ble
mi sog'a my
mi sog'y ny
mi sol'o gy
mis"o ne'ism
mis"o pe'di a
mis"o psy'chi a
mis'tle toe
mi'tis
mit"o chon'dri a
mit"o chon'dri on

mit"o gen'e sis
mi'tome
mi to'sis
mi tot'ic
mit'o some
mi'tral
mi'troid
mit'tel schmerz
mix"o sco'pi a
mne"mas the'ni a
mne"mo der'mia
mne mon'ics
mne'mo tech"ny
mo bil'i ty
mo"bi li za'tion
Möbius' sign
mo dal'i ty
mod'el
mod'er a tor
mo di'o lus
mod'u la"tor
mod'u lus
mo'dus
mog"i graph'i a
mog"i la'li a
mog"i pho'ni a
moi'e ty
mo'lal
mo'lar
mo las'ses
mold
mold'ing
mole
mo lec'u lar
mol'e cule
mo li'men
mol li'ti es
mol lus'cum
molt

mo lyb′de num
mo lys″mo pho′bi a
mo men′tum
mon′ad
mon ar′thric
mon″ar thri′tis
mon″ar tic′u lar
mon as′ter
mon″a the to′sis
mon″a tom′ic
Monckeberg's dis ease′
mo nes′trus
mon′go lism
mon′go loid
Mo nil′i a
mo″ni li′a sis
mo nil′i form
mo nil′i id
mon′i tor ing
mon″o am′ine
mo″no a′mine ox i′dase
mon″o ar tic′u lar
mon″o bas′ic
mon′o blast
mon″o blep′si a
mon″o bra′chi us
mon″o car′di an
mon″o car′di o gram
mon″o cell′u lar
mon″o ceph′a lus
mon′o chord
mon″o cho re′a
mon″o chor i on′ic
mon″o chro′ma sy
mon″o chro′mat
mon″o chro mat′ic
mon″o chro mat′o phil
mon″o chro′ma tor
mon″o clin′ic

mon″o coc′cus
mon″o cra′ni us
mon″o crot′ic
mon oc′u lar
mon oc′u lus
mon″o cy e′sis
mon″o cys′tic
mon′o cyte
mon″o cy te′mic
mon″o cy to′ma
mon″o cy″to pe′ni a
mon″o cy to′sis
mon″o dac′ty lism
mon″o di plo′pi a
mon″o dro′mi a
mo nog′a my
mon″o gas′tric
mon″o ger′mi nal
mo nog′o ny
mon″o hy′brid
mon″o hy′drate
mon″o-i de′ism
mon″o ma′ni a
mon″o mel′ic
mon′o mer
mon″o mer′ic
mon″o mo′ri a
mon″o mor′phic
mon″o mor′phous
mo nom′pha lus
mon″o neph′rous
mon″o neu′ral
mon″o neu ri′tis
mon″o nu′cle ar
mon″o nu cle o′sis
mon″o pha′gi a
mo noph′a gism
mon″o pha′si a
mon″o pha′sic

181

mon"o pho'bi a
mon"oph thal'mi a
mon"o phy'o dont
mon"o ple'gi a
mon"o po'di a
mon"o psy cho'sis
mon"o pty'chi al
mon'o pus
mon"o ra dic'u lar
mon or'chid
mon"o rrhi'nous
mon"o sac'cha ride
mon"o scel'ous
mon"o som'a tous
mon'o some
mon'o stot'ic
mon'o stra'tal
mon"o symp"to mat'ic
mon"o ther'mi a
mon o'tic
mo not'o cous
mon ox'ide
mon"o zy got'ic
mons
mon'ster
mon'stri cide
mon strip'a ra
mon stros'i ty
mon tic'u lus
mor'bi
mor'bid
mor bid'i ty
mor"cel la'tion
mor da'cious
mor'dant
Morgagni, Giovanni B.
morgue
mor'i bund
Moro re'flex

mo'ron
mo ron'i ty
mor'phine
mor'phin ism
mor"pho gen'e sis
mor phol'gy
Morquio's dis ease'
mor'sal
mor tal'i ty
mor'tar
mor'tu ar"y
mor'u la
mo sa'ic
mo'tile
mo til'i ty
mou"lage'
mu'cin
mu'co cele
mu"co cu ta'ne ous
mu"co en"ter i'tis
mu"co hem"or rhag'ic
mu'coid
mu"co per"i os'te um
mu"co poly"sac'cha ride
mu"co pro'tein
mu"co pu'ru lent
mu"cor my'co sis
mu co'sa
mu"co san guin'e ous
mu"co se'rous
mu cos'i ty
mu'cous
mu"co vis ci do'sis
mu'cro nate
mu'cus
mu"li eb'ri ty
Müllerian duct
mul tan'gu lum
mul'ti cap'su lar

mul″ti cel′lu lar
mul″ti cos′tate
mul″ti cus′pid
mul″ti den′tate
mul″ti dig′i tate
mul″ti fa mil′i al
mul′ti fid
mul tif′i dus
mul′ti form
mul″ti gan′gli on ate
mul″ti glan′du lar
mul″ti grav′i da
mul″ti in fec′tion
mul″ti lo′bar
mul″ti lob′u lar
mul″ti loc′u lar
mul″ti mam′mae
mul″ti nod′u lar
mul″ti nu′cle ar
mul tip′a ra
mul″ti par′i ty
mul tip′a rous
mul″ti po′lar
mul″ti va′lent
mul ti vi′ta min
mum″mi fi ca′tion
mum′mi fied
mumps
mu′ral
mu″ri at′ic
mu′rine ty′phus
mur′mur
mus′ca rine
mus′cle
mus″cu lar′is
mus″cu lar′i ty
mus′cu la ture
mus″cu lo ap″o neu rot′ic
mus″cu lo cu ta′ne ous

mus″cu lo fas′ci al
mus″cu lo fi′brous
mus″cu lo phren′ic
mus″cu lo skel′e tal
mus″cu lo spi′ral
mus″cu lo ten′di nous
mu″si co ma′ni a
mu″si co ther′a py
mu′tant
mu ta′tion
mu″ti la′tion
mu′tism
my al′gi a
my″as the′ni a
my″a to′ni a
my ce′li oid
my ce′li um
my ce′tes
my″ce to′ma
My″ci fra′din
my″co an″gi o neu ro′sis
My″co bac te′ri um
my′coid
my col′o gy
my″coph thal′mi a
my co′sis
My″co spo′rum
My″co stat′in
my co′tic
my cot″i za′tion
myc″ter o pho′ni a
my de′sis
my dri′a sis
myd″ri at′ic
my ec′to my
my″e lat′ro phy
my″e len ceph′a lon
my el′ic
my′e lin

my"e li nat'ed
my"e li na'tion
my"e li ni za'tion
my"e lin o cla'sis
my"e li no gen'e sis
my"e li nop'a thy
my"e li no'sis
my"e li'tis
my'e lo blast"
my"e lo blas te'mi a
my'e lo blas'tic
my"e lo blas to'ma
my"e lo blas to'sis
my'e lo cele"
my"e lo cys'to cele
my'e lo cyte"
my'e lo cyt'ic
my'e lo cy to'sis
my"e lo dys pla'si a
my"e lo en ceph"a li'tis
my"e lo fi bro'sis
my"el o gen'e sis
my"e lo gen'ic
my'e lo gram
my"e log'ra phy
my'e loid
my"e lo lym'pho cyte"
my"e lo'ma
my"e lo ma la'ci a
my"e lo ma to'sis
my"e lo men"in gi'tis
my"e lo me nin'go cele"
my'e lo mere"
my"e lo mon'o cyte"
my'el on
my"e lo neu ri'tis
my"e lo pa ral'y sis
my"e lo path'ic
my"e lop'a thy

my"e lop'e tal
my"e loph'thi sic
my"e loph'thi sis
my'e lo plast"
my'e lo ple'gi a
my'e lo poi e'sis
my'e lo pore"
my"e lo pro lif'er a tive
my'e lo ra dic"u li'tis
my"e lo ra dic"u lo dys pla'si a
my"e lo ra dic"u lop'a thy
my'e lo rrha'gi a
my'e lo sar co'ma
my'e los'chi sis
my"e lo scin to'gram
my"e lo scin tog'ra phy
my"e lo scle ro'sis
my'e lo'sis
my en'ta sis
my"en ter'ic
my en'ter on
my'es the'si a
my'ia sis
my"la ceph'a lus
my lo'dus
my"lo glos'sus
my"lo hy'oid
my"lo phar yn'ge al
my'o blast
my'o blast o'ma
my"o car'di al
my"o car di'tis
my"o car'di um
my"o car do'sis
my"o clo'ni a
my"o clo'nic
my"o clo'nus
my'o cyte
my"o dys to'ni a

my"o dys'tro phy
my"o e de'ma
my"o e las'tic
my"o ep"i the'li al
my"o ep"i the"li o'ma
my"o fas'ci al
my"o fas ci'tis
my"o fi'bril
my"o fi"bro sar co'ma
my"o fi"bro si'tis
my"o ge lo'sis
my'o gen
my"o gen'ic
my"o glo'bin
my"o glo"bin u'ri a
my"o gnath'us
my'o gram
my'o graph
my"o he'ma tin
my"o he"mo glo'bin
my"o ki ne'si o gram"
my"o kin"es i og'ra phy
my"o ky mi a
my ol'o gy
my o'ma
my"o ma la'ci a
my"o mec'to my
my"o me tri'tis
my"o me'tri um
my"o neu'ral
my"o pal'mus
my"o pa ral'y sis
my"o pa re'sis
my"o path'i a
my op'a thy
my'ope
my"o per"i car di'tis
my o'pi a
my o'pic

my'o plasm
my'o plas"ty
my"o por tho'sis
my"o psy chop'a thy
my or'rha phy
my"o sar co'ma
my"o scle ro'sis
my'o sin
my"o sit'ic
my"o si'tis
my"o stat'ic
my"o su'ture
my"o syn"o vi'tis
my"o tac'tic
my ot'a sis
my"o ten"o si'tis
my"o te not'o my
my'o tome
my ot'o my
my"o to'ni a
my"ot'ro phy
myr'i a gram
myr"i a li'ter
myr"i a me'ter
my rin'ga
myr"in gec'to my
myr"in gi'tis
my rin"go dec'to my
my rin"go my co'sis
my rin'go plas"ty
my rin'go tome
myr"in got'o my
myr'ti form
My'so line
my"so pho'bi a
myth"o ma'ni a
myth"o pho'bi a
myx ad"e ni'tis
myx"as the'ni a

myx″e de′ma
myx id′i o cy
myx″i o′sis
myx″o ad″e no′ma
myx″o chon″dro
   fi″bro sar co′ma
myx″o chon″dro sar co′ma
myx″o fi bro′ma
myx″o fi″bro sar co′ma

myx″o gli o′ma
myx′oid
myx o′ma
myx″o ma to′sis
myx o′ma tous
myx″o neu ro′ma
myx″or rhe′a
myx″o sar co′ma
myx″o vi′rus

N

na bo′thi an
nail
na′ked
Nal′line
na′nism
na″no ceph′a lus
na′noid
na nom′e lus
nan″oph thal′mi a
na″no so′ma
na″no so′mus
na′nus
nape
na′pex
naph′tha
naph′tha lene
nar′can
nar cis′sism
nar cis′sist
nar″cis sis′tic
nar″co an al′y sis
nar″co hyp′ni a
nar″co hyp no′sis
nar′co lep″sy
nar″co lep′tic
nar co′ma
nar″co ma′ni a

nar co′sis
nar′co spasm
nar cot′ic
nar′co tism
nar′co tize
na res′
na′ris
na′sal
na sa′lis
nas′cent
na″si o al ve′o lar
na′si on
na si′tis
na″so cil′i ar″y
na″so fron′tal
na″so gen′i tal
na″so la′bi al
na″so la bi a′lis
na″so lac′ri mal
na″so max′il lar y
na″so pal′a tine
na″so phar yn gi′tis
na″so pha ryn′go scope
na″so phar′ynx
na″so-spi na′le
na″so tur′bi nal
na′sus

na'tal
na tal'i ty
na tal'o in
na'tant
nat re'mi a
na"tri u ret'ic
nat'u ar"y
nat'u ral
na'tur o path"
nau pa'thi a
nau'se a
nau'se ant
nau'se ous
na'vel
na vic'u lar
na vic"u lar thri'tis
na vic"u lo cu'boid
na vic"u lo cu ne'i form
ne"ar thro'sis
neb'u la
ne bu'li um
neb"u li za'tion
neb'u lize
neb'u li"zer
Ne ca'tor , a mer"i can'us
nec"ro bi o'sis
nec"ro cy to'sis
nec"ro cy"to tox'in
nec"ro gen'ic
nec"ro ma'ni a
nec"ro mi me'sis
ne croph'a gous
nec'ro phile
nec"ro phil'i a
ne croph'il ism
ne croph'i lous
nec"ro pho'bi a
nec'rop sy
ne crose'

nec'ro sin
ne cro'sis
nec"ro sper'mi a
nec"ro zo o sper'mi a
nee'dle
ne"en ceph'a lon
ne'frens
neg'a tive
neg'a tiv ism
neg'a tron
neg'li gence
Negri bo'dies
Neis se'ri a
nem"a thel'minth
Nem"a to'da
nem"a to sper'mi a
Nem'bu tal
ne"o ars"phen a mine'
ne"ar thro'sis
ne"o blas'tic
ne"o cer"e bel'lum
ne"o cor'tex
ne"o cys tos'to my
ne"o gen'e sis
Ne"o hy'drin
ne ol'o gism
ne"o mor'phism
ne"o my'cin
ne'on
ne"o na'tal
ne"o na tol'o gy
ne"o na to'rum
ne"o na'tus
ne"o-ol'ive
ne"o pal'li um
ne oph'il ism
ne"o pho'bi a
ne"o phren'i a
ne"o pla'si a

ne′o plasm
ne″o plas′tic
ne″o stig′mine
ne″o stri a′tum
Ne′o-sy neph′rin
neph″e lom′e ter
ne phral′gi a
ne″phrec ta′si a
ne phrec′to mize
ne phrec′to my
neph′ric
ne phrid′i um
ne phrit′i des
ne phrit′ic
ne phri′tis
neph″ro ab dom′i nal
neph″ro cal″ci no′sis
neph″ro cap sec′to mv
neph″ro cap″su lot′o my
neph″ro car′di ac
neph′ro coele
neph″ro col′o pex″y
neph″ro co″lop to′sis
neph″ro cys″tan as″to mo′sis
neph″ro cys ti′tis
neph″ro gen′ic
ne phrog′e nous
neph′roid
neph′ro lith
neph″ro li thi′a sis
neph″ro lith′ic
neph″ro li thot′o my
ne phrol′y sin
ne phrol′y sis
neph ro′ma
neph′ron
neph″ro path′ic
ne phrop′athy
neph′ro pex″y

neph″ro poi′e tin
neph″rop to′sis
neph″ro py″e li′tis
neph″ro py′e lo plas″ty
neph ror′rha phy
neph′ros
neph″ro scle ro′sis
ne phro′sis
neph′ro stome
ne phros′to my
neph rot′ic
neph′ro tome
ne phrot′o my
neph″ro tox′ic
neph″ro tox′in
neph″ro tro′ pic
neph″ro tu ber″cu lo′sis
neph″ro u″re ter ec′to my
nep″i ol′o gy
nerve
nerv′ine
ner vos′i ty
nerv′ous
nerv′ous ness
ner′vus
nes tei′a
nes″ti at′ri a
nes″ti os′to my
nes′tis
neu′ral
neu ral′gi a
neu ral′gic
neu ral′gi form
neu ram′e bim′e ter
neu″ra a min′ni dase
neu″ra poph′y sis
neu″ra prax′i a
neu″ras the′ni a
neu rax′is

neu"rax i'tis
neu"rec ta'si a
neu rec'to my
neu"rec to'pi a
neu"ren ter'ic
neu rer'gic
neur"ex e re'sis
neu ri'a sis
neu ri'a try
neu"ri lem'ma
neu"ri lem mi'tis
neu"ri lem mo'ma
neu"ri lem"mo sar co'ma
neu"ri no'ma
neu rit'ic
neu ri'tis
neu"ro ab"i ot'ro phy
neu"ro a nas"to mo'sis
neu"ro a nat'o my
neu"ro ar'thri tism
neu"ro ar throp'a thy
neu"ro as"tro cy to'ma
neu"ro bi ol'o gy
neu"ro bi"o tax'is
neu'ro blast
neu"ro blas to'ma
neu"ro cal"o rim'e ter
neu'ro ca nal'
neu'ro cele
neu"ro chem'is try
neu"ro cho"ri o ret"i ni'tis
neu"ro cho"roid i'tis
neu"ro cir'cu la to"ry
neu roc'la dism
neu"ro cra'ni um
neu"ro cu ta'ne ous
neu'ro cyte"
neu"ro cy to'ma
neu"ro de al'gi a

neu"ro de"a tro'phi a
neu"ro den'drite
neu"ro der"ma ti'tis
neu"ro der"ma to my"o si'tis
neu"ro der"ma to'sis
neu"ro der"ma tro'phi a
neu"ro di as'ta sis
neu"ro dy nam'i a
neu"ro e lec"tro ther"a peu'tics
neu"ro en'do crine
neu"ro ep"i der'mal
neu"ro ep"i the li o'ma
neu"ro ep"i the'li um
neu"ro fi'bril
neu"ro fi bro'ma
neu"ro fi bro"ma to'sis
neu"ro fi"bro sar co'ma
neu"ro fi"bro si'tis
neu"ro gan gli i'tis
neu"ro gas'tric
neu"ro gen'e sis
neu"ro gen'ic
neu rog'e nous
neu rog'li a
neu rog"li a cyte"
neu rog"li o'ma
neu rog"li o'sis
neu'ro gram
neu"ro his tol'o gy
neu"ro hu'mor
neu"ro hu'mor al
neu"ro hyp nol'o gy
neu"ro hy poph'y sis
neu'roid
neu"ro in duc'tion
neu"ro in'su lar
neu"ro ker'a tin
neu rol'o gist
neu rol'o gy

neu″ro lu′es
neu′ro lymph″
neu rol′y sis
neu ro′ma
neu″ro ma la′ci a
neu″ro ma to′sis
neu″ro mech′a nism
neu′ro mere
neu rom′er y
neu″ro mi me′sis
neu″ro mus′cu lar
neu″ro my′al
neu″ro my″e li′tis
neu″ro my′on
neu″ro my″o path′ic
neu″ro my″o si′tis
neu′ron
neu″ro ni′tis
neu″ro nog′ra phy
neu ro″no pha′gi a
neu′ro path
neu″ro path″o gen′e sis
neu″ro pa thol′o gy
neu rop′a thy
neu″ro phleg′mon
neu″ro pho′ni a
neu″ro phys″i ol′o gy
neu′ro pil
neu′ro plasm
neu′ro plas″ty
neu″ro po′di um
neu′ro pore
neu″ro psy chi′a try
neu″ro psy chol′o gy
neu″ro psy chop′a thy
neu″ro ra″dic u′lar
neu″ro re lapse′
neu″ro ret″i ni′tis
neu ror′rha phy

neu″ror rhex′is
neu″ror rhyc′tes
neu″ro sar co′ma
neu″ro scle ro′sis
neu″ro se cre′tion
neu ro′sis
neu′ro sism
neu″ro skel′e tal
neu′ro somes
neu′ro spasm
neu″ro spon′gi um
neu″ro ste ar′ic
neu″ro sur′geon
neu″ro sur′ger y
neu″ro su′ture
neu″ro syph′i lis
neu″ro the ci′tis
neu″ro ther′a py
neu rot′ic
neu rot′i ca
neu rot′i cism
neu rot″i za′tion
neu″rot me′sis
neu″ro tol′o gy
neu′ro tome
neu rot′o my
neu″ro ton′ic
neu″ro tox′in
neu′ro trau′ma
neu″ro trip′sy
neu″ro troph′ic
neu″ro trop′ic
neu rot′ro pism
neu″ro var″i co′sis
neu″ro vas′cu lar
neu′ru la
neu′tral
neu″tra li za′tion
neu′tral lize

neut′ro clu″sion
neu′tro cyte
neu′tron
neu″tro pe′ni a
neu′tro phil
neu″tro phil′i a
ne′vose
ne″vo xan″tho en″do the″li o′ma
ne′vus
new′born′
nex′us
ni′a cin
niche
nick′el
nic″o tin am′ide
nic′o tine
nic″o tin′ic ac′id
nic′ti ta″ting
nic″ti ta′ti o
nic″ti ta′tion
ni da′tion
ni′dus
nig′ri cans
ni gri′ti es
ni′hil ism
ni keth′a mide″
niph″a blep′si a
niph″o typh lo′sis
nip′ple
ni′sus
ni′trate
Ni′tra zine
ni′trite
ni″tri tu′ri a
ni′tro gen
ni trog′e nous
ni″tro glyc′er in
ni′trous
Nobel, Alfred

no″car di o′sis
no″ci cep′tive
no″ci fen′sor
no″ci per cep′tion
no″ci per cep′tion
noc″tal bu″mi nu′ri a
noc tam″bu la′tion
noc″ti pho′bi a
noc tu′ri a
noc tur′nal
noc′u ous
nod′al
node
no′dose
no dos′i ty
nod′u lar
nod′ule
nod′u lus
no″e gen′e sis
no″e mat″a chym′e ter
no′ma
no mad′ic
no′men cla ture
nom′o graph
nom″o top′ic
non ac′cess
non″ad he′rent
non″al ler′gic
no′nan
non a′que ous
non com′pos men′tis
non″con duc′tor
non″dis junc′tion
non″e lec′tro lyte
no″ni grav′i da
no nip′a ra
non″lu et′ic
non″ma lig′nant
non med′ul la″ted

non mo'tile
non my el'i na"ted
non par'ous
non"py o gen'ic
non re"a gin'ic
non"re frac'tive
non"re straint'
non sex'u al
non'spe cif'ic
non sup'pu ra"tive
non sur'gi cal
non vi'a ble
no'o psy"che
nor ep"i neph'rine
nor'mo blast
nor"mo chro mat'ic
nor"mo chro'mi a
nor"mo chro'mic
nor'mo cyte
nor"mo cy to'sis
nor"mo gly ce'mi a
nor"mo ten'sive
nor"mo ther'mi a
nor"mo ton'ic
nor"mo to'pi a
nor"mo vo le'mi a
nos er"es the'si a
nos"o co'mi a
no sog'e ny
no sol'o gy
nos"o ma'ni a
nos"o par'a sites
nos"o pho'bi a
nos'o phyte
nos"o tax'y
nos tal'gi a
nos"to ma'ni a
nos top'a thy
nos"to pho'bi a

nos'tras
nos'trate
nos'tril
nos'trum
nos tal'gi a
no"tan ce pha'li a
no"tan en"ce pha'li a
no ta'tion
notch
no"ten ceph'a lo cele
no"ten ceph'a lus
no'to chord
no"to gen'e sis
no tom'e lus
No vo bi o'cin
No'vo caine
nox'ious
Ntaya vi'rus
nu'bile
nu cel'lus
nu'ces
nu'cha
nu'cle ar
nu'cle ase
nu'cle a"ted
nu"cle a'tion
nu'cle i
nu'cle i form"
nu"cle o al bu'min
nu"cle o chy le'ma
nu'cle o chyme
nu"cle o cy"to plas'mic
nu"cle of'u gal
nu'cle oid
nu cle'o li form
nu cle'o loid
nu cle'o lus
nu"cle o mi"cro so'ma
nu'cle on

nu''cle on'ics
nu''cle op'e tal
nu'cle o plasm
nu''cle o pro'te in
nu''cle o re tic'u lum
nu'cle o tide
nu''cle o tox'in
nu'cle us
nud'ism
nul lip'a ra
numb
numb'ness
num'mi form
num'mu lar
nun na'tion
Nu'per caine
nurs'ling
nu ta'tion
nu'tri ent
nu'tri ment
nu tri'tion
nu tri'tious
nu'tri tive
nu'tri ture
nyc tal'gi a

nyc'to lope
nyc''to lo'pi a
nyc'ter ine
nyc''to phil'i a
nyc''to pho'bi a
nyc''to pho'ni a
nyc''to typh lo'sis
Ny'dra zid
Ny'lon
nymph
nym'pha
nym phec'to my
nym phi'tis
nym'pho lep'sy
nym''pho ma'ni a
nym''pho ma'ni ac
nym phon'cus
nym phot'o my
nys tag'mic
nys tag'mi form
nys tag'mo graph
nys''tag mog'ra phy
nys tag'moid
nys tag'mus
Ny stat'in
nyx'is

O

oa'kum
o''a ri al'gi a
o a'sis
ob''dor mi'tion
ob duc'tion
o be'li on
Obermayer's re a'gent
o bese'
o be'si ty
o'bex

ob''fus ca'tion
ob jec'tive
ob'li gate
ob lique'
ob liq'ui ty
ob li'quus
ob lit''er a'tion
ob''mu tes'cence
ob nu''bi la'tion
ob ses'sion

ob ses'sive
ob"so les'cence
ob"ste tri'cian
ob stet'rics
ob"sti pa'tion
ob struc'tion
ob'stru ent
ob tund'
ob tund'ent
ob"tu ra'tion
ob'tu ra"tor
ob tuse'
ob tu'sion
oc cip'i tal
oc cip"i ta'lis
oc cip'i tal ize
oc cip"i to an te'ri or
oc cip"i to ax'i al
oc cip"i to fron'tal
oc cip"i to fron ta'lis
oc cip"i to pos te'ri or
oc cip"i to scap"u lar'is
oc'ci put
oc clu'sion
oc clu'sive
oc cult'
oc"cu pa'tion al
och le'sis
och"lo pho'bi a
o chrom'e ter
o"chro no'sis
Ochsner, Alton
oc'tan
oc"ti grav'i da
oc tip'a ra
oc"to roon'
oc'u lar
oc"u len'tum
oc'u list

oc"u lo ce phal'ic
oc"u lo ce re"bro re'nal
oc"u lo gy ra'tion
oc"u lo gy'ric
oc"u lo mo'tor
oc"u lo my co'sis
oc"u lo phar yn ge'al
oc"u lo phren"i co re cur'rent
oc"u lo zy"go mat'ic
oc'u lus
o"cy o din'ic
o"dax es'mus
o"don tag'ra
o"don tal'gi a
o"don tal'gic
o"don tec'to my
o don'ter ism
o"don tex e'sis
o dont"he mo'di a
o"don thy'a lus
o don'ti a
o"don ti'a sis
o"don ti'a try
o don'tic
o don'tin oid
o"don ti'tis
o don'to blast
o don"to blas to'ma
o don"to bo thri'tis
o don"to both'ri um
o don"to cele
o don"to ce ram'ic
o"don to'cha lix
o don"to chi rur'gi cal
o don to cla'sis
o don'to clast
o don"toc ne'sis
o don"to dyn'i a
o don"to gen'e sis

o"don tog'e ny
o don'to glyph
o don'to gram
o don'to graph
o"don tog'ra phy
o don"to hy"per es the'si a
o don'toid
o don'to lith
o"don tol'o gist
o"don tol'o gy
o don"to lox'i a
o"don tol'y sis
o"don to'ma
o don"to ne cro'sis
o don"to neu ral'gi a
o don"to par"al lax'is
o"don top'a thy
o don"to pho'bi a
o don'to plast
o don"to pri'sis
o don"top to'si a
o don"to ra'di o graph
o don"for rha'gi a
o"don tos'chi sis
o don'to schism
o don'to scope
o"don tos'co py
o don"to sei'sis
o"don to'sis
o don"to ste re'sis
o don"to syn"er is'mus
o don"to the'ca
o don"to ther'a py
o"don tot'o my
o don"to trip'sis
o"don tot'ry py
o'dor
o"dor if'er ous
o"do rim'e try

o dyn"a cou'sis
o dyn"o pha'gi a
o dyn"o pho'bi a
o"dy nu'ri a
oed'i pal
oes'trus
of'fal
ohm
ohm'me"ter
o id"i o my co'sis
O id'i um
oi"ko pho'bi a
oint'ment
o"le ag'i nous
o"le an do my'cin
o"le cra"nar thri'tis
o"le cra"nar throc'a ce
o"le cra"nar throp'a thy
o lec'ra noid
o lec'ra non
o le'ic ac'id
o"le o mar'ga rine
o"le om'e ter
o"le o res'in
o"le o ther'a py
o"le o tho'rax
ol fac'tion
ol"fac tom'e ter
ol fac'to rv
ol"i ge'mi a
ol"i ger ga'si a
ol"ig hid'ri a
ol"ig hy'dri a
ol"i go am'ni os
ol"i go ceph'a lon
ol"i go cho'li a
ol"i go chro ma'si a
ol"i go chro me'mi a
ol"i go chy'li a

ol''i go cy the'mi a
ol''i go dac'ry a
ol''i go dac tyl'i a
ol''i go den''dro blas to'ma
ol''i go den drog'li a
ol''i go den''dro gli o'ma
ol''i go den''dro gli o''ma to'sis
ol''i go don'ti a
ol''i go dy nam'ic
ol''i go el'e ment
ol''i go ga lac'ti a
ol''i go gen'ic
ol''i go hy dram'ni os
ol''i go hy dru'ri a
ol''i go ma'ni a
ol''i go me'lus
ol''i go men''or rhe'a
ol''i go phos''pha tu'ri a
ol''i go phre'ni a
ol''i gop noe'a
ol''i go psy'chi a
ol''i gop ty'a lism
ol''i go py'rene
ol''i go'ri a
ol''i go si a'li a
ol''i go sper'mi a
ol''i go trich'i a
ol''i go zo''o sper'mi a
ol''i gu'ri a
o lis''ther o chro'ma tin
o lis''ther o zone'
ol''i vif'u gal
ol''i vip'e tal
ol''i vo pon''to cer e bel'lar
ol''o pho'ni a
o''ma ceph'a lus
o ma'gra
o''mar thral'gi a
o''mar thri'tis

o''mar throc'a ce
o ma'sum
om''bro pho'bi a
o''men tec'to my
o men'to pex y
o''men tor'rha phy
o men'tum
o men''tum ec'to my
o mi'tis
om''ma tid'i um
om niv'o rous
o''mo cer''vi ca'lis
o''mo hy'oid
o''mo ver'te bral
om''pha lec'to my
om phal'ic
om''pha li'tis
om phal'o cele
om''pha lo cho'ri on
om''pha lo cra''ni o did'y mus
om''pha lo did'y mus
om''pha lo gen'e sis
om''pha lo mes''en ter'ic
om''pha lo mon''o did'y mus
om''pha lop'a gus
om phal'o pleure
om''pha lo prop to'sis
om'pha los
om phal'o site
om''pha lo so'tor
om''pha lo tax'is
om phal'o tome
om''pha lot'o my
om''pha lo trip''sy
o'nan ism
o'nan ist
On''cho cer'ca
on''cho cer ci'a sis
on''cho cer co'ma

on"cho der ma ti'tis
on"cho my co'sis
on'to cyte
on"co cy to'ma
on"co gen'e sis
on'co graph
on cog'ra phy
on col'o gy
on com'e ter
on co'sis
o nei"ro dyn'i a
o"nei rog'mus
o"nei rol'o gy
o"nei ron'o sus
o"nei ros'co py
o"ni o ma'ni a
on kin'o cele
on"o mat"o ma'ni a
on"o mat"o pho'bi a
on"o mat"o poi e'sis
on tog'e ny
on"y chal'gi a
on"y cha tro'phi a
on"y chaux'is
on"y chec'to my
on"y chex"al lax'is
o nych'i a
on'y chin
on"y choc'la sis
on"y cho cryp to'sis
on"y cho dys'tro phy
on"y cho gen'ic
on"y cho gry po'sis
on"y cho hel co'sis
on"y cho het"er o to'pi a
on'y choid
on"y chol'y sis
on"y cho'ma
on"y cho ma de'sis

on"y cho ma la'ci a
on"y cho my co'sis
on"y cho pac'i ty
on"y chop'a thy
on"y cho pha'gi a
on"y choph'a gist
on"y cho phy'ma
on"y chop to'sis
on"y chor rhex'is
on"y chor rhi'za
on"y cho schiz'i a
on"y cho stro'ma
on"y chot"il lo ma'ni a
on"y chot'o my
on'yx
o"nyx i'tis
o"o ceph'a lus
o'o cyst
o'o cyte
o"o gen'e sis
o"o go'ni um
o"o ki ne'sis
o"o pho rec'to my
o"o pho ri'tis
o oph"o ro cys tec'to my
o oph"o ro cys to'sis
o oph"o ro hys"ter ec'to my
o oph"o ro ma la'ci a
o oph"o ro ma'ni a
o oph'o ron
o oph"o ro path'i a
o oph'o ro pex"y
o oph'o ro plas"ty
o oph"o ro sal"pin gec'to my
o oph"o ro sal"pin gi'tis ·
o"o pho ros'to my
o"o phor'rha phy
o'o plasm
o'o sperm

o pac''i fi ca'tion
o pac'i ty
o''pal es'cent
o paque'
o pei'do scope
op''er a bil'i ty
op'er a ble
op'er ant
op''e ra'tion
op'er a''tive
o phi'a sis
o phid''i o pho'bi a
o'phid ism
oph'i o phobe''
oph''i o'sis
oph''ry i'tis
oph'ry on
oph''ry o'sis
oph''ryph thei ri'a sis
oph'rys
oph thal''ma cro'sis
oph''thal ma'gra
oph''thal mal'gi a
oph''thal mec''chy mo'sis
oph''thal mec'to my
oph''thal men ceph'a lon
oph thal'mi a
oph thal'mi a''ter
oph thal''mi at'rics
oph thal'mic
oph''thal mi'tis
oph thal''mo blen''nor rhe'a
oph''thal moc'a ce
oph thal'mo cele
oph thal''mo cen te'sis
oph thal''mo co'pi a
oph thal''mo di''ag no'sis
oph thal''mo di''a phan'
  o scope

oph thal''mo di''a stim'e ter
oph thal''mo do ne'sis
oph thal''mo dy''na mom'e ter
oph thal''mo dyn'i a
oph thal''mo fun'do scope
oph''thal mog'ra phy
oph thal''mo gy'ric
oph thal''mo i''co nom'e ter
oph thal''mo leu'ko scope
oph thal'mo lith''
oph''thal mol'a gist
oph''thal mol'o gy
oph thal''mo ly'ma
oph thal''mo ma cro'sis
oph thal''mo ma la'ci a
oph thal''mo mel''a no'ma
oph thal''mo mel''a no'sis
oph''thal mom'e ter
oph thal''mo my co'sis
oph thal''mo my'ia sis
oph thal''mo my i'tis
oph thal''mo my ot'o my
oph thal''mo neu ri'tis
oph''thal mop'a thy
oph thal''mo pha com'e ter
oph thal''mo phan'tom
oph thal''mo phas''ma tos'co py
oph thal''mo pho'bi a
oph''thal moph'thi sis
oph thal''mo phy' ma
oph thal''mo plas''ty
oph thal''mo ple'gi a
oph thal''mop to'sis
oph thal'mo-re ac'tion
oph thal''mor rha'gi a
oph thal''mor rhe'a
oph thal''mor rhex'is
oph thal'mos
oph thal'mo scope

oph"thal mos'co pist
oph"thal mos'co py
oph thal'mo spasm
oph thal"mo spin'ther ism
oph"thal mos'ta sis
oph thal'mo stat
oph thal"mo sta tom'e ter
oph thal"mo sta tom'e try
oph thal"mo ste re'sis
oph thal"mo syn'chy sis
oph thal"mo ther mom'e ter
oph"thal mot'o my
oph thal"mo to nom'e ter
oph thal"mo to nom'e try
oph thal'mo trope
oph thal"mo tro pom'e ter
oph thal"mo tro pom'e try
oph thal"mo vas'cu lar
oph thal"mo xy'sis
oph thal"mox ys'ter
oph thal'mu la
oph thal'mus
o'pi ate
o"pi o ma'ni a
o"pi o pha'gi a
o'pi o phile
o pis'the nar
o pis'thi on
o pis"tho cra'ni on
op"is thog'na thism
o pis"tho neph'ros
o pis"tho po rei'a
op"is thot'o nos
o'pi um
op"o ceph'a lus
op"o del'doc
op"o did'y mus
op"pi la'tion
op po'nens

op por tu'nist
op sig'e nes
op"si o no'sis
op"si u'ri a
op so clo'nus
op"so ma'ni a
op'so nin
op son"i za'tion
op"so no cy"to pha'gic
op"so nom'e try
op son"o ther'a py
op"tes the'si a
op'tic
op'ti cal
op ti'cian
op ti'cian ry
op"ti co chi"as mat'ic
op"ti co cil'i ar"y
op'ti coele
op"ti co pu'pil lar"y
op'tics
op tim'e ter
op'ti mum
op'to gram
op tom'e ter
op tom'e trist
op tom'e try
op"to my om'e ter
op'to type
o'ra
o'rad
o'ral
o ra'le
or bic'u lar
or bic"u la're
or bic"u lar'is
or'bit
or'bi tal
or"bi ta'le

or''bi to na'sal
or''bi to nom'e ter
or''bi to nom'e try
or''bi to sphe'noid
or''bi tot'o my
or'chic
or''chi dop'a thy
or chid''o plas''ty
or''chi dot'o my
or''chi ec'to my
or''chi en ceph''a lo'ma
or''chi ep''i did''y mi'tis
or''chi o ca tab'a sis
or'chi o cele
or''chi op'a thy
or'chi o pex''y
or'chi o plas''ty
or'chis
or chi'tis
or'der ly
or'di nate
o rex'is
or'gan
or gan'ic
or'gan ism
or''gan i za'tion
or'gan i''zer
or''ga no gen'e sis
or''ga nog'e ny
or'gan oid
or''ga nol'o gy
or''ga nos'co py
or''ga no ther'a py
or''ga no troph'ic
or''ga no trop'ic
or''gan ot'ro pism
or'gasm
or gas'mo lep''sy
o''ri en ta'tion

or'i fice
or''i fi'ci um
Or''ni tho do'ra
or''ni tho'sis
O ro'ya
o''ro phar'ynx
or''rho men''in gi'tis
or'ris
or''thi auch'e nus
or''thi o chor'dus
or''thi o cor'y phus
or' thi o don'tus
or''thi o me to'pus
or''thi o pis'thi us
or''thi o pis tho cra'ni us
or''thi o pro so'pus
or''thi op'y lus
or''thi or rhi'nus
or''thi u ra nis'cus
or''tho ceph'a ly
or''tho cho re'a
or''tho chro mat'ic
or''tho cra'si a
or''tho dac'ty lous
or''tho di'a gram
or''tho di'a graph
or''tho di ag'ra phy
or''tho dol''i cho ceph'a lous
or''tho don'ti a
or''tho don'tics
or''tho dont'ist
or''tho gen'e sis
or''thog nath'ic
or'tho grade
or''tho mes''o ceph'a lous
or thom'e ter
or''tho pe'dic
or''tho pe'dist
or''tho per cus'sion

or''tho pho'ri a
or''thop ne'a
or''tho prax'is
or''tho psy chi'a try
Or thop'ter a
or''thop'tic
or thop'to scope
or''tho roent''gen og'ra phy
or'tho scope
or''tho scop'ic
or thos'co py
or tho'sis
or''tho stat'ic
or'tho tast
or''tho ter'i on
or thot'o nus
or thot'ro pism
os
o'sa zone
os'che a
os''cil la'tion
os'cil la''tor
os'cil lo graph''
os''cil lom'e ter
os''cil lom'e try
os''cil lop'si a
os cil'lo scope
os'ci tan cy
os''ci ta tion
os'cu lum
Osler, William
os mat'ic
os me'sis
os''mes the'si a
os''mo dys pho'ri a
os'mol
os''mo lar'i ty
os mol'o gy
os mom'e ter

os''mo pho'bi a
os'mo phor
os''mo re cep'tors
os''mo reg''u lar'i ty
os mo'sis
os mot'ic
os phre''si ol'o gy
os phre''si om'e ter
os phre'sis
os''phy al'gi a
os''phy o my''e li'tis
os'sa
os'se in
os'se let
os''se o al bu'mi noid
os''se o car''ti lag'i nous
os''se o fi'brous
os''se o mu'coid
os'se ous
os'si cle
os''si cu lec'to my
os''si cu lot'o my
os sif'er ous
os sif'ic
os''si fi ca'tion
os sif'lu ence
os sif'lu ent
os'si form
os si fy
os tal'gi a
os''tal gi'tis
os'te al
os''te al''le o'sis
os''te an''a gen'e sis
os''te a naph'y sis
os tec'to my
os tec'to py
os''te i'tis
os''tem py e'sis

os"te o an"a gen'e sis
os"te o an'eu rysm
os"te o ar threc'to my
os"te o ar thri'tis
os"te o ar throp'a thy
os"te o ar thro'sis
os"te o ar throt'o my
os'te o blast
os"te o camp'si a
os"te o car"ci no'ma
os"te o car"ti lag'i nous
os"te o chon'dral
os"te o chon dri'tis
os"te o chon"dro dys pla'si a
os"te o chon"dro dys tro'phi a
os"te o chon dro'ma
os"te o chon"dro ma to'sis
os"te o chon"dro myx o'ma
os"te o chon"dro myx"o
    sar co'ma
os"te o chon"dro sar co'ma
os"te o chon dro'sis
os"te o chon'drous
os"te oc'la sis
os'te o clast"
os"te o clas to'ma
os"te o cra'ni um
os"te o cys to'ma
os'te o cyte"
os"te o den'tin
os"te o der"ma to plas'tic
os"te o der'mi a
os"te o di as'ta sis
os"te o dyn'i a
os"te o dys tro'phi a
os"te o dys'tro phy
os"te o fi"bro chon dro'ma
os"te o fi"bro li po'ma
os"te o fi bro'ma

os"te o fi"bro sar co'ma
os"te o fi bro'sis
os'te o gen
os"te o gen'e sis
os"te o gen'ic
os"te og'e nous
os"te o ha lis"ter e'sis
os"te o hy"per troph'ic
os'te oid
os"te o lip"o chon dro'ma
os'te o lith
os"te ol'o gy
os"te ol'y sis
os"te o'ma
os"te o ma la'ci a
os"te om'e try
os"te o my"e li'tis
os"te o my"e log'ra phy
os"teo my e'lo scle ro'sis
os"te o myx"o chon dro'ma
os'te on
os"te o ne cro'sis
os"te o neph rop'a thy
os"te o neu ral'gi a
os"te o ny"cho dys pla'sia
os'te o path
os"te o path'i a
os"te o pe'di on
os"te o per"i os ti'tis
os"te o pe tro'sis
os'te o phage
os"te oph'o ny
os'te o phyte"
os'te o plaque"
os"te o plas'tic
os"te o plas"ty
os"te o poi"ki lo'sis
os"te o po ro'sis
os"te o ra"di o ne cro'sis

os"te or rha'gi a
os"te or'rha phy
os"te o sar co'ma
os"te o scle ro'sis
os"te o'sis
os"te o spon"gi o'ma
os"te o stix'is
os"te o su'ture
os"te o syn"o vi'tis
os"te o syn'the sis
os"te o ta'bes
os"te o throm bo'sis
os"te o tome"
os"te o to"mo cla'si a
os"te ot'o my
os'te o tribe
os"te ot'ro phy
os'ti um
os"tre o tox is'mus
o tal'gi a
o"tan tri'tis
o"thel co'sis
o the"ma to'ma
ot"hem or rha'gi a
ot"hem or rhe'a
o'tic
o"ti co din'i a
o ti'tis
o"to blen"or rhe'a
o"to ca tarrh'
o"to ceph'a lus
o"to clei'sis
o"to co'ni um
o'to cyst
o"to dyn'i a
o"to gen'ic
o"to hem"i neur"as the'ni a
o"to lar"yn gol'o gist
o"to lar"yn gol'o gy

o'to lith
o tol'o gist
o tol'o gy
o"to my"as the'ni a
O"to my'ces
o"to my co'sis
o"to neur"as the'ni a
o"to pha ryn'ge al
o'to pol'y pus
o"to py"or rhe'a
o"to py o'sis
o"to rhi nol'o gy
o"tor rha'gi a
o"tor rhe'a
o"to sal'pinx
o"to scle ro'sis
o"to scle rot'ic
o'to scope
o tos'co py
o tot'o my
oua ba'in
ou'loid
ou"lor rha'gi a
ounce
out'let
out'pa"tient
o'va
o'val
o val'o cyte
o"va lo cy to'sis
o va'ri a
o"va ri al'gi a
o va'ri an
o va"ri ec'to my
o va'ri o cele"
o va"ri o cen te'sis
o va"ri o cy e'sis
o va"ri o dys neu'ri a
o va"ri o gen'ic

o va"ri o hys"ter ec'to my
o va"ri o lyt'ic
o va"ri on'cus
o va"ri or rhex'is
o va"ri o ste re'sis
o va"ri ot'o my
o va"ri o tu'bal
o va'ri um
o'va ry
o"va tes'tis
o'ver bite"
o"ver cor rec'tion
o'ver de pen'den cy
o'ver de ter"mi na'tion
o"ver ex ten'sion
o"ver max'i mal
o'ver tone"
o"vi cap'sule
o'vi duct
o vif'er ous
o"vi fi ca'tion
o'vi form
o"vi gen'e sis
o vig'e nous
o'vi germ
o vig'er ous
o vip'a rous
o"vi po si'tion
o"vi pos'i tor
o'vi sac
o'vo plasm
o"vo tes'tis
ov'u lar
ov"u la'tion
ov'ule

o'vum
ox'a late
ox al'ic
ox"al o'sis
ox"a lu'ri a
ox'i dase
ox"i da'tion
ox'ide
ox'i dize
ox im'e ter
ox"y a'phi a
ox"y blep'si a
ox"y ceph'a ly
ox"y ci ne'sis
ox"y es the'si a
ox'y gen
ox'y gen ase"
ox'y ge na'tion
ox"y geu'si a
ox"y hem'a tin
ox"y hem"a to por'phy rin
ox"y he"mo glo'bin
ox"y o'pi a
ox"y op'ter
ox"y os phre'si a
ox"y pho'ni a
ox"y tet"ra cy'cline
ox"y to'ci a
ox"y to'cic
ox"y to'cin
Ox"y u'ris ver mic"u la'ris
o ze'na
o'zone
o"zos to'mi a

P

pab'u lum

pace'mak"er

pach″y ac′ri a
pach″y bleph′a ron
pach″y bleph″a ro′sis
pach″y ceph′a ly
pach″y chi′li a
pach″y chro mat′ic
pach″y dac tyl′i a
pach″y der′ma tous
pach″y der′mi a
pach″y der mo per″i os ti′tis
pach″y glos′si a
pach″y gy′ri a
pach″y hem′a tous
pach″y hy men′ic
pach″y lep″to men″in gi′tis
pach″y lo′sis
pach″y men″in gi′tis
pach″y men″in gop′a thy
pach″y me′ninx
pa chyn′sis
pach″y o nych′i a
pach″y o′ti a
pach″y pel″vi per″i to ni′tis
pach″y per″i os to′sis
pach″y per″i to ni′tis
pa chyp′o dous
pach″y rhi nic
pach″y sal pin′go-o″va ri′tis
pach′y tes
pa chyt′ic
pach″y vag″i ni′tis
pac′i fi″er
pack′er
Paget's dis ease′
pa″go plex′i a
pai dol′o gy
pain
pal′a dang″
pal′a tal

pal′ate
pa lat′ic
pa lat′i form
pal′a tine
pal″a ti′tis
pal″a to glos′sal
pal″a to glos′sus
pal′a to graph″
pal″a to max′il lar″y
pal″a to na′sal
pal″a to pha ryn′ge al
pal″a to pha ryn′ge us
pal′a to plas″ty
pal″a to ple′gi a
pal″a to pter′y goid
pal″a tor′rha phy
pal″a to sal pin′ge us
pal″a tos′chi sis
pal′a tum
pa″le en ceph′a lon
pa″le o cer″e bel′lum
pa″le o ki net′ic
pa″le on tol′o gy
pa″le o-ol′ive
pa″le o pal′li um
pa″le o pa thol′o gy
pa″le o stri a′tum
pa″le o thal′a mus
pal″i ki ne′si a
pal″i la′li a
pal″in dro′mi a
pal″in gen′e sis
pal″i op′si a
pal″i phra′si a
pal″ir rhe′a
pal la′di um
pal″lan es the′si a
pal″les the′si a
pal′li ate

pal"li a'tion
pal'li a"tive
pal'li dum
pal'lor
pal'mar
pal ma'ris
pal'ma ture
pal'mi ped
pal'mi tate
pal mit'ic
pal'mi tin
pal mod'ic
pal"mo plan'tar
pal'mus
pal'pa ble
pal'pate
pal pa'tion
pal"pa to per cus'sion
pal'pe bra
pal'pe brae
pal'pe bral
pal'pe brate
pal"pe bra'tion
pal'pi tate
pal"pi ta'tion
pal'sy
pal'u dal
pan"a ce'a
pan"ar te ri'tis
pan"ar thri'tis
pan at'ro phy
pan"car di'tis
Pancoast syn'drome
pan"co lec'to my
pan'cre as
pan"cre a tec'to my
pan"cre at'ic
pan"cre at"i co du"o de'nal
pan"cre at"i co en"ter os'to my

pan"cre at"i co gas tros'to my
pan"cre at"i co je"ju nos'to my
pan"cre at"i co li thot'o my
pan"cre at"i co splen'ic
pan'cre a tin
pan"cre a ti'tis
pan"cre a to du"o de nec'to my
pan"cre a to du"o de nos'to my
pan"cre a to en"ter os'to my
pan"cre a tog'e nous
pan"cre a to li'pase
pan"cre at'o lith
pan"cre a to li thec'to my
pan"cre a to li thot'o my
pan"cre a tol'y sis
pan"cre a tot'o my
pan"cre op'a thy
pan"cre o zy'min
pan"cy to pe'ni a
pan de'mi a
pan dem'ic
pan dic"u la'tion
Pandy's test
pan"e lec'tro scope
pan en'do scope
pan en dos'co py
pan"es the'si a
pan gen'e sis
pan glos'si a
pan hem"at o pe'ni a
pan"hi dro'sis
pan hy'grous
pan hy"po pi tu'i ta rism
pan"hys ter ec'to my
pan hys"ter o col pec'to my
pan hys"ter o-o"o pho rec'to my
pan hys"ter o sal"pin gec'to my
pan hys"ter o sal pin"go-
    o"o pho rec'to my

pan′ic
pan″im mu′ni ty
pa niv′o rous
pan″me tri′tis
pan mne′si a
Pan my′cin
pan″my e loph′thi sis
pan my″e lo tox″i co′sis
pan nic″u li′tis
pan nic′u lus
pan′nus
pan″oph thal mi′tis
pan″os te i′tis
pan″o ti′tis
pan phar′ma con
pan″phle bi′tis
pan″scle ro′sis
pan si′nus i′tis
pan″ta mor′phi a
pan″tan en ce pha′li a
pan″tan en ceph′a lus
pan tan′ky lo bleph′a ron
pan″ta pho′bi a
pan″ta som′a tous
pan″ta tro′phi a
pan′to graph″
Pan to′paque
pan″to pho′bi a
Pan to′pon
pan″top to′sis
pan″to som′a tous
pan″ta tro′phi a
pan′to graph″
Pan to′paque
pan″to pho′bi a
Pan to′pon
pan″top to′sis
pan″to som′a tous
pan″to then′ic ac′id

pan trop′ic
pa′nus
pan″zo ot′ic
Papanicolau tech nique′
pa pav′er ine
pa pa′ya
pa pes′cent
pa pil′la
pap′il lary
pap′il late
pap″il lec′to my
pa pil″le de′ma
pap″il lif′er ous
pa pil′li form
pap″il li′tis
pap″il lo′ma
pap″il lo″ma to′sis
pa pil″lo ret″i ni′tis
pa″po va vi′rus
pap′pose
pap′pus
pap″u la′tion
pap′ule
pap″u lif′er ous
pap″u lo er″y them′a tous
pap″u lo pus′tu lar
pap″u lo squa′mous
pap″u lo ve sic′u lar
pap″y ra′ce ous
par″a-a mi″no ben zo ′ic ac′id
par″a-an″al ge′si a
par″a-an″es the′si a
par″a-ap pen″di ci′tis
par″a bi o′sis
par″a bi ot′ic
par″a blep′sis
par″a bu′li a
par ac″an tho′ma
par ac″an tho′sis

par''a ca ri'nal
par''a cen te'sis
par''a cen'tral
par''a ceph'a lus
par''a chol'er a
par''a cho'li a
par''a chor'dal
par''a chro'ma
par''a chro'ma tism
par''a chro'mo phore
par ac'me
par''a coc cid''i oi''do my co'sis
par''a co li'tis
par''a co'lon
par''a col pi'tis
par''a col'pi um
par''a con'dy lar
par'a cone
par''a con'id
par''a cu'si a
par''a cy e'sis
par''a cys'tic
par''a cys ti'tis
par''a cy'tic
par''a de ni'tis
par''a den'tal
par''a di''ag no'sis
par''a did'y mis
Par a di'one
par''a dox'i a sex''u al'is
par''a dox'ic
par''a du''o de'nal
par''a dys'en ter''y
par''a ep'i lep''sy
par''a-e ryth'ro blast
par'af fin
par''af fi no'ma
par''a gan''gli o'ma
par''a gan'gli ons

par''a gen''i tal'is
par''a geu'si a
par''a geu'sic
par''ag glu''ti na'tion
par''a glos'sa
par''a glos'si a
par''a gnath'ous
par''a gnath'us
par''a gom pho'sis
par''a go''ni mi'a sis
Par''a gon'i mus
par''a gram'ma tism
par''a graph'i a
par''a he''mo phil'i a
par''a he pat'ic
par''a hep'a ti'tis
par''a hor'mone
par''a hyp no'sis
par''a in''flu en'za
par''a ker''a to'sis
par''a la'li a
par al'de hyde
par''a lep ro'sis
par'a lep''sy
par'a le re'ma
par'a le re'sis
par'a lex'i a
par''al ge'si a
par al'gi a
par'al lax
par'al lei ism
par''al lei om'e ter
par''a lo'gi a
pa ral'y sis
par''a lyt'ic
par'a ly''zant
par'a ly''zer
par''a mag net'ic
par''a mas ti'tis

par"a mas"toid i'tis
Par"a me'ci um
par"a me'di an
par"a me'ni a
par"a met'ric
par"a met'rism
par"a me tri'tis
par"a me'tri um
par"a me trop'a thy
par"a mim'i a
par"a mi'tome
par"am ne'si a
par"a mo'lar
par"a mor'phism
par"a mu'si a
par"a my'e lo blast"
par am'y loid
par"a my oc'lo nus mul'ti plex
par"a my"o to'ni a
par"a na'sal
par"a ne phri'tis
par"a neu'ral
par"a noi'a
par"a noi'ac
par'a noid
par'a noid ism
par an'tral
par"a nu'cle us
par"a pan"cre at ic
par"a pa re'sis
par"a per tus'sis
par"a pha'si a
par"a phe'mi a
pa ra'phi a
par"a phil'i a
par"a phi mo'sis
par"a pho'bi a
par"a pho'ni a
pa raph'o ra

par"a phra'si a
par"a phre ne'sis
par"a phre ni'tis
pa raph'y sis
par'a plasm
par"a plas'tic
par"a plec'tic
par"a ple'gi a
par'a pneu mo'ni a
pa rap'o plex"y
par"a prax'i a
par"a proc ti'tis
par"a proc'ti um
par"a pros"ta ti'tis
pa"ra pro"tein e'mi a
par"a pso ri'a sis
par"a psy chol'o gy
par"a pyk"no mor'phous
par"a rec'tal
par"a sa'cral
par"a sag'it tal
par"a sal"pin gi'tis
par"a se cre'tion
par"a sex u al'i ty
par'a site
par"a sit'ic
par"a sit'i cide
par"a sit ism
par'a sit tize
par"a si"to gen'ic
par"a si tol'o gy
par"a si"to pho'bi a
par"a si to'sis
par"a si"to trop'ic
par"a small'pox
par'a some
par"a spa'di as
par'a spasm
par"a ste"a to'sis

par"a ster'nal
par"a sym"pa thet'ic
par"a sym"pa tho lyt'ic
par"a sym"pa tho mi met'ic
par"a syn ap'sis
par"a syph'i lis
par"a sys'to le
par"a te re"si o ma'ni a
par"a ter'mi nal
par"a the li o'ma
Par" a thi'one
par"a thor'mone
par"a thy'mi a
par"a thy'roid
par"a thy"roid ec'to my
par"a thy"ro pri'val
par"a thy"ro tro'pic
par"a ton'sil lar
par"a tri cho'sis
par"a trip'sis
par"a troph'ic
pa rat'ro phy
par"a typh li'tis
par"a ty'phoid
par"a u re'thral
par"a u'ter ine
par"a vac cin'i a
par"a vag'i nal
par"a vag"i ni'tis
par"a ver'te bral
par"a ves'i cal
par"a vi"ta min o'sis
par ax'i al
par ec'ta sis
Par'e drine
par"e gor'ic
pa ren'chy ma
pa ren chy'mal
par en'ter al

par"ep i thym'i a
par"e reth'i sis
par"er ga'si a
pa re'sis
par"es the'si a
pa reu'ni a
par fo'cal
par"hi dro'sis
pa'ri es
pa ri'e tal
pa ri"e to fron'tal
pa ri"e to mas'toid
pa ri"e to-oc cip'i tal
pa ri"e to squa mo'sal
Parinaud's syn'drome
par'i ty
par'kin son ism
Parkinson's dis ease'
par"o don ti'tis
par"o don'ti um
par"o dyn'i a
par'ol i var"y
par"o ni'ri a
par"o nych'i a
par"o nych"o my co'sis
par"o ny cho'sis
par"o oph"o ri'tis
par"o oph'o ron
par"oph thal'mi a
par"oph thal mon'cus
pa ro'pi a
pa ro'pi on
par op'si a
par op'tic
par"o ra'sis
par"o rex'i a
par os'mi a
par"os ti'tis
par"os to'tis

pa ro'tic
pa rot'id
pa rot''id ec'to my
pa rot''i do scle ro'sis
par''o ti'tis
par'ous
par''o va'ri an
par''o var''ri ot'o my
par''o va ri'tis
par''o va'ri um
par'ox ysm
par''ox ys'mal
pars'ley
par''the no gen'e sis
par'tial
par'ti cle
par tic'u late
par ti'tion
par tu'ri en cy
par tu'ri ent
par tu''ri fa'cient
par tu''ri om'e ter
par''tu ri'tion
par'tus
pa ru'lis
par''um bil'i cal
par''vi cel'lu lar
par'vule
pas'sion
pas'siv ism
Pasteur, Louis
Pas''teur el'la
pas''teur i za'tion
pa tel'la
pa tel'la pex''y
pa tel'lar
pat''el lec'to my
pa'ten cy
path''er ga'si a

path'er gy
pa thet'ic
path'e tism
path'e tist
path''o don'ti a
path'o gen
path''o gen'e sis
path''o gen'ic
path''o ge nic'ity
pa thog''no mon'ic
path''o le'si a
path''o log'ic
pa thol'o gist
pa thol'o gy
path''o ma'ni a
pa thom'e try
path''o mi me'sis
path''o pho'bi a
path''o psy chol'o gy
pa tho'sis
pat''re lin'e al
pat'u lous
pau''lo car'di a
Pav'a trine
pave'ment ing
Pavlov, I.
pa'vor
pec'ten
pec'tin
pec tin o'sis
pec'to ral
pec''to ra'lis
pec''to ril'o quy
pec'tus
pe''dar throc'a ce
pe dat'ro phy
ped'er as''ty
pe de'sis
ped''i al'gi a

pe"di at'rics
pe"di at'rist
ped'i at"ry
ped'i cel late
ped'i cle
pe dic'te rus
pe dic'u lar
pe dic"u la'tion
pe dic'u li cide
pe dic"u lo pho'bi a
pe dic"u lo'sis
pe dic'u lous
Pe dic'u lus
ped'i cure
pe di'tis
pe"do bar"o ma crom'e ter
pe"do ba rom'e ter
pe"do don'tics
pe"do don'tist
pe dol'o gist
pe dol'o gy
pe dom'e ter
pe dop'a thy
pe"do phil'i a
pe"do pho'bi a
pe dun'cle
peel'ing
pel'age
pel"i o'sis
pel lag'ra
pel'let
pel'li cle
pel lic'u la
pel ol'o gy
pe lop'si a
pel"o ther'a py
pel'vic
pel"vi en ceph"a lom'e try
pel vim'e ter

pel vim'e try
pel"vi o li thot'o my
pel"vi o ne"o cys tos'to my
pel"vi o ra"di og'ra phy
pel"vi ot'o my
pel"vi rec'tal
pel'vis
pel'vi scope
pel'vi sec'tion
pem'mi can
pem'phi goid
pem'phi gus
pen"al ge'si a
pen'du lous
pen'e tra"ting
pen'e tra'tion
pen'e trom'e ter
pen"i cil'li form
pen"i cil'lin
pen"i cil'lin ase
pen"i cil"li o'sis
Pen"i cil'li um
pe'nis
pen'nate
pen'ni form
pen'ny weight"
pe nol'o gist
pe nol'o gy
pe"no scro'tal
Penrose drain
pen"ta ba'sic
pen"ta dac'tyl
pen'tane
pen"ta va'lent
pen'tose
pen"to su'ri a
Pen'to thal so'di um
pe"o til"lo ma'ni a
pep'per mint

pep'si gogue
pep'sin
pep sin'o gen
pep'tic
pep'tide
pep'tone
pep''to ne'mi a
pep'to nize
pep''to nol'y sis
pep''to nu'ri a
per''a ceph'a lus
per''ac'id
per''a cid'i ty
per''a cute'
per''a to dyn'i a
per bo'rate
per cent
per cen'tile
per cep'tion
per''cep tiv'i ty
per clu'sion
per'co la''tor
per cus'sion
per cus'sor
per''cu ta'ne ous
per'for ans
per'fo ra''ted
per'fo ra'tion
per'fo ra''tor
per''fo ra to'ri um
per''fri ca'tion
per fu'sion
per''i ad''e ni'tis
per''i a''lien i'tis
per''i a'nal
per''i an''gi i'tis
per''i an''gi o cho li'tis
per''i a''or ti'tis
per''i ap'i cal

per''i ap pen''di ce'al
per''i ap pen''di ci'tis
per''i ap''pen dic'u lar
per''i ar te'ri al
per''i ar''te ri'tis
per''i ar thri'tis
per''i ar tic'u lar
per''i a.tri al
per''i au ric'u lar
per''i ax'i al
per''i blep'sis
per''i bron'chi al
per''i bron''chi o'lar
per''i bron''chi o li'tis
per''i bron chi'tis
per''i bro'sis
per''i cap'il lar''y
per''i car'di al
per''i car''di ec'to my
per''i car''di o cen te'sis
per''i car''di ol' y is
per''i car''di o pleu'ral
per''i car''di or'rha phy
per''i car''di os'to my
per''i car''di ot'o my
per''i car di'tis
per''i car'di um
per''i ce'cal
per''i ce ci'tis
per''i cel'lu lar
per''i ce''men ti'tis
per''i ce men''to cla'si a
per''i ce men'tum
per''i cha rei'a
per''i chol''an gi'tis
per''i chol''e cys ti'tis
per''i chon dri'tis
per''i chon'dri um
per''i chon dro'ma

per''i chord
per''i cho'roid
per''i col'ic
per''i co li'tis
per''i con'chal
per''i con chi'tis
per''i cor'ne al
per''i cor''o ni'tis
per''i cow''per i'tis
per''i cra'ni um
per''i cys'tic
per''i cys ti'tis
per''i cys'ti um
per'i cyte
per''i cy'ti al
per'i del
per''i den drit'ic
per''i den'tal
per''i den ti'tis
per'i derm
per''i di''ver tic''u li'tis
per''i du''o de ni'tis
per''i du'ral
per''i en ceph''a li'tis
per''i en ter'ic
per''i en''ter i'tis
per''i ep en'dv mal
per''i e''so phag'e al
per''i e soph''a gi'tis
per''i fis'tu lar
per''i fol lic'u lar
per''i fol lic''u li'tis
per''i gan''gli i'tis
per''i gan''gli on'ic
per''i gas'tric
per''i glan'du lar
per''i glot'tic
per''i gnath'ic
per''i he pat'ic

per''i her'ni al
per''i hi'lar
per''i hys ter'ic
per''i je''ju ni'tis
per''i kar'y on
per''i ker at'tic
per''i lab''y rin thi'tis
per''i la ryn'ge al
per''i lar''yn gi'tis
per''i lu'nar
per'i lymph
per''i lym phan'ge al
per''i lym'phan gi'tis
per''i lym phat'ic
per''i mas ti'tis
per im'e ter
per''i met'ric
per''i me tri'tis
per''i me'tri um
per''i met''ro sal''pin gi'tis
per im'e try
per im'i trist
per im'i try
per''i my''e li'tis
per''i my''o si'tis
per''i mys'i um
per''i ne''o col''po
    rec''to my''o mec'to my
per''i ne om'e ter
per''i ne'o plas''ty
per''i ne or'rha phy
per''i ne''o scro'tal
peri''ne''o syn'the sis
per''i ne ot'o my
per''i ne''o vag'i nal
per''i ne''o va gi''no rec'tal
per''i neph'ric
per''i ne phri'tis
per''i neph'ri um

per"i ne'um
per"i neu'ral
per"i neu ri'tis
per"i neu'ri um
per"i nu'cle ar
per"i oc'u lar
per"ri o dic'i ty
per"i o don'tal
per"i o don'tics
per"i o don'tist
per"i o don ti'tis
per"i o don'ti um
per"i o don"to cla'si a
per"i o don tol'o gy
per"i o don to'sis
pe"ri od'o scope
per"i o dyn'i a
per"i om phal'ic
per"i o nych'i a
per"i o nych'i um
per"i o"o pho ri'tis
per"i o oph"or o sal"pin gi'tis
per'i o"ple
per"i op tom'e try
per"i or'al
per"i or'bit
per"i or'bi tal
per"i or"bi ti'tis
per"i os'te o phyte"
per"i os"te ot'o my
per"i os'te um
per"i os ti'tis
per"i os to'ma
per"i os to'sis
per"i o'tic
per"i o'vu lar
per"i pach"y men"in gi'tis
per"i pan"cre a ti'tis
per"i pap'il lar"y

per"i phak'us
per"i pha ryn'ge al
pe riph'er al
pe riph'er a phose"
pe riph'er y
per"i phle bi'tis
per"i pleu ri'tis
per"i por'tal
per"i proc'tal
per"i proc ti'tis
per"i pro stat'ic
per"i py"e li'tis
per"i py e'ma
per"i py"le phle bi'tis
per"i py lor'ic
per"i rec'tal
per"i re'nal
per"i rhi'nal
per"i sal"pin gi'tis
per"i sal'pinx
per"i sig"moid i'tis
per"i sin'u ous
per"i si"nus i'tis
per"i sper"ma ti'tis
per"i splen'ic
per"i sple ni'tis
per"i spon dyl'ic
per"i spon"dy li'tis
per"i stal'sis
per"i stal'tic
per"i staph'y line
per"i sta'sis
per'i stome
per"i syn o'vi al
per"i tec'to my
per"i ten din'e um
per"i ten"di ni'tis
per"i ten'on
per"i the'li um

per"i thy"roid i'tis
per rit'o my
per"i to ne'al
per"i to ne'a tome
per"i to ne"o cen te'sis
per"i to ne op'a thy
per"i to ne"o per"i car'di al
per"i to ne'o pex"y
per"i to ne'o scope
per"i to ne ot'o my
per"i to ne'um
per"i to ni'tis
per'i to nize
per"i ton'sil lar
per"i ton"sil li'tis
per"i tra'che al
per"i tra"che i'tis
per"i trich'i al
per"i trun'cal
per"i typh'lic
per"i typh li'tis
per"i um bil'i cal
per"i un'gual
per"i u"re ter'ic
per"i u re"ter i'tis
per"i u re'thral
per"i u"re thri'tis
per"i u'ter ine
per"i u'vu lar
per"i vag'i nal
per"i vas'cu lar
per"i vas"cu li'tis
per"i ve'nous
per"i ves'i cal
per"i ve sic"u li'tis
per"i vis'cer al
per"i vis"cer i'tis
per"i vit'el line
per"i xe ni'tis

perle
per lèche'
per'ma nent
per man'ga nate
per"me a bil'i ty
per'me a ble
per"me a'tion
per ni'cious
per"ni o'sis
per noc ta'tion
pe"ro bra'chi us
pe"ro chi'rus
pe"ro cor'mus
pe"ro dac tyl'i a
pe"ro dac'ty lus
pe"ro hep"a ti'tis
pe"ro me'li a
pe rom'e lus
pe rom'e ly
per"o ne'al
per"o ne"o cal ca'ne us
per"o ne"o cu boi'de us
per"o ne"o tib"ia'lis
per"o ne'us
pe ro'ni a
pe"ro pla'si a
pe'ro pus
per o'ral
per os
pe ro'sis
pe"ro so'mus
pe"ro splanch'ni ca
per os'se ous
per ox'ide
per"pen dic'u lar
per rec'tum
per sev"er a'tion
per'son al
per"son al'i ty

per"spi ra'tion
per spire'
per"tur ba'tion
per tus'al
per tus'sis
per ver'sion
pes'sa ry
pes'ti cide
pes'tis
pes'tle
pe te'chi a
pe te'chi al
pe ti'o lus
pe tit' mal'
pet"ri fac'tion
pe"tris sage'
pet"ro bas'i lar
pet"ro la'tum
pe tro'le um
pet"ro mas'toid
pet"ro-oc cip'i tal
pet"ro pha ryn'ge us
pe tro'sa
pe tro'sal
pet"ro si'tis
pet"ro sphe'noid
pet"ro squa'mous
pet'rous
Peutz-Jeghers syn'drome
Peyer's patch'es
Pfannenstiel's in ci'sion
pha cen'to cele
pha ci'tis
phac"o-an"a phy lax'is
phac'o cyst
phac"o cys tec'to my
phac"o er'i sis
phac"o hy"men i'tis
pha'coid

pha col'y sis
phac"o ma to'sis
phac"o met"a cho re'sis
phac"o met"e ce'sis
pha com'e ter
phac"o pla ne'sis
phac"o scle ro'sis
phac'o scope
phac"o sco tas'mus
phag'o cyte
phag"o cy'to blast
phag"o cy tol'y sis
phag"o cy to'sis
pha gol'y sis
phag"o ma'ni a
phag"o ther'a py
pha"ko ma to'sis
pha lan'ge al
phal"an gec'to my
pha lan'ges
phal"an gi'tis
pha lan"gi za'tion
pha lan"go pha lan'ge al
pha'lanx
phal'lic
phal'lo plas ty
phal'lus
phan"er o ma'ni a
phan"er o'sis
phan'tasm
phan tas"ma to mo'ri a
phan'ta sy
phan'tom
phar'ci dous
phar'ma cal
phar"ma ceu'tic
phar'ma cist
phar"ma co dy nam'ics
phar"ma cog'no sy

phar''ma col'o gist
phar'' ma col'o gy
phar''ma co ma'ni a
phar''ma co pe'ia
phar''ma co pho'bi a
phar''ma co psy cho'sis
phar''ma co ther'a py
phar'ma cy
phar''yn gal'gi a
phar''yn ge'al
phar''yn gec'to my
phar''yn gis'mus
phar''yn gi'tis
pha ryn'go cele
pha ryn''go dyn'i a
pha ryn''go ep''i glot'tic
phar ryn''go ep''i glot'ti cus
pha ryn''go e soph'a ge''al
pha ryn''go e soph'a gus
pha''ryn''go glos'sal
pha ryn''go glos'sus
pha ryn''go ker''a to'sis
pha ryn''go la ryn'ge al
pha ryn''go lar''yn gi'tis
pha ryn'go lith
phar''yn gol'y sis
pha ryn''go max'il lar''y
pha ryn''go my co'sis
pha ryn''go na'sal
pha ryn''go pal'a tine
phar''yn gop'a thy
pha ryn'go plas''ty
pha ryn''go ple'gi a
pha ryn''go rhi ni'tis
pha ryn''gor rha'gi a
pha ryn''gor rhe'a
pha ryn''go scle ro'ma
pha ryn'go scope
pha ryn'go spasm

pha ryn''go ste'ni a
pha ryn''go ther'a py
pha ryn'go tome
phar''yn got'o my
pha ryn''go ton''sil li'tis
pha ryn''go xe ro'sis
phar'ynx
phase
phat''nor rha'gi a
phe nac'e tin
phen''go pho'bi a
phe''no bar'bi tal
phen'o cop''y
phe'nol
phe''nol phthal'ein
phen''nol sul fon phthal'ein
phe''no lu'ri a
phe nom'e non
phe''no thi'a zine
phe'no type
phen tol'a mine
phen''yl al'a nine
phen''yl ke''to nu'ri a
phen''yl pu ru'vic ac'id
phe''o chro''mo blas to'ma
phe''o chro''mo cy to'ma
phi li'a ter
phil''o ne'ism
phil''o pa trid''o ma'ni a
phil'ter
phil'trum
phi mo'sis
phi mot'ic
phleb an''gi o'ma
phleb''ar te''ri ec ta'si a
phleb''ar te''ri o di al'y sis
phleb''ec ta'si a
phle bec'to my
phleb''ec to'pi a

phleb"em phrax'is
phleb"ep a ti'tis
,phleb"ex ai re'sis
phle bis'mus
phle bi'tis
phleb"o car"ci no'ma
phle boc'ly sis
phleb'o gram
phleb'o graph
phle bog'ra phy
phleb'oid
phleb'o lith
phleb"o li thi'a sis
phleb"o ma nom'e ter
phleb"o phle bos'to my
phleb'o plas"ty
phleb"o ple ro'sis
phleb"or rha'gi a
phle bor'rha phy
phleb"or rhex'is
phleb"o scle ro'sis
phle bos'ta sis
phleb"o ste no'sis
phleb"o strep'sis
phleb"o throm bo'sis
phleb'o tome
Phle bot'o mus
phle bot'o my
phlegm
phleg mat'ic
phleg'mon
phlog"o gen'ic
phlyc te'na
phlyc ten'u lar
phlyc ten'ule
pho'bi a
pho'bic
pho"bo pho'bi a
pho"co me'li a

pho"na the'ni a
pho na'tion
pho'na to"ry
phon au'to gram
pho'neme
pho nen'do scope
pho net'ic
pho'ni ca
phon'ics
pho'nism
pho"no car'di o gram"
pho"no car'di o graph"
pho"no chor'da
pho'no gram
pho'no graph
pho"no ma'ni a
pho"no mas sage'
pho nom'e ter
pho"no my oc'lo nus
pho"no my og'ra phy
pho nop'a thy
pho"no pho'bi a
pho"no pho tog'ra phy
pho nop'si a
phor'o blast
phor'o cyte
pho rom'e ter
phor op'ter
phor'o scope
phos'gene
phos'pha tase
phos'phate
phos"pha te'mi a
phos"pha tu'ri a
phos"pho lip'id
phos"pho res'cence
phos"phor hi dro'sis
phos phor'ic ac'id
phos"phor ol'y sis

phos'pho rus
pho tal'gi a
pho tau''gi o pho'bi a
phote
pho'tech''y
pho''tes the'si a
pho'tic
pho'tism
pho''to ac tin'ic
pho''to bi ot'ic
pho'to chrome
pho''to col''or im'e ter
pho''to con''duc tiv'i ty
pho''to der''ma to'sis
pho''to dy nam'ic
pho''to dyn'i a
pho''to dys pho'ri a
pho''to flu''or os'co py
pho'to gene
pho'to gen'ic
pho''to ki net'ic
pho''to ky'mo graph
pho tol'y sis
pho''to ma'ni a
pho tom'e ter
pho''to mi'cro graph
pho''to mo'tor
pho ton'o sus
pho''to path''o log'ic
pho''to per cep'tive
pho''to phil'ic
pho''to pho'bi a
pho''toph thal'mi a
pho top'si a
pho''top tom'e ter
pho''to ra''di om'e ter
pho''to re cep'tive
pho''to sen'si tive
pho''to shock'

pho''to syn'the sis
pho''to tax'is
pho''to ther'a py
pho'to ti''mer
pho''to to'pi a
pho''to troph'
phre nal'gi a
phren''as the'ni a
phren''a tro'phi a
phren''em phrax'is
phre ne'sis
phren'ic
phren''i cec'to my
phren''i co ex er'e sis
phren''i cot'o my
phren''i co trip'sy
phre ni'tis
phren''o bla'bi a
phren''o car'di a
phren''o col'ic
phren''o gas'tric
phren''o glot'tic
phren''o glot tis'mus
phren''o he pat'ic
phren''o lep'si a
phre nol'o gy
phren'o path
phren''o ple'gi a
phren''o splen'ic
phric''to path'ic
phron''e mo pho'bi a
phro ne'sis
phryn''o der'ma
phthi ri'a sis
phthis''i o pho'bi a
phthi'sis
Phy''co my ce'tes
phy''co my co'sis
phyg''o ga lac'tic

phy lax'is
phy log'e ny
phy'ma
phy''ma tor rhy'sin
phy''ma to'sis
phys co'ni a
phys''i at'rics
phys''i at'rist
phys'ic
phy si'cian
phys'i cist
phys''i co chem'i cal
phys''i co gen'ic
phys''i co py rex'i a
phys'ics
phys''i no'sis
phys''i og'no my
phys''i og no'sis
phys''i o log'ic
phys''i o log''i co an''a tom'ic
phys''i ol'o gist
phys''i ol'o gy
phys''i o pa thol'o gy
phys''i o ther'a py
phy sique'
phy''so hem''a to me'tra
phy''so hy''dro me'tra
phy''so me'tra
phy''so py''o sal'pinx
phy''so stig'ma
phy''so stig'mine
phy'tase
phy'tin
phy''to be'zoar
phy''to chem'is try
phy''to gen'e sis
phy tog'e nous
phy'toid
phy''to path''o gen'ic

phy''to pa thol'o gy
phy toph'a gous
phy''to pho''to der''ma to'sis
phy''to pneu''mo no co''ni o'sis
phy to'sis
phy''to tox'ic
phy''to tox'in
pi'a ma'ter
pi an'
pi''a rach'noid
pi blok'to
pi'ca
pic'e ous
Pickwickian syn'drome
pi cor''na vi'rus
pic'ric ac'id
pic''ro tox'in
pie'bald ism
pie'dra
pig'ment
pig''men ta'tion
pig men'to phage
pig men'tum
pig'weed
pile
pi'le ous
pi''li a'tion
pil'i form
pill
pil'lar
pil'le us
pi''lo car'pine
pi''lo cys'tic
pi''lo e rec'tion
pi''lo mo'tor
pi''lo ni'dal
pi'lose
pi''lo se ba'ceous
pi lo'sis

221

pil'u la
pi'lus
pim"e li'tis
pim"e lo pte ryg'i um
pim"e lor rhe'a
pim"e lor thop'ne a
pim"e lu'ri a
pim'ple
pin'e al
pin"e a lec'to my
pin'e al ism
pin"e a lo'ma
pin gue'cu la
pin'na
pi'no cyte
pi"no cy to'sis
pin'ta
pin'worm"
pi"or thop ne'a
pi per'a zine
pi pet'
pip"to nych'i a
pir'i form
pir"i for'mis
Pirquet test
pis'i form
pi"si met"a car'pus
pi"si un"ci na'tus
pith'i a tism
pith"i at'ric
Pi to'cin
Pi tres'sin
pi tu'i tar"y
Pi tu'i trin
pit"y ri'a sis
pla ce'bo
pla cen'ta
plac"en ta'tion
pla cen'tin

plac"en ti'tis
plac"en tog'ra phy
plac"en to'ma
plad"a ro'ma
pla"gi o ce phal'ic
pla"gi o ceph'a ly
plague
pla'ni ceps
plank'ton
pla"no cel'lu lar
pla"no con'cave
pla"no con'ic
pla"no con'vex
plan'o cyte
pla'no gram
plan"o ma'ni a
plan'ta
plan'tar
plan tar'is
plan'ti grade
pla'num
plaque
plasm
plas'ma
plas'ma blast
plas'ma cyte
plas"ma cy to'sis
plas'ma gel
plas"ma lem'ma
plas"ma pher'e sis
plas'ma some
plas mat'ic
plas"ma to sis
plas"mo cy to'ma
Plas mo'di um
plas mol'y sis
plas'mo lyze
plas'mo some
plas"mo trop'ic

plas′ter
plas′tic
plas″ti ciz′er
plas′tid
plas″to dy na′mi a
pla teau′
plate′let
plat′i num
plat″o nych′i a
plat″y ba′si a
plat″y ce′li an
plat″y ce phal′ic
plat″yc ne′mi a
plat″y co′ri a
plat″y hi er′ic
plat″y mer′ic
plat″y mor′phi a
plat″y o′pi a
plat″y o′pic
plat″y pel′lic
pla tys′ma
plat″ys ten″ce pha′li a
pledg′et
ple′gia
ple′gic
ple″o cy to′sis
ple″o mor′phism
ple′o nasm
ple″o nec′tic
ple″o nex′ia
ple″on os″te o′sis
ple″o no′tus
ple op′tics
ple ro′sis
ple″si o gnath′us
ple″si o mor′phism
ple″si o′pi a
pless″es the′si a
pleth′o ra

ple thys′mo graph
pleu′ra
pleu″ra cot′o my
pleu′ral
pleu ral′gi a
pleu ram′ni on
pleu″ra poph′y sis
pleur′a tome
pleu rec′to my
pleu′ri sy
pleu rit′ic
pleu ri′tis
pleu″ro cen te′sis
pleu″ro cen′trum
pleu″ro chol″e cys ti′tis
pleu″ro cu ta′ne ous
pleu″ro dont
pleu″ro dy′ni a
pleu″ro gen′ic
pleu″ro hep a ti′tis
pleu″ro lith
pleu rol′y sis
pleu ro′ma
pleu″ro me′lus
pleu″ro per″i car′di al
pleu″ro per″i car di′tis
pleu″ro pneu mo′ni a
pleu″ro pneu″mo ni′tis
pleu″ro pros″o pos′chi sis
pleu″ro pul′mo nar″y
pleu ros′co py
pleu″ro so′ma
pleu″ro so″ma tos′chi sis
pleu″ro so′mus
pleu′ro spasm
pleu″ro thot′o nos
pleu rot′o my
pleu″ro ty′phoid
pleu″ro vis′cer al

plex'i form
Plex'i glas
plex im'e ter
plex'or
plex'us
pli'ca
pli cot'o my
plomb
plom bage'
plo ra'tion
plum ba'go
plum'bism
plu"ri glan'du lar
plu"ri grav'i da
plu"ri loc'u lar
plu rip'a ra
plu"ri par'i ty
plu"to ma'ni a
plu to'ni um
pne"o dy nam'ics
pne'o graph
pneu"mar thro'sis
pneu mat'ic
pneu"ma ti za'tion
pneu"ma to car'di a
pneu'ma to cele"
pneu"ma to dysp ne'a
pneu'ma to gram"
pneu"ma tol'o gy
pneu"ma tom'e ter
pneu"ma tor'ra chis
pneu"ma to'sis
pneu"ma tu'ri a
pneu'ma type
pneu"mo an"gi og'ra phy
pneu"mo-ar throg'ra phy
pneu"mo ba cil'lus
pneu"mo bul'bar
pneu"mo cen te'sis

pneu"mo ceph'a lus
pneu"mo chol"e cys ti'tis
pneu"mo coc'cal
pneu"mo coc ce'mi a
pneu"mo coc'cus
pneu"mo co'lon
pneu"mo co"ni o'sis
pneu"mo cra'ni um
pneu"mo cys tog'ra phy
pneu"mo der'ma
pneu"mo dy nam'ics
pneu"mo en ceph'a lo gram"
pneu"mo en"ter i'tis
pneu"mo gas'tric
pneu'mo graph
pneu mog'ra phy
pneu"mo he"mo per"i car'di um
pneu"mo he"mo tho'rax
pneu"mo hy"dro per"i car'di um
pneu"mo hy"po der'ma
pneu'mo lith
pneu"mo li thi'a sis
pneu"mo me"di as ti'num
pneu mom'e try
pneu"mo nec'to my
pneu mo'ni a
pneu mon'ic
pneu"mo ni'tis
pneu"mo no coc'cic
pneu"mo nol'y sis
pneu"mo no my co'sis
pneu"mo nop'a thy
pneu mo'no pex"y
pneu"mo nor'rha phy
pneu"mo no'sis
pneu"mo not'o my
pneu mop'a thy
pneu"mo per"i car di'tis
pneu"mo per"i car'di um

pneu″mo per″i to ne′um
pneu″mo per″i to ni′tis
pneu″mo py el′o gram″
pneu″mo py″o per″i car′di um
pneu″mo ra′chis
pneu″mo ra″di og′ra phy
pneu″mo roent″gen og′ra phy
pneu″mo scle ro′sis
pneu″mo tax′is
pneu″mo tho′rax
pneu″mo tox′in
pneu″mo ty′phus
pneu″mo ven′tri cle
pneu″mo ven tric″u log′ra phy
pneu′sis
pnig′ma
pni″go pho′bi a
pock
po dag′ra
po dal′gi a
po dal′ic
pod″ar thri′tis
pod″ar throc′a ce
pod″e de′ma
pod″el co′ma
pod″en ceph′a lus
po di′a trist
po di′a try
pod″o brom″hi dro′sis
pod′o derm
pod″o dyn′i a
po dom′e ter
po doph′yl lin
pod″o phyl′lum
po go′ni on
po″i kil o ther′mi a
poi′ki lo blast″
poi′ki lo cyte″
poi″ki lo cy to′sis

poi″ki lo der′ma
poi″ki lo der″ma to my″o si′tis
poi″ki lo throm′bo cyte
poi″ki lo zo o sper′mi a
poi′son
poi′son ous
po′lar
po″lar im′e ter
po lar′i scope
po lar′i ty
po″lar i za′tion
po′lar ize
po lar′o gram
po″lar og′ra phy
Po′la roid
pole
po′li o
po′li o en ceph″a li′tis
po′li o en ceph″a lo
    me nin″go my″e li′tis
po′li o en ceph″a lo my″e li′tis
po′li o en ceph″a lop′a thy
po′li o my″e len ceph″a li′tis
po′li o my″e li′tis
po′li o my″e lop′a thy
po′li o′sis
po lit′zer i za″tion
pol″la ki u′ri a
pol′len
pol″le no′sis
pol′lex
pol lu′tion
pol toph′a gy
pol″y ar″te ri′tis
pol″y ar′thric
pol″y ar thri′tis
pol″y ar tic′u lar
pol″y ba′sic
pol′y blast

pol''y bleph'a ron
pol''y cel'lu lar
pol''y cen'tric
pol''y chei'ri a
pol''y cho'li a
pol''y chro mat'ic
pol''y chro''ma to phil'i a
pol''y chro''ma to phil'ic
pol''y chro'mi a
pol''y chy'li a
pol''y clin'ic
pol''y clo'ni a
pol''y co'ri a
pol''y cy'clic
pol''y cy e'sis
pol''y cys'tic
pol''y cy the'mi a
pol''y dac'ty ly
pol''y de fi'cien cy
pol''y dip'si a
pol''y em'bry o ny
poly''men or rhe'a
pol''y e'mi a
pol''y es the'si a
pol''y es'trus
pol''y ga lac'ti a
po lyg'a mous
po lyg'a my
pol''y gas'tri a
pol''y a gen'ic
pol''y glan'du lar
pol''y gnath'us
po lyg'o nal
pol'y graph
pol'y gyr'i a
pol''y he'dral
pol''y hy'brid
pol''y hy dram'ni os
pol''y hy dru'ri a

pol''y in fec'tion
pol''y lep'tic
pol''y mas'ti a
pol''y me'li a
pol''y me'lus
pol''y me'ni a
pol'y mer
pol''y me'ri a
pol''y mer'ic
po lym'er ism
pol''y mer i za'tion
pol''y mi cro'bic
pol'y morph
pol'y mor'phic
pol''y mor''pho cel'lu lar
pol''y mor'pho cyte
pol''y mor''pho nu'cle ar
pol''y my''o si'tis
pol''y myx'in
pol''y ne'sic
pol''y neu'ral
pol''y neu ral'gi a
pol''y neu ri'tis
pol''y neu''ro my''o si'tis
pol''y neu rop'a thy
pol''y o don'ti a
pol''y o nych'i a
pol''y o'pi a
pol''y or'chid ism
pol''y or'chis
pol''y o rex'i a
pol''y o stot'ic
pol''y o'ti a
pol'yp
pol''y pa re'sis
pol''y path'i a
pol''y pep'tide
pol''y pha'gi a
pol''y pha lan'gism

pol"y pho'bi a
pol"y phy let'ic
pol"y phy'o dont
pol"y pif'er ous
pol'y plast
pol'y ploid
pol"yp ne'a
pol"y po'di a
pol'yp oid
po lyp'o rous
pol"y po'sis
pol"y pty'chi al
pol"y ra dic"u li'tis
pol"y sac'cha ride
pol"y sce'li a
po lys'ce lus
pol"y se"ro si'tis
pol"y si"nus i'tis
pol"y som'a tous
pol"y sper'mi a
pol'y sper"my
pol"y sphyg'mo graph
pol"y stich'i a
pol"y stom'a tous
pol"y sty'rene
pol"y symp"to mat'ic
pol"y the'li a
po lyt'o cous
pol"y trich'i a
pol"y trop'ic
pol"y un'gui a
pol"y u'ri a
pol"y va'lent
pom"pho ly he'mi a
pon"o pal mo'sis
pons
pon'tic
pon'tine
pon"to bul'bar

Pont'o caine
pop"li te'al
pop"li te'us
pore
po ren"ce pha'li a
po"ren ceph"a li'tis
po"ren ceph'a lus
po"ri o ma'ni a
po'ri on
por nog'ra phy
por"o ceph"a li'a sis
po ro'ma
po ro'sis
po ros'i ty
po'rous
por"pho bi lin'o gen
por phy'ri a
por'phy rin
por"phy rin'o gen
por"phy ri nu'ri a
por'ta
por ta ca'val
por'tal
por'ti o
po'rus
po"si o ma'ni a
po si'tion
pos'i tive
pos'i tron
po sol'o gy
post a'nal
post"an es thet'ic
post"ap o plec'tic
post au'di to"ry
post ax'i al
post bra'chi al
post cap'il lar"y
post car'di nal
post ca'va

post cen'tral
post ci'bal
post"cla vic'u lar
post co'i tal
post"con nu'bi al
post"con vul'sive
post cor'di al
post"di crot'ic
post"di ges'tive
post"diph the rit'ic
post"em bry on'ic
post"en ceph"a lit'ic
post"ep i lep'tic
pos te'ri ad
pos te'ri or
pos te'ri or ly
pos"ter o an te'ri or
pos"ter o ex ter'nal
pos"ter o in ter'nal
pos"ter o lat'er al
pos"ter o me'di al
pos"ter o me'di an
pos"ter o su pe'ri or
post"e rup'tive
post"e so phag'e al
post fe'brile
post"gan gli on'ic
post"gas trec'to my
post gle'noid
post"hem i pleg'ic
post"hem or rhag'ic
pos thet'o my
pos thi'tis
pos'tho lith
post'hu mous
post"hyp not'ic
post ic ter'ic
post"in flu en'zal
post"mor'tem

post na'ris
post na'sal
post na'tal
post"ne crot'ic
post"neu rit'ic
post nod'u lar
post oc'u lar
post op'er a"tive
post o'ral
post pal'a tine
post"pa lu'dal
post"par a lyt'ic
post-par'tum
post"pha ryn'ge al
post"phle bi'tic
post pran'di al
post"pu bes'cent
post"pyc not'ic
post"py ram'i dal
post ro'ta to"ry
post"scar la ti'nal
post"ste not'ic
post"syph i lit'ic
post"trau mat'ic
post ty'phoid
pos'tu late
pos'tur al
pos'ture
post vac'ci nal
po'ta ble
pot"a mo pho'bi a
pot'ash"
pot as se'mi a
po tas'si um
po'ten cy
po ten'tial
po ten"ti a'tion
po'tion
po"to ma'ni a

pouch
poul'tice
pound
pow'der
pox
prag''mat ag no'si a
prag''mat am ne'si a
pran'di al
pra tique'
prax in'o scope
prax''i ol'o gy
pre ag'o nal
pre am'pul lar y
pre a'nal
pre''an es thet'ic
pre''an ti sep'tic
pre''a or'tic
pre''a sep'tic
pre''a tax'ic
pre''au ric'u lar
pre ax'i al
pre can'cer ous
pre cap'il lar''y
pre car'di ac
pre car'di al
pre car'ti lage
pre ca'va
pre cen'tral
pre chor'dal
pre cip'i tant
pre cip'i tate
pre cip''i ta'tion
pre cip'i ta''tor
pre cip'i tin
pre clin'i cal
pre co'cious
pre coc'i ty
pre cog ni'tion
pre''con vul'sant

pre''con vul'sive
pre cor'di al
pre cor'di um
pre cos'tal
pre cu'ne us
pre den'tin
pre''di crot'ic
pre''di gest'ed
pre''dis po'sing
pre''dis po si'tion
pred nis'o lone
pred'ni sone
pre''dor mi'tion
pre''ec lamp'si a
pre ep''i glot'tic
pre''e rup'tive
pre fron'tal
pre''gan gli on'ic
pre glob'u lin
preg'nan cy
preg na'no lone
preg'nant
pre hal'lux
pre''hem i pleg'ic
pre hen'sile
pre hen'sion
pre''in farc'tion al
pre''lo co mo'tion
pre'lum
pre''ma lig'nant
pre''ma ni'a cal
Pre'ma rin
pre''ma ture'
pre''max il'la
pre''med i ca'tion
pre men'stru al
pre mo'lar
pre''mo ni'tion
pre mon'i to''ry

pre"mu ni'tion
pre my'e lo blast"
pre my'e lo cyte"
pre"nar co'sis
pre na'tal
pre"ne o plas'tic
pre nid'a to"ry
pre"oc cip'i tal
prep"a ra'tion
pre"pa tel'lar
pre pol'lex
pre pon'der ance
pre po'ten cy
pre po'tent
pre"psy chot'ic
pre pu'ber al
pre"pu bes'cent
pre'puce
pre"pu cot'o my
pre pu'tial
pre"py lor'ic
pre"ra chit'ic
pre rec'tal
pre re'nal
pre"re pro duc'tive
pre ret'i nal
pre sa'cral
pres"by at'rics
pres"by card'ia
pres"by a cu'sis
pres"by der'ma
pres"by o phre'ni a
pres"by o'pi a
pres"by o sphac'e lus
pres byt'
pre"schiz o phren'ic
pre"scle ro'sis
pre scribe'
pre scrip'tion

pre"se nil'i ty
pres"en ta'tion
pre sphe'noid
pre sphyg'mic
pres'sor
pres"so re cep'tor
pres"so sen'si tive
pres'sure
pre sta'sis
pre su bic'u lum
pre sup'pu ra"tive
pre sys'to le
pre"sys tol'ic
pre"thy rog'e nous
pre"thy roid'e an
pre"trans fer'ence
pre u"re thri'tis
prev'a lence
pre"ven to'ri um
pre"ven tric"u lo'sis
pre"ver tig'i ncus
pre ves'i cal
pre'vi a
pre vil'lous
pre zo'nu lar
pre"zy ga poph'y sis
pri'a pism
pri'ma ry
Pri'mates
pri"mi grav'i da
pri mip'a ra
pri"mi par'i ty
pri mi'ti ae
prim'i tive
pri mor'di al
pri mor'di um
prin'ceps
prin'ci ple
prism

pris mat'ic
pris'moid
pris"mop tom'e ter
pris'mo sphere
pro"ag glu'ti noid
pro'al
pro am'ni on
pro at'las
pro'bang
probe
pro'bit
pro bos'cis
pro'caine
pro cal'lus
pro ce'lous
pro"ce phal'ic
pro cer'coid
pro ce'rus
pro ces"so ma'ni a
pro ces'sus
pro chei'li a
pro chei'lon
pro chon'dral
pro chor'dal
pro"cho re'sis
proc"i den'ti a
pro"con'dy lism
pro"con ver'tin
pro"cre a'tion
proc ta'gra
proc tal'gi a
proc"ta tre'si a
proc"tec ta'si a
proc"tec'to my
proc ten'cli sis
proc"teu ryn'ter
proc ti'tis
proc'to cele
proc toc'ly sis

proc to co li'tis
proc"to co"lon os'co py
proc"to col'po plas"ty
proc"to cys'to plas"ty
proc"to de'um
proc"to dyn'i a
proc tol'o gist
proc tol'o gy
proc"to pa ral'y sis
proc'to pex"y
proc"to pho'bi a
proc'to plas"ty
proc"to ple'gi a
proc"top to'si a
proc tor'rha phy
proc"tor rhe'a
proc'to scope
proc tos'co py
proc"to sig"moid ec'to my
proc"to sig"moid i'tis
proc"to sig"moid os'co py
proc'to spasm
proc tos'ta sis
proc"to ste no'sis
proc tos'to my
proc tot'o my
pro cum'bent
pro cur'sive
pro"cur va'tion
pro cu'tin
prod'ro mal
pro'drome
pro duc'tive
pro"en ceph'a lus
pro en'zyme
pro'e ryth'ro blast
pro es'tro gen
pro es'trus
Proetz's treat'ment

231

pro fes'sion al
pro"fi brin"o ly'sin
pro flu'vi um
pro fun'da
pro fun'dus
pro gen'er ate
pro gen'e sis
pro gen'i tor
prog'e ny
pro ge'ri a
pro ges'ter one
Pro ges'tin
pro glot'tid
pro gnath'ic
prog'na thism
prog nose'
prog no'sis
prog nos'ti cate
prog"nos ti'cian
pro"gon o'ma
pro grav'id
pro gres'sion
pro gres'sive
pro"i o sys"to le
pro"i o'ti a
pro jec'tion
pro la'bi um
pro lac'tin
pro'lan A or B
pro lapse'
pro lep'sis
pro leu'ko cyte
pro lif'er ate
pro lif"er a'tion
pro lif'ic
pro lig'er ous
pro lym'pho cyte
pro meg"a kar'y o cyte"
Pro'min

prom'i nence
pro mon'o cyte
prom'on to ry
pro my'e lo cyte
pro'nate
pro na'tion
pro na'tor
prone
pro neph'ros
prong
pro'no grade
pro nor'mo blast
pro nu'cle us
pro o'tic
pro"pae deu'tics
prop'a gate
pro pal'i nal
pro'pane
pro"per i to ne'al
pro'phase
pro"phy lac'tic
pro"phy lax'is
pro plas'ma cyte
pro pri'e tar"y
pro"pri o cep'tion
pro"pri o cep'tor
pro'pri us
prop tom'e ter
prop to'sis
pro pul'sion
pro'pyl
pro'pyl ene
pro"pyl thi"o u'ra cil
pro re na'ta
pro se'cre tin
pro sect'
pro sec'tor
pros"en ceph'a lon
pros"o dem'ic

pros''op ag no'si a
pros''o pal'gi a
pro sop'ic
pros''o po''a nos'chi sis
pros''o po''di ple'gi a
pros''o po dyn'i a
pros''o pop'a gus
pros''o po ple'gi a
pros''o pos'chi sis
pros'o po spasm
pros''o po thor''a cop'a gus
pros''o po to'ci a
pros'o pus va'rus
pros'tate
pros''ta tec'to my
pros'ta tism
pros''ta ti'tis
pros''ta to cys ti'tis
pros tat'o gram
pros''ta tog'ra phy
pros tat'o lith
pros''ta to li thot'o my
pros''ta tor rhe'a
pros''ta tot'o my
pros''ta to ve sic''u lec'to my
pros''ta to ve sic''u li'tis
pro ster'num
pros'the sis
pros thet'ics
pros'the tist
pros'thi on
pros''tho don'ti a
pros''tho don'tist
pro stig'mine
pros''ti tu'tion
pros'trate
pros'trat ed
pros tra'tion
pro'ta mine

pro''tan o'pi a
pro tar'gin
pro'te an
pro'te ase
pro tec'tive
pro te'ic
pro te'i form
pro' te in
pro'te in ase
pro''te in e'mi a
pro''te in o'sis
pro''te in u'ri a
pro''te ol' y sis
pro'te ose
Pro'teus
pro throm'bin
pro throm''bi ne'mi a
pro throm''bi no pe'ni a
pro throm''bo ki'nase
pro thy'mi a
pro''tis tol'o gist
pro'to blast
pro'to col
pro''to di''as tol'ic
pro''to gas'ter
pro'to gen
pro''to leu'ko cyte
pro tol'y sis
pro''to met'ro cyte
pro'ton
pro''to path'ic
pro''to pep'si a
pro'to plasm
pro''to plas'mic
pro'to plast
pro''to por phy'ri a
pro''to por phy'rin
pro''to spasm
pro''to troph'ic

pro"to tro'py
Pro"to zo'a
pro"to zo'an
pro"to zo'on
pro"to zo'o phage
pro trude'
pro tru'sion
pro tu'ber ance
pro vi'ta min
pro voc'a tive
prox'i mal
prox'i mate
prox"i mo a tax'i a
prox"i mo buc'cal
prox"i mo la'bi al
prox"i mo lin'gual
pru'i nate
pru ri'go
pru ri'tus
prus'sic ac'id
psam'mism
psam mo'ma
psam"mo sar co'ma
psam'mous
psel'lism
pseu dac"ro meg'a ly
pseu"da cu'sis
pseu"da graph'i a
pseu"dal bu"mi nu'ri a
pseu"dam ne'si a
pseu"dan ky lo'sis
pseu"dar thro'sis
pseu"den ceph'a lus
pseu"des the'si a
pseu"do a ceph'a lus
pseu"do ag glu"ti na'tion
pseu"do al bu"mi nu'ri a
pseu"do al ve'o lar
pseu"do an"a phy lac'tic

pseu"do a ne'mi a
pseu"do an gi'na
pseu"do an"gi o'ma
pseu"do an"o rex'i a
pseu"do a or'tic
pseu"do ap'o plex"y
pseu"do ap pen"di ci'tis
pseu"do ath"er o'ma
pseu"do a tro"pho der'ma
 col'li
pseu"do blep'si a
pseu"do bulb'ar
pseu"do car'ti lage
pseu'do cast
pseu'do cele
pseu"do chan'cre
pseu"do cho les"te a to'ma
pseu"do cho"li nes'ter ase
pseu"do cho re'a
pseu"do chrom"es the'si a
pseu"do chrom"hi dro'sis
pseu"do chro'mi a
pseu"do cir rho'sis
pseu"do claud i ca'tion
pseu"do col'loid
pseu"do col'o bo'ma
pseu"do cri'sis
pseu'do croup"
pseu"do cryp tor'chid ism
pseu"do cy e'sis
pseu"do cyl'in droid
pseu'do cyst"
pseu"do de men'ti a
pseu"do di"a bet'ic
pseu"do di"ver tic'u lum
pseu"do e de'ma
pseu"do en"do me tri'tis
pseu"do ep'i lep"sy
pseu"do ep"i the li om'a tous

pseu"do fluc"tu a'tion
pseu"do gan'gli on
pseu"do geu"ses the'si a
pseu"do geu'si a
pseu"do gli o'ma
pseu"do glob'u lin
pseu"do gon"or rhe'a
pseu"do hal lu"ci na'tion
pseu"do hem"i car'di us
pseu"do he"mo phil'i a
pseu"do her maph'ro dite
pseu"do her maph'ro dit ism
pseu"do hy"dro ne phro'sis
pseu"do hy"dro pho'bi a
pseu"do hy"per troph'ic
pseu"do hy per'tro phy
pseu"do hy po par"a thy'roid ism
pseu"do il'e us
pscu"do in'ti ma
pseu"do i"so chro mat'ic
pseu"do jaun'dice
pseu"do li thi'a sis
pseu"do lo'gi a fan tas'ti ca
pseu"do lys'sa
pseu"do ma lar'i a
pseu"do mam'ma
pseu"do ma'ni a
pseu"do mel"a no'sis
pseu"do mem'brane
pseu"do men"in gi'tis
pseu"do me'ninx
pseu"do men"stru a'tion
pseu"do mi"cro ceph'a lus
Pseu"do mo'nas ae"rug i no'sa
pseu"do mu'cin
pseu"do my o to'ni a
pseu"do myx o'ma
pseu"do nar'co tism

pseu"do ne'o plasm
pseu"do neu ri'tis
pseu"do neu ro'ma
pseu"do nu cle'o lus
pseu"do nys tag'mus
pseu"do oph thal"mo ple'gi a
pseu"do os"te o ma la'ci a
pseu"do pa ral'y sis
pseu"do par"a ple'gi a
pseu"do par'a site
pseu"do pa re'sis
pseu"do pho"tes the'si a
pseu"do ple'gi a
pseu"do po'di um
pseu"do pol y po'sis
pseu"do pseu"do hy"po par a
    thy'roid ism
pseu dop'si a
pseu"do pte ryg'i um
pseu"dop to'sis
pseu'do pus"
pseu"do re ac'tion
pseu"do rhon'cus
pseu"do scar"la ti'na
pseu"do scle ro'sis
pseu"do small'pox
pseu dos'mi a
pseu"do sto'ma
pseu"do strat'i fied
pseu"do ta'bes
pseu"do tet'a nus
pseu"do tho'rax
pseu"do trun'cus ar ter"i o'sus
pseu"do tu ber"cu lo'sis
pseu"do tu'mor
pseu"do ty'phoid
pseu"do vac'u oles
pseu"do ven'tri cle

pseu″do vom′it ing
pseu″do xan tho′ma
   e las′ti cum
psil o cy′bin
psi lo′sis
psit″ta co′sis
pso′as
psod′y mus
pso i′tis
pso″mo pha′gi a
pso″ri as′i form
pso ri′a sis
pso″ri at′ic
pso″roph thal′mi a
psy′cha go″gy
psy chal′gi a
psy cha′li a
psy″chas the′ni a
psy″cha tax′i a
psych au′di to″ry
psy′che
psy″che de′lic
psy′che ism
psy″chen to′ni a
psy chi′a ter
psy″chi at′ric
psy chi′a trist
psy chi′a try
psy′chic
psy′chi no′sis
psy chlamp′si a
psy″cho an″al ge′si a
psy″cho a nal′y sis
psy″cho an′a lyst
psy″cho bi ol′o gy
psy″cho co′ma
psy″cho cor′ti cal
psy″cho di″ag nos′tic
psy″cho dom′e ter

psy″cho dra′ma
psy″cho dy nam′ics
psy″cho gal″va nom′e ter
psy″cho gen′e sis
psy″cho gen′ic
psy chog′e ny
psy″cho geu′sic
psy chog′no sis
psy′cho gram
psy″cho ki ne′si a
psy″cho ki ne′sis
psy″cho lag′ny
psy′cho lep″sy
psy″cho log′ic
psy″cho log′i cal
psy chol′o gist
psy chol′o gy
psy cho′ma
psy″cho math″e mat′ics
psy″cho met′rics
psy chom′e try
psy″cho mo′tor
psy″cho neu″ro log′ic
psy″cho neu ro′sis
psy″cho neu rot′ic
psy″cho nom′ics
psy chon′o my
psy″cho no se′ma
psy″cho pa re′sis
psy′cho path
psy″cho pa thol′o gist
psy″cho pa thol′o gy
psy chop′a thy
psy″cho pho″nas the′ni a
psy″cho phys′ics
psy″cho phys″i o log′ic
psy″cho phys″i ol′o gy
psy″cho ple′gi a
psy″cho ryth′mi a

psy"chor rha'gi a
psy"cho sen'so ry
psy"cho sex'u al
psy cho'sis
psy"cho so mat'ic
psy"cho sur'ger y
psy"cho tech'nics
psy"cho ther'a py
psy chot'ic
psy chral'gi a
psy"chro es the'si a
psy"chro lu'si a
psy chrom'e ter
psy"chro pho'bi a
psy'chro phore
psy"chro ther'a py
ptar'mic
ptar'mus
ptel'e or rhine
pter'i on
pter"o yl glu tam'ic ac'id
pte ryg'i um
pter'y goid
pter"y go man dib'u lar
pter"y go max'il lar"y
pter"y go pal'a tine
pter"y go pha ryn'ge us
pter"y go spi'nous
pti lo'sis
pto'sis
pty al'a gogue
pty"a lec'ta sis
pty'a lin
pty'a lism
pty'a lo cele
pty"a lo gen'ic
pty al'o gogue
pty"a log'ra phy
pty'a lo lith

pty"a lo li thi'a sis
pty"a lor rhe'a
pty'a lose
pty"a lo'sis
pty'sis
ptys'ma
ptys'ma gogue
pu bar'che
pu'ber
pu'ber ty
pu'bes
pu bes'cence
pu bes'cent
pu"be trot'o my
pu'bic
pu"bi ot'o my
pu'bis
pu"bo cap'su lar
pu"bo cav"er no'sus
pu"bo coc cyg'e al
pu"bo coc cyg'e us
pu"bo fem'o ral
pu"bo per"i to ne al'is
pu"bo pro stat'ic
pu"bo rec tal'is
pu"bo rec tal'is
pu"bo ves'i cal
pu"bo ves i cal'is
pu"den dag'ra
pu'den da
pu den'dal
pu den'dum
pu'er i cul"'ture
pu'er il ism
pu"er i'ti a
pu er'per a
pu er'per al
pu er'per al ism
pu er'per ant

pu''er pe'ri um
Pu'lex ir'ri tans
pu'li cide
pul'lu late
pul'mo nar''y
pul mon'ic
pul'mo''tor
pulp
pul pal'gi a
pul pa'tion
pul pec'to my
pulp''i fac'tion
pulp'i form
pulp'i fy
pulp i'tis
pulp ot'o my
pulp'y
pul'sate
pul'sa tile
pul sa'tion
pul sa'tor
pulse
pul sim'e ter
pul'sion
pul'sus
pul ta'ceous
pul'ver ize
pul vi'nar
pul'vule
pum'ice
punc'tate
punc tic'u lum
punc'ti form
punc'to graph
punc'tum
punc'ta do''lo ro'sa
pun'gent
pu'pa
pu'pal

pu'pil
pu pil'la
pu'pil la ry
pu''pil lom'e ter
pu''pil lo sta tom'e ter
pur ga'tion
pur'ga tive
purge
pu'ri fied
pu'ri form
pu'rine
pu''ro hep''a ti'tis
pu''ro mu'cous
pu''ro thi'o nin
pur'pu ra
pu'ru lence
pu'ru lent
pu'ru loid
pus
pus'tu lant
pus'tu lar
pus'tule
pus'tu li form''
pus''tu lo der'ma
pus''tu lo'sis
pu ta'men
pu''tre fac'tion
pu''tre fac'tive
pu'tre fy
pu tres'cent
pu'trid
py''ar thro'sis
pyc nom'e ter
pyc''no mor'phous
pyc''no phra'si a
pyc no'sis
pyc not'ic
py ec'chy sis
py''e lec ta'si a

py″e li′tis
py″e lo cys ti′tis
py′e lo gram″
py″e log′ra phy
py″e lo li thot′my
py′e lo ne phri′tis
py′e lo plas″ty
py″e lo pli ca′tion
py″e los′co py
py″e los′to my
py″e lot′o my
py″e lo ve′nous
py em′e sis
py e′mi a
py″en ceph′a lus
py gal′gi a
pyg ma′li on ism
pyg′my
py″go a mor′phus
py″go did′y mus
py gom′e lus
py gop′a gus
py″go par″a si′tus
py″go ter″a toi′des
py′ic
pyk′nic
pyk′no cy to″sis
pyk′no lep″sy
py″lem phrax′is
py″le phle bec′ta sis
py″le phle bi′tis
py″le throm″bo phle bi′tis
py″le throm bo′sis
py″lo ral′gi a
py″lo rec′to my
py lor′ic
py lor″i ste no′sis
py″lor i′tis
py lor″o col′ic

py lor″o di′la tor
py lor″o di o′sis
py lor″o gas trec′to my
py lor″o my ot′o my
py lor′o plas″ty
py lor″op to′sis
py lor″o sche′sis
py″lor os′co py
py lor′o spasm″
py lor″o ste no′sis
py″lor os′to my
py″lor ot′o my
py lo′rus
py″o ceph′a lus
py″o che′zi a
py″o coc′cus
py″o col′po cele
py″o col′pos
py″o cy an′ic
py′o cyst″
py″o der′ma
py″o der″ma ti′tis
py″o der″ma to′sis
py og′e nes
py″o gen′e sis
py″o gen′ic
py″o he″mo tho′rax
py′oid
py″o lab″y rin thi′tis
py″o me′tra
py″o my″o si′tis
py″o ne phri′tis
py″o neph″ro li thi′a sis
py″o ne phro′sis
py″o-o va′ri um
py o pa′gus
py″o per″i car di′tis
py″o per″i car′di um
py″o per″i to ne′um

239

py"o per"i to ni'tis

py"o pha'gi a

py"oph thal'mi a

py"o phy lac'tic

py"o phy"so me'tra

py"o pneu"mo per"i car di'tis

py"o pneu"mo per"i car'di um

py"o pneu"mo per"i to ne'um

py"o pneu"mo per"i to ni'tis

py"o pneu"mo tho'rax

py"o poi e'sis

py op'ty sis

py"or rhe'a

py"o sal"pin gi'tis

py"o sal pin"go-o"o pho ri'tis

py"o sal'pinx

py o'sis

py"o sper'mi a

py"o stat'ic

py"o ther'a py

py"o tho'rax

py"o u'ra chus

py"o u re'ter

pyr'a mid

py ram"i da'lis

pyr"a mid ot'o my

py re'thrum

py ret'ic

py ret'o gen

pyr"e to ge ne'si a

pyr"e to gen'ic

pyr"e tog'ra phy

pyr"e tol'o gist

pyr"e tol'o gy

pyr"e tol'y sis

pyr"e to ther'a py

py rex"e o pho'bi a

py rex'i a

pyr he"li om'e ter

Pyr"i benz'a mine

Py rid'i um

py"ro gal'lol

py"ro gen

py"ro gen'ic

py"ro glob"u li ne'mi a

py"ro glos'si a

py"ro lag'ni a

py"ro lig'ne ous

py rol'y sis

py"ro ma'ni a

py rom'e ter

py"ro pho'bi a

py'ro punc"ture

py ro scope

py ro'sis

py"ro tox'in

py ru'vic ac'id

py u'rĭ a

Q

quack'er y

quad ran'gu lar

quad'rant

quad"ran ta no'pi a

quad'rate

quad ra'tus

quad'ri ceps

quad"ri cus'pid

quad"ri gem'i na

quad"ri gem'i nal

quad rip'a ra

quad"ri ple'gi a

quad"ri tu ber'cu lar

quad"ri va'lent

quad roon'
quad'ru plet
qua lim'e ter
qual'i ta"tive
quan tim'e ter
quan'ti ta"tive
quan'tum
quar'an tine
quar'tan
quar tip'a ra
quartz
Queckenstedt's test
Quervain's dis ease'

quin'a crine
Quincke's dis'ease
quin'i dine
qui'nine
quin'o line
qui none'
quin'sy
quin'tan
quin tip'a ra
quin'tu plet
quit'tor
quo tid'i an
quo'tient

R

ra'bi ate
rab'id
rab'ies
ra ce'mic
rac'e mose
ra"chi an"al ge'si a
ra"chi an"es the'si a
ra"chi as'mus
ra'chi cele
ra"chi cen te'sis
ra chil'y sis
ra"chi o camp'sis
ra"chi o dyn'i a
ra"chi om'e ter
ra"chi op'a thy
ra"chi o ple'gi a
ra"chi o sco"li o'sis
ra'chi o tome"
ra"chi ot'o my
ra chip'a gus
ra"chi re sis'tance
ra'chis
ra chis'chi sis

ra"chi ter'a ta
ra chit'ic
ra chi'tis
ra'chi tism
rach"i to gen'ic
ra clage'
ra dec'to my
ra'di al
ra"di a'lis
ra'di an
ra'di ant
ra"di a'tion
rad'i cal
ra dic'u lar
ra dic"u lec'to my
ra dic"u li'tis
ra dic"u lo my"e lop'a thy
ra dic"u lo neu ri'tis
ra dic"u lo neu rop'a thy
ra dic"u lop'a thy
ra"di o ac tin'i um
ra"di o ac'tive
ra"di o ac tiv'i ty

ra''di o au'to graph
ra'di obe
ra''di o bi ol'o gy
ra''di o car'pe us
ra''di o cir''cu log'ra phy
ra''di o co'balt
ra''di o cur a bil'i ty
ra''di o cys ti'tis
ra'di ode
ra''di o der''ma ti'tis
ra''di o di''ag no'sis
ra''di o don'ti a
ra''di o don'tist
ra'di o graph''
ra''di og'ra pher
ra''di og'ra phy
ra''di og'ra phy
ra''di o hu'mer al
ra''di o i'o dine
ra''di o i'so tope
ra''di o ky mog'ra phy
ra''di ol'o gist
ra''di ol'o gy
ra''di o lu'cent
ra''di o lu''mi nes'cence
ra''di o man om'e try
ra''di o mi crom'e ter
ra''di o mi met'ic
ra'di on
ra''di o ne cro'sis
ra''di o neu ri'tis
ra''di o paque'
ra''di o par'ent
ra''di o pel vim'e try
ra''di o pho to scan'ning
ra''di o prax'is
ra''di o re sist'ance
ra''di os'co py
ra''di o sen''si tiv'i ty

ra''di o ther''a peu'tic
ra''di o ther'a py
ra''di o ther'my
ra''di o tox e'mi a
ra''di o trans par'ent
ra''di o ul'nar
ra'di um
ra'di us
ra'dix
ra'don
ra'fle
rag'weed''
rale
ra'mi
ram''i fi ca'tion
ram'i fy
ra'mose
ram'u lus
ra'mus
ran'cid
ran'u la
rape
ra pha'ni a
ra'phe
rap'tus
rar''e fac'tion
rar'e fy
rash
ra'tio
ra'tion al
ra''tion al i za'tion
Rau wol'fi a
Raynaud's dis ease'
re ac'tion
re ac'ti vate
re a'gent
re'a gin
re al'gar
re''am pu ta'tion

re"at tach'ment
re bound'
re cal"ci fi ca'tion
re"ca pit"u la'tion
rec"ep tac'u lum
re cep'tive
re cep'tor
re cess'
re ces'sion
re ces'sive
re cid'i va'tion
re cid'i vism
rec"i div'i ty
Recklinghausen,
    Friedrich D. von
rec"li na'tion
re"com po si'tion
re"com pres'sion
re"con stit'u ent
re"con struc'tion
re co'ver y
rec're ment
re"cru des'cence
re cruit'ment
rec'tal
rec tal'gi a
rec"ti fi ca'tion
rec"to ab dom'i nal
rec'to cele
rec toc'ly sis
rec"to coc cyg'e al
rec"to coc cyg'e us
rec"to co li'tis
rec"to co lon'ic
rec"to cys tot'o my
rec"to fis'tu la
rec"to gen'i tal
rec"to la'bi al
rec'to pex"y

rec"to rec tos'to my
rec"to ro man'o scope
rec'to scope
rec tos'co py
rec"to sig'moid
rec"to sig"moid ec'to my
rec"to ste no'sis
rec"to u re'thral
rec"to u'ter ine
rec"to vag'i nal
rec"to vag"i no ab dom'i nal
rec"to ves'i cal
rec"to ves i ca'lis
rec'tum
rec'tus
re cum'ben cy
re cum'bent
re cu'per ate
re cu'per a"tive
re cur'rence
re cur'rent
re"cur va'tion
re dresse'ment
re duce'
re duc'tion
re du'pli ca"ted
re du"pli ca'tion
re"ed u ca'tion
re"ev o lu'tion
re"ex ci ta'tion
re fec'tion
re flect'ed
re flec'tor
re'flex
re flex"o gen'ic
re"flex om'e ter
re'flux
re fract'
re frac'ta do'si

re frac'tion
re frac'tion ist
re frac'tive
re"frac tiv'i ty
re frac tom'e ter
re frac'to ry
re frac'ture
re frig'er ant
ref'use
re gen'er ate
reg'i men
re'gion
reg'is ter
reg'is try
reg"le men ta'tion
re gres'sion
re gres'sive
reg"u la'tion
reg'u la"tive
re gur'gi tant
re gur"gi ta'tion
re"ha bil"i ta'tion
re"ha la'tion
re"in fec'tion
re"in force'ment
re"in fu'sion
re"in ner va'tion
re"in oc"u la'tion
re in"te gra'tion
re"in ver'sion
Reiter's syn'drome
re ju"ve nes'cence
re lapse'
re la'tion
re lax'
re"lax a'tion
re me'di al
rem'e dy
re"min er al i za'tion

re mis'sion
re mit'tance
re mit'tence
re'nal
ren'i form
re'nin
ren'in ism
ren'net
ren'nin
re pel'lent
re"per co la'tion
re"per cus'sion
re place'ment
re"plan ta'tion
re ple'tion
re"pli ca'tion
re po"lar i za'tion
re pos'i tor
re pous"soir'
re pres'sion
re"pro duc'tion
re pul'sion
re sect'
re sec'tion
re sec'to scope
re serve'
re sid' u al
res'i due
re sid'u um
re sil'i ence
re sil'i ent
res'in
re sist'ance
res"o lu'tion
re sol'vent
res'o nance
res'o nant
res'o na"tor
re sorb'ent

re sor′cin ol
re sorp′tion
re spir′a ble
res″pi ra′tion
res′pi ra″tor
res pi′ra tory
res″pi rom′e ter
res″pi rom′e try
re sponse′
res′ti form
res″ti tu′ti o ad in′te grum
res″ti tu′tion
res″to ra′tion
re stor′a tive
re straint′
re sul′tant
re su′pi nate
res″ur rec′tion ist
re sus″ci ta′tion
re sus′ci ta″tor
re su′ture
re tard′er
retch
re′te
re ten′tion
re tic′u la
re tic′u lar
re tic′u la″ted
re tic′u lin
re tic″u lo cyte″
re tic″u lo cy″to pe′ni a
re tic″u lo cy to′sis
re tic″u lo en″do the′li al
re tic″u lo en″do the″li o′ma
re tic″u lo en″do the″li o′sis
re tic″u lo′sis
re tic′u lum
re′ti fism
ret′i na

ret″i nac′u lum
ret′i nal
ret′i nene
ret′i ni′tis
ret″i no blas to′ma
ret″i no cho″roid i′tis
ret″i no cy to′ma
ret″i no pap″il li′tis
ret″i nop′a thy
ret″i nos′co py
re tort′
re tract′
re″trac til′i ty
re trac′tion
re trac′tor
ret″ro ac′tion
ret″ro an″ter o am ne′si a
ret″ro an′ter o grade
ret″ro bul′bar
ret″ro car′di ac
ret″ro ce′cal
ret′ro cele
ret″ro chei′li a
ret″ro col′ic
ret″ro con′dy lism
ret″ro cop″u la′tion
ret″ro de″vi a′tion
ret″ro dis place′ment
ret″ro e″so phag′e al
ret′ro flex
ret″ro flex′ion
ret″ro gas se′ri an
ret″ro gnath′ism
ret′ro grade
re trog′ra phy
ret″ro gres′sion
ret″ro jec′tion
ret″ro len′tal
ret″ro lin′gual

ret"ro mor'pho sis
ret"ro na'sal
ret"ro per"i to ne'al
ret"ro per"i to ni'tis
ret"ro pha ryn'ge al
ret"ro phar"yn gi'tis
ret"ro phar'ynx
ret"ro pla cen'tal
ret"ro pla'si a
ret'ro posed
ret"ro po si'tion
ret"ro pul'sion
ret"ro stal'sis
ret'ro tar'sal
ret"ro ton'sil lar
ret"ro tra'che al
ret"ro vac"ci na'tion
ret"ro ver"si o flex'ion
ret"ro ver'sion
ret"ro vert'ed
re trude'
re tru'sion
re"vac ci na'tion
re ver"ber a'tion
rev'er ie
re ver'sal
re ver'sion
re"vi tal i za'tion
re vive
re viv"i fi ca'tion
rev'o lute
re vul'sant
re vul'sive
Rh
rhab"do my o'ma
rhab"do my"o sar co'ma
rhab"do pho'bi a
rhab"do vi'rus
rha'cous

rhag'a des
rhag'i o crin
rhag'oid
rhan'ter
rhe"bo sce'li a
rheg'ma
rhe'o base
rhe'o car"di og'ra phy
rhe'o cord
rhe ol'o gy
rhe om'e ter
rhe'o nome
rhe'o pex"y
rhe'o phore
rhe'o scope
rhe'o stat
rhe"o ta chyg'ra phy
rhe"o tax'is
rhe'o tome
rhe'o trope
rheu mat'ic
rheu'ma tism
rheu'ma toid
rheu"ma tol'o gy
rheu"mo crin ol'o gy
rhex'is
rhic no'sis
rhi'nal
rhi nal'gi a
rhi"nan tral'gi a
rhi nel'cos
rhi"nen ceph'a lon
rhi"nen chy'sis
rhi"neu ryn'ter
rhin he"ma to'ma
rhin'i on
rhi'nism
rhi ni'tis
rhi"no an tri'tis

rhi″no by′on
rhi″no ceph′a lus
rhi″no ceph′a ly
rhi″no chei′sis
rhi″noc nes′mus
rhi″no dac′ry o lith
rhi″no dym′i a
rhi nog′e nous
rhi″no ky pho′sis
rhi″no la′li a
rhi″no lar″yn gi′tis
rhi″no lar″yn gol′o gy
rhi′no lith
rhi″no li thi′a sis
rhi nol′o gist
rhi nol′o gy
rhi″no ma nom′e ter
rhi″no mi o′sis
rhi″nom mec′to my
rhi″no my co′sis
rhi″no ne cro′sis
rhi nop′a thy
rhi″no pha ryn′ge al
rhi″no phar″yn gi′tis
rhi″no pha ryn′go lith
rhi″no pho′ni a
rhi″no phy′ma
rhi″no plas′tic
rhi′no plas″ty
rhi″no pol′yp
rhi nop′si a
rhi″nor rha′gi a
rhi nor′rha phy
rhi″nor rhe′a
rhi nos′chi sis
rhi″no scle ro′ma
rhi′no scope
rhi″no si″nus o path′i a
Rhi″no spo rid′i um

rhi″no ste no′sis
rhi′no thrix
rhi not′o my
Rhi″pi ceph′a lus
rhi″zo don′tro py
rhi′zoid
rhi′zome
rhi′zo neure
rhi″zo nych′i a
rhi zot′o my
rho″do gen′e sis
rho″do phy lax′is
rho dop′sin
rhom″ben ceph′a lon
rhom′bo coele
rhom′boid
rhom boi′de us
rhon′chus
Rhus
rhythm
rhyth′mic
rhyth′mi cal
rhyth mic′i ty
rhyt″i do plas′ty
rhyt″i do′sis
rib
ri″bo fla′vin
ri″bo nu′cle ase
ri″bo nu cle′ic
ri″bo nu″cleo pro′tein
ri′bose
rick′ets
Rick ett′si a
rick ett′si al
rick ett′si al pox
Riedel's stru′ma
ri gid′i ty
rig′or
ri′ma

ri'mose
Rinne's test
ri so'ri us
ri'sus sar don'i cus"
rob'o rant
ro'dent
ro den'ti cide
roent'gen
roent"gen i za'tion
roent'gen o gram"
roent'gen o graph"
roent"gen og'ra phy
roent"gen o ky'mo gram
roent"gen o ky mog'ra phy
roent"gen ol'o gist
roent"gen ol'o gy
roent"gen o lu'cent
roent"gen om'e try
roent"gen o paque'
roent"gen os'co py
roent"gen ther'a py
Rikitansky, Carl von
Rolando's a're a
Romberg's sign
Rorschach test
ro sa ce'a
ro sa'ce i form"
Rosenmuellar, John C.
ro se'o la
ro se'o lous
ro sette'

ros'trum
ro'ta me"ter
ro ta'tion
ro ta to'res
ru be'do
ru"be fa'cient
ru"be fac'tion
ru bel'la
ru be'o la
ru"be o'sis i'rid is
ru'ber
ru bes'cence
ru'bor
ruc ta'tion
ruc'tus
ru'di ment
ru"di men'ta ry
ru"di men'tum
ru'ga
ru gi'tus
ru'gose
ru gos'i ty
ru'men
ru"men ot'o my
ru'mi nant
ru"mi na'tion
rup'ti o
rup'ture
ru'tin
rye

S

Sabin vac'cine
Sabouraud's me'di a
sab'u lous
sac
sac'cha ride

sac"cha rim'e ter
sac'cha rin
sac"cha ro ga lac"tor rhe'a
sac"cha ro me tab'o lism
Sac"cha ro my'ces

sac'cha rose
sac''cha ro su'ri a
sac'cu lar
sac'cule
sac''cu lo coch'le ar
sac'cu lus
sa'cral
sa cral'gi a
sa''cral i za'tion
sa crec'to my
sa''cro an te'ri or
sa''cro coc cyg'e al
sa''cro coc cyg'e us
sa''cro dyn'i a
sa''cro il'i ac
sa''cro lum'bar
sa''cro pos te'ri or
sa''cro sci at'ic
sa''cro spi na'lis
sa''cro u'ter ine
sa'crum
sad'ism
sad'ist
sad''o mas'o chism
sa'fu
sag'it tál
sa'go
sag'u lum
Saint Vitus' dance
sal
sal'i cyl''ate
sal''i cyl'ic ac'id
sal'i cyl ism
sa lim'e ter
sa'line
sa li'va
sal'i vant
sal'i vary
sal''i va'tion

sal'i va''tor
sal''i vo li thi'a sis
Salk vac'cine
Sal''mo nel'la
sal''mo nel lo'sis
sal''pin gec'to my
sal''pin gem phrax'is
sal ''pin gi'tis
sal pin''go cath'e ter ism
sal pin'go cele
sal pin''go cy e'sis
sal''pin gol'y sis
sal pin''go-o''o pho rec'to my
sal pin''go-o''pho ri'tis
sal pin''go-o oph'o ro cele
sal pin''go pal'a tine
sal pin''go per''i to ni'tis
sal pin'go pex''y
sal pin''go pha ryn'ge al
sal pin''go phar''yn ge'us
sal pin'go plas''ty
sal''pin gor'rha phy
sal pin''go sal''pin gos'to my
sal pin'go scope
sal pin''go sten''o cho'ri a
sal''pin gos'to my
sal''pin got'o my
sal''pin gys''ter o cy e'sis
sal'pinx
sal ta'tion
sa lu'bri ty
Sal'var san
salve
sal'vi a
san''a to'ri um
sane
san guic'o lous
san''gui fi ca'tion
san'guine

san guin'e ous
san guin'o lent
san'guis
sa'ni es
san"i ta'ri an
san"i tar'i um
san'i tar"y
san"i ta'tion
san'i tize
san'i ty
san'to nin
Santorini's duct
sa phe'na
sa phe'nous
sa'po
sap"o na'ceous
sa pon"i fi ca'tion
sa pon'i form
sap'o nin
sap'phism
sa pre'mi a
sa pre'mic
sap"ro gen'ic
sa proph'a gous
sap'ro phyte
sap"ro zo'ic
sar'a pus
sar ci'tis
sar"co bi'ont
sar'co blast
sar'co cele
sar"co en"do the li o'ma
sar'coid o'sis
sar"co lem'ma
sar co'ma
sar co"ma to'sis
sar co'ma tous
sar'co mere
sar"co mes"o the li o'ma

sar"co my'ces
sar'co plasm
sar"co poi et'ic
Sar cop'tes
sar"co spo rid"i o'sis
sar'cous
sar"sa pa ril'la
sar to'ri us
sas'sa fras
sat'el lite
sat"el li to'sis
sa ti'e ty
sat'u ra"ted
sat'ur nism
sat"y ri'a sis
sau'cer ize
sau ri'a sis
sau'sar ism
sa'vo ry
scab
scab'bard
sca'bi es
sca"bi o pho'bi a
sca'bi ous
sca bri'ti es
sca'la
sca lene'
sca"le nec'to my
sca"le not'o my
sca le'nus
sca'ler
sca'ling
scalp
scal'pel
sca'ly
scan sor'i us
Scanzoni's ma neu'ver
sca'pha
scaph"o ceph'a ly

scaph'oid
scap'u la
scap"u lal'gi a
scap'u lar
scap"u lec'to my
scap"u lo cla vic"u la'ris
scap'u lo cos"tal
scap"u lo hu'mer al
scap'u lo pex"y
scar"a bi'a sis
scarf'skin"
scar"i fi ca'tion
scar'i fi ca"tor
scar"la ti'na
scar"la ti nel'la
scar"la ti'ni form
scar"la ti'noid
scar'let fe'ver
Scarpa's fas'ci a
scat"o lo'gi a
sca to'ma
sca toph'a gous
sca tos'co gy
scav'en ger
sche'ma
sche'mo graph
Schick test
Schilder's dis ease'
Schiötz
schis"to ceph'a lus
schis"to cor'mus
schis"to cys'tis
schis'to cyte
schis"to glos'si a
schis tom'e lus
schis tom'e ter
schis"to pro so'pi a
schis tor'rha chis
schis to'sis

Schis"to so'ma
Schis"to so'ma hae"ma to'bi um
Schis"to so'ma ja po'ni cum
Schis"to so'ma man so'ni
schis"to so mi'a sis
schis"to so'mus
schis"to ster'ni a
schis"to tho'rax
schis"to tra'che lus
schiz am'ni on
schiz ax'on
schiz"o ble pha'ri a
schiz"o gen'e sis
schiz"o gnath'ism
schi zog'o ny
schiz"o gy'ri a
schiz'oid
schiz"o ma'ni a
schiz'ont
schiz"o nych'i a
schiz"o pha'si a
schiz"o phre'ni a
schiz"o phren'ic
schiz"o so'ma
schiz"o thy'mic
schiz"o trich'i a
schiz'o type
Schrimer's dis ease'
schwan no'ma
sci age'
sci ap'o dy
sci at'ic
sci at'i ca
sci"e ro'pi a
scil'lism
scil"lo ceph'a ly
scin'ti gram
scin til'la scope
scin"til la'tion

scin'ti scan'ner
scir'rhoid
scir'rhous
scir'rhus
scis'sion
scis'sors
scis su'ra
scle''ec ta'si a
scle rec''to ir''i dec'to my
scle rec'to my
scler''e de'ma
scle re'ma
scle''ren ce pha'li a
scle ren'chy ma
scle rit'ic
scle ri'tis
scle''ro a troph'ic
scle''ro blas te'ma
scle''ro cat''a rac'ta
scle''ro cho''roid i'tis
scle''ro con''junc ti'val
scle''ro cor'ne a
scle''ro dac tyl'i a
scle''ro der'ma
scle''ro der''ma ti'tis
scle rog'e nous
scle'roid
scle''ro i ri'tis
scle''ro ker''a ti'tis
scle''ro ker''a to i ri'tis
scle ro'ma
scle''ro ma la'ci a
scle rom'e ter
scle''ro nych'i a
scle''ro nyx'is
scle''ro-o'' pho ri'tis
scle'ro plas''ty
scle rose'
scle ros'ing

scle ro'sis
scle''ro ste no'sis
scle ros'to my
scle''ro thrix
scle rot'ic
scle rot''i cec'to my
scle'ro tome
scle rot'o my
scle''ro to nyx'is
scle''ro trich'i a
scle'rous
sco'bi nate
sco lec'i form
sco'lex
sco''li o lor do'sis
sco''li o si om'e try
sco''li o'sis
sco''li o som'e ter
sco'li o tone''
scoop
sco pol'a mine
sco pom'e ter
sco pom'e try
sco''po pho'bi a
scor''a cra'ti a
scor bu'tic
scor'pi on
scot''o din'i a
scot'o gram
sco to'ma
sco to'ma graph
sco tom'e ter
sco''o pho'bi a
scours
scra'per
scrof'u la
scrof''u lo der'ma
scro tec'to my
scro'to plas''ty

scro'tum
scru''pu los'i ty
scu'ba di'ving
scur'vy
scu'tum
scyb'a lum
scy'phi form
scy ti'tis
se ba''ce o fol lic'u lar
se ba'ceous
se bas''to ma'ni a
se bip'a rous
seb'o lith
seb''or rhe'a
se'bum
sec'o dont
Se'co nal
se cre'ta
se cre'ta gogue
se crete'
se cre'tin
se cre'tion
se cre'tor
se cre'to ry
sec'tile
sec'tion
sec to'ri al
se cun''di grav'i da
sec'un dines
sec''un dip'a ra
se da'tion
sed'a tive
sed'en tar''y
sed''i ment
sed'i men ta'tion
seg'ment
seg men'tal
seg''men ta'tion
seg''re ga'tion

seg're ga''tor
Seitz fil'ter
sei'zure
se''la pho bi a
se lec'tion
se lec'tor
se le'ne
se le'nic
se le'ni um
se le'no dont
se le''no gam'i a
sel'la tur'ci ca
se man'tics
se'men
sem''i ca nal'
sem'i car''ti lag'i nous
sem''i co'ma
sem''i com'a tose
sem''i con'scious
sem''i lu'nar
sem''i lux a'tion
sem''i mem''bra no'sus
sem''i mem'bra nous
sem'i nal
sem''i na'tion
sem''i nif'er ous
sem''i no'ma
sem''i nu'ri a
sem''i pro na'tion
sem''i pto'sis
sem''i so'por
sem''i spi na'lis
sem''i su''pi na'tion
sem''i ten''di no'sus
sem''i ten'di nous
se nec'ti tude
se nes'cence
se'nile
se'nil ism

se'ni um
sen'na
se no'pi a
sen sa'tion
sense
sen'si ble
sen sim'e ter
sen"si tiv'i ty
sen"si ti za'tion
sen'si tized
sen"so mo'tor
sen"so pa ral'y sis
sen"so ri mo'tor
sen so'ri um
sen'so ry
sen'su al ism
sen'sus
sen'tient
sen'ti ment
sep'a ra"tor
sep'sis
sep'tal
sep tec'to my
sep'tic
sep"ti ce'mi a
sep"ti co phle bi'tis
sep"ti grav'i da
sep"ti me tri'tis
sep tip'a ra
sep"to mar'gi nal
sep tom'e ter
sep'to tome
sep tot'o my
sep'tu lum
sep'tum
sep'tu plet
sep'ul ture
se que'la
se'quence

se ques'ter
se"ques tra'tion
se"ques trec'to my
se ques'trum
se'ries
ser'i flux
se"ro co li'tis
se'ro cul"ture
se"ro der"ma ti'tis
se"ro der"ma to'sis
se"ro di"ag no'sis
se"ro en"ter i'tis
se"ro fi'brin ous
se"ro lem'ma
se"ro li'pase
se"ro log'ic
se rol'o gist
se rol'o gy
se rol'y sin
se ro'ma
se"ro mem'bra nous
se"ro mu'cous
se"ro per"i to ne'um
se"ro prog no'sis
se"ro pu'ru lent
se"ro re ac'tion
se"ro re sis'tance
se ro'sa
se ro"sa mu'cin
se"ro san guin'e ous
se"ro se'rous
se"ro si'tis
se"ro syn"o vi'tis
se"ro ther'a py
ser"o to'nin
se'rous
ser pig'i nous
ser ra'tion
ser ra'tus

Sertoli cells
se'rum
ses'a moid
ses"a moid i'tis
ses'sile
se'ta
se'ton
se'vum
sew'age
sex"i dig'i tal
sex'-in'ter grade"
sex'o-es thet'ic
sex ol'o gy
sex re ver'sal
sex"ti grav'i da
sex tip'a ra
sex'tu plet
sex'u al
sha'king
sheath
shed'ding
shield
Shi gel'la
shi"gel lo'sis
shiv'er
shoul'der
shunt
Shwartzman re ac'tion
si"a go nag'ra
si al'a den
si"al ad"e ni'tis
si al'a gogue
si"al a po'ri a
si al'ic
si"a li thot'o my
si"a lo ad"e nec'to my
si"a lo ad"e ni'tis
si"a lo ad"e not'o my
si"a lo a"er oph'a gy

si"a lo an gi'tis
si"a lo do chi'tis
si"a lo do'chi um
si"a lo do'cho plas"ty
si"a log'e nous
si al'o gram
si"a log'ra phy
si'a loid
si al'o lith"
si"a lo li thi'a sis
si"a lo li thot'o my
si"al'o mu"cins
si"a lor rhe'a
si"a los'che sis
si"a lo se"mei ol'o gy
si"a lo ste no'sis
si"a lo syr'inx
sib'i lant
sib'ling
sib"i la'tion
sib"i lis'mus
sib'i lus
sib'ship
sic'cant
sic cha'si a
sic'cus
sickle cell
sick le'mi a
sick'ness
sid'er ism
sid"e ro blas'tic
sid"er o dro"mo pho'bi a
sid"er o fi bro'sis
sid"er o pe'ni a
sid'er o phil
sid"er oph'i lous
sid'er o scope"
sid"er o sil"i co'sis
sid"er o'sis

sigh
sig'ma tism
sig'moid
sig'moid ec'to my
sig''moid i'tis
sig moi'do pex''y
sig moi''do proc tos'to my
sig moi''do rec tos'to my
sig moi'do scope
sig''moid os'co py
sig moi''do sig''moid os'to my
sig''moid os'to my
sig''moid ot'o my
sign
sig'na
sig nif'i cant
sig'num
sil'i ca
sil''i ca to'sis
si li'ceous
sil'i con
si''li co si''der o'sis
sil''i co'sis
sil''i co tu ber''cu lo'sis
sil'ver
sim'i an
Simmond's dis ease'
sim'ple
si'mul
sim''u la'tion
sin'a pis'co py
sin'a pism
sin'ci put
sin'ew
sin gul'tus
sin'is ter
sin'is trad
sin is tral
sin'is tra'tion

sin''is trau'ral
sin''is tro car'di al
sin''is tro cer'e bral
sin''is troc'u lar
sin''is tro gy ra'tion
sin''is tro man'u al
sin''is trop'e dal
sin''is tro'sis
sin''is tro tor'sion
sin'is trous
si''no a'tri al
si''no bron chi'tis
sin'u ous
si'nus
si''nus i'tis
si'nus oid
si''nus oi'dal
si''nus oi''dal i za'tion
si''nus ot'o my
si'phon
si'phon age
Sippy di'et
si''re no me'li a
si''ren om'e lus
si ri'a sis
site
sit'fast''
sit''i eir'gi a
si tol'o gy
si''to ma'ni a
si''to pho'bi a
si''to ther'a py
si'tus in ver'sus
skat'ole
ske lal'gi a
skel'e tal
skel''e ti za'tion
skel'e ton
Skene's gland

ske nei′tis
skene′o scope″
ski′a gram
ski ag′ra phy
ski am′e try
ski′a scope
ski as′co py
skin
skin′ny
Ski′o dan
skull
sli′cer
slough
slum′ber
small′pox″
smear
smeg′ma
smell
Smithwick's op″er a′tion
smudg′ing
smut
snap
sneeze
snore
soap
so″ci ol′o gy
so″ci o med′i cal
sock′et
so cor′di a
so′di um
sod′om ite
sod′om y
sof′ten ing
sol
so″lar i za′tion
so′lar plex′us
sole-plate
so′le us
so lid″i fi ca′tion

sol′i ped
sol′ip sism
sol′i tar″y
sol′-lu′nar
sol″u bil′i ty
sol′u ble
so′lum tym′pa ni
sol′ute
so lu′tion
sol′vate
sol va′tion
sol′vent
so′ma
so″ma tes the′si a
so mat′ic
so mat″i co vis′cer al
so′ma tist
so″ma ti za′tion
so mat′o chrome″
so″ma to did′y mus
so″ma to dym′i a
so″ma tog′e ny
so″ma tol′o gy
so″ma to mam″mo tro′pin
so′ma tome
so″ma to meg′a ly
so″ma tom′e try
so″ma top′a gus
so′ma to path′ic
so′ma to plasm″
so′ma to pleure″
so″ma to psy′chic
so″ma to splanch″no pleu′ric
so″ma to to′ni a
so″ma to top″ag no′si a
so″ma to top′ic
so″ma to trid″y mus
so″ ma to trop′ic
so″ma to tro′pin

257

so'ma to type"
so"mes the'si a
so"mes thet'ic
so"mes the"tog no'sis
so"mes the"to psy'chic
so'mite
som nam'bu lism
som nam'bu list
som'ni al
som'ni a"tive
som nic'u lous
som"ni fa'cient
som nif'er ous
som nif'ic
som nif'u gous
som nil'o quism
som nil'o quist
som nip'a thist
som nip'a thy
som"no cin"e mat'o graph
som'no lence
som"no len'ti a
som"no les'cent
som'no lism
sone
so no'gra phy
so nom'e ter
so phis"ti ca'tion
soph"o ma'ni a
so'por
sop'o rate
so"po rif'ic
sop'o rose
sor'bi tol
sor'des
sor'did
so ro"ri a'tion
souf'fle
sou'ma

sound
soy'bean
spa
space
span"i o car'di a
spar'a drap
spar ga no'sis
spar go'sis
Spa'rine
spasm
spas mod'ic
spas mol'o gy
spas"mo lyt'ic
spas"mo phe'mi a
spas"mo phil'i a
spas'mus nu'tans
spas'tic
spas tic'i ty
spa'ti um
spat'u la
spav'in
spay
spe'cial ist
spe'cial ty
spe'cies
spe cif'ic
spec"i fic'i ty
spec'ta ces
spec'ta cles
spec"tro col"or im'e ter
spec'tro gram
spec'tro graph
spec trom'e ter
spec"tro pho"te lom'e ter
spec"tro pho tom'e ter
spec"tro po"lar im'e ter
spec'tro scope
spec tros'co py
spec'trum

spec'u lum
speech
sperm
sper''ma cet'i
sperm as'ter
sper''ma ta cra'si a
sper mat'ic
sper'ma tid
sper''ma to cele''
sper''ma to ce lec'to my
sper''ma to ci'dal
sper'ma to cide''
sper''ma to cys ti'tis
sper''ma to cys tot'o my
sper''ma to cyte''
sper''ma to cy to'ma
sper''ma to gen'e sis
sper''ma to gen'ic
sper''ma to go'ni um
sper'ma toid
sper''ma tol'y sin
sper''ma tol'y sis
sper''ma top'a thy
sper'ma to phore''
sper''ma tor rhe'a
sper''ma to zo'i cide
sper''ma to zo'on
sper''ma tu'ri a
sper mec'to my
sper'mi cide
sperm'ism
sper'mo lith
sper mol'y sin
sphac''e la'tion
sphac'e lism
sphac''e lo der'ma
sphac'e lus
spha''gi as'mus
spha gi'tis

sphe'ni on
sphe''no bas'i lar
sphe''no ceph'a lus
sphe''no ceph'a ly
sphe''no eth'moid
sphe'noid
sphe''noid i'tis
sphe''noid ot'o my
sphe''no man dib'u lar
sphe''no max'il lar''y
sphe''no-oc cip'i tal
sphe''no pal'a tine
sphe''no pa ri'e tal
sphe''no pe tro'sal
sphe no'sis
sphe''no tre'si a
sphe'no tribe
sphe'no trip''sy
sphere
sphe''res the'si a
sphe''ro ceph'a lus
sphe''ro cyl'in der
sphe'ro cyte
sphe''ro cy'tic
sphe''ro cy to'sis
sphe'roid
sphe rom'e ter
spher'ule
sphinc'ter
sphinc''ter al'gi a
sphinc''ter ec'to my
sphinc''ter is'mus
sphinc''ter i'tis
sphinc''ter ol'y sis
sphinc'ter o plas''ty
sphinc''ter ot'o my
sphin''go li pi do'ses
sphin''go my'e lin
sphyg'mic

sphyg"mo bo lom'e ter
sphyg"mo chron'o graph
sphyg"mo chro nog'ra phy
sphyg mod'ic
sphyg"mo dy"na mom'e ter
sphyg'mo gram"
sphyg'mo graph"
sphyg mog'ra phy
sphyg'moid
sphyg"mo ma nom'e ter
sphyg"mo-os"cil lom'e ter
sphyg"mo pal pa'tion
sphyg'mo phone
sphyg'mo scope
sphyg mos'co py
sphyg"mo sys'to le
sphyg'mo tech"ny
sphyg"mo to'no graph
sphyg"mo to nom'e ter
sphyg'mus
spi'ca
spic'ule
spi lo'ma
spi"lo pla'ni a
spi'lus
spi'na bi'fi da
spi'nal
spi na'lis
spin'dle
spine
spi"no cel'lu lar
spi"no gal"va ni za'tion
spi'no graph"
spi"no tec'tal
spin thar'i scope
spin'ther ism
spi'ral
spi'reme
spir"il li ci'dal

spir"il lo'sis
Spi ril'lum
Spi"ro chae'ta
spi"ro chet'al
spi'ro chete
spi"ro che te'mi a
spi"ro che'ti cide
spi"ro che tol'y sis
spi"ro che to'sis
spi'ro gram"
spi'ro graph"
spi rom'e ter
spis'sa ted
spis'si tude
splanch'na
splanch"nec to'pi a
splanch"nem phrax'is
splanch"nes the'si a
splanch"neu rys'ma
splanch'nic
splanch"ni cec'to my
splanch"ni cot'o my
splanch'no cele
splanch"no di as'ta sis
splanch nog'ra phy
splanch'no lith
splanch"no li thi'a sis
splanch nol'o gy
splanch"no meg'a ly
splanch"no mi'cri a
splanch nop'a thy
splanch'no pleure
splanch"nop to'sis
splanch"no scle ro'sis
splanch nos'co py
splanch"no skel'e ton
splanch"no so mat'ic
splanch not'o my
splanch'no tribe

spleen
sple nal'gi a
sple nec'to my
splen''ec to'pi a
sple net'ic
splen'ic
splen''i co pan''cre at'ic
splen'i form
sple ni'tis
sple'ni um
sple'ni us
splen''i za'tion
sple'no cele
sple''no clei'sis
sple'no cyte
sple''no dyn'i a
sple''no hep''a to meg'a ly
sple'noid
sple nol'y sis
sple''no ma la'ci a
sple''no meg'a ly
sple nop'a thy
sple'no pex''y
sple''no pneu mo'ni a
sple''no por'tal
sple''no por''to'graph y
sple''nop to'sis
sple''no re'nal
sple nor'rha phy
sple not'o my
sple''no tox'in
splen'u lus
splice
splint
splint'age
splin'ter
splint'ing
spon''dy lal'gi a
spon''dy lar throc'a ce

spon''dy li'tis
spon''dy lo ar thri'tis
spon''dy lo di dym'i a
spon''dyl od'y mus
spon''dy lo dyn'i a
spon''dy lo lis the'sis
spon''dyl ol'y sis
spon''dyl op'a thy
spon''dy lo py o'sis
spon''dy lo'sis
spon''dy lo syn de'sis
spon''dy lot'o my
sponge
spon'gi o blast''
spon''gi o blas to'ma
spon'gi o cyte''
spon'gi oid
spon'gi o plasm
spon'gi ose
spon''gi o'sis
spon''gi o si'tis
spon'gy
spon ta'ne ous
spo rad'ic
spore
spo'ri cide
spo'ro cyte''
spo''ro gen'e sis
spo'ro phyte
spo''ro tri cho'sis
Spo''ro zo'a
spor'u late
sprain
sprue
spur'gall''
spu'tum
squa'ma
squame
squa''mo-oc cip'i tal

squa mo'sa
squa''mo sphe'noid
squa''mo tym pan'ic
squa'mous
squint
sta'bi li''zer
sta'ble
stac ca'to
stag'gers
stag na'tion
stain
stal''ag mom'e ter
sta'ling
stalk
sta'men
stam'i na
stam'mer ing
stand'ard
stand''ard i za'tion
sta''pe dec'to my
sta'pe des
sta pe'di al
sta pe''di o te not'o my
sta pe''di o ves tib'u lar
sta pe'di us
sta pe''do plas'ty
sta'pes
Staph cil'lin
staph''y lec'to my
staph''yl e de'ma
staph''y le'us
staph''yl he''ma to'ma
sta phyl'i on
staph''y li'tis
staph''y lo coc'cal
staph''y lo coc ce'mi a
staph''y lo coc'cic
Staph''y lo coc'cus
staph''y lo der''ma ti'tis

staph''y lol'y sin
staph''y lo'ma
staph''y lo phar''yn gor'rha phy
staph'y lo plas''ty
staph''y lop to'sis
staph''y lor'rha phy
staph''y los'chi sis
staph'y lo tome''
staph''y lot'o my
staph''y lo tox'in
starch
star va'tion
stas''i bas''i pho'bi a
stas''i pho'bi a
sta'sis
stat'ic
stat'ics
stat''i den sig'ra phy
stat'im
sta tis'ti cal
sta tis'tics
stat''o ki net'ic
stat'o lith
sta tom'e ter
stat'ure
sta'tus asth ma'ti cus''
sta'tus epi lep'ti cus''
sta'tus thym''i co''lym phat'i cus
sta''tu vo'lence
stau'ri on
steap'sin
stear'ate
ste ar'ic ac'id
stear''o der'mi a
ste''ar rhe'a
ste'a tin
ste''a ti'tis
ste''a to cryp to'sis
ste''a to cys to'ma

ste″a tog′e nous
ste″a tol′y sis
ste″a to′ma
ste″a to py′gi a
ste″a tor rhe′a
steg no′sis
stel′la len′tis hy″a loi′de a
stel′la len′tis i rid′i ca
stel′late
ste nag′mus
ste′ni on
sten″o car′di a
sten″o ceph′a ly
sten″o chas′mus
sten″o cho′ri a
sten″o co ri′a sis
sten″o crot′a phy
sten′o dont
sten′o mer′ic
sten′o pe′ic
ste nosed′
ste no′sis
sten″o sto′mi a
ste nos′to my
sten″o ther′mal
sten″o tho′rax
stent
sten″to roph′o nous
ste pha′ni on
step′page gait
ster″co bi′lin
ster″co bi lin′o gen
ster′co lith
ster″co ra′ceous
ster′co rar″y
ster″co ro′ma
ster′cus
ster″e o an″es the′si a
ster″e o ar throl′y sis

ster″e o cam pim′e ter
ster″e o chem′is try
ster″e o cil′i a
ster″e o en ceph′a lo tome
ster″e o en ceph″a lot′o my
ster″e og no′sis
ster′e o gram″
ster′eo o graph″
ster″e og′ra phy
ster″e o phor′o scope
ster″e op′sis
ster′e op″ter
ster″e o ra′di og′ra phy
ster″e o roent″gen og′ra phy
ster′e o scope
ster″e o stro′bo scope
ster″e o tax′i a
ster″e o tax′is
ster″e ot′ro pism
ster′e o ty″py
ster″e o vec″tor
   car′di o graph″
ster′ile
ste ril′i ty
ster″i li za′tion
ster′i lize
ster′i li″zer
ster nal′gi a
ster na′lis
ster″no chon″dro scap″u lar′is
ster″no cla vic′u lar
ster″no cla vic″u lar′is
ster″no clei″do mas′toid
ster″no dym′i a
ster nod′y mus
ster″no dyn′i a
ster″no hy′oid
ster″no hy oid′e us a zy′gos
ster″no mas′toid

ster″no-om phal″o dym′i a
ster″no per″i car′di al
ster nos′chi sis
ster″no thy′roid
ster not′o my
ster′num
ster″nu ta′tion
ster′nu ta″tor
ster′oid
ster′ol
steth ar″te ri′tis
steth″o pol′y scope
steth′o scope
steth″o scop′ic
ste thos′co py
sthe′ni a
sthen′ic
sti′fle
stig′ma
stig′ma tism
stil bam′i dine
stil bes′trol
still′birth″
stim′u lant
stim′u late
stim″u la′tion
stim′u li
stim′u lus
stip′pling
stock″i net′
sto′ma
sto mac′a ce
stom′ach
sto mach′ic
sto″ma tal′gi a
sto mat′ic
sto″ma ti′tis
sto″ma toc′a ce
sto″ma to dyn′i a

sto″ma to dy so′di a
sto″ma to gas′tric
sto″ma tol′o gy
sto″ma to ma la′ci a
sto″ma to me′ni a
sto″ma to′mi a
sto mat′o my
sto″ma to no′ma
sto″ma top′a thy
sto′ma to plas″ty
sto″ma tor rha′gi a
sto′ma to scope″
sto″ma to′sis
sto″ma tot′o my
sto men″or rha′gi a
sto″mo de′um
sto mos′chi sis
stool
stop′cock″
stra bis′mus
stra bom′e ter
stra bom′e try
strag′u lum
strait
stra mo′ni um
stran′gle
stran′gles
stran″gu la′tion
stran′gu ry
strat″i fi ca′tion
strat′i fied
stra tig′ra phy
strat′um
streph″o sym bo′li a
strep′i tus
strep″ti ce′mi a
strep″to ba cil′lus
strep″to coc′cal
strep″to coc ce′mi a

strep''to coc'ci
Strep''to coc'cus
strep''to der''ma ti'tis
strep''to dor'nase
strep''to ki'nase
strep''to ly'sin
Strep''to my'ces
strep''to my'cin
strep''to sep''ti ce'mi a
Strep'to thrix
stretch'er
stri'a
stri'ae
stri'a ted
stri a'tum
stric'ture
stri'dor
strid'u lous
strin'gent
string''halt''
strip
strob'ic
stro bi'la
strob''i la'tion
stro'bo csope
stro'ma
Stron''gy loi'des
stron'ti um
stro phan'thin
stroph''o ceph'a lus
stroph''o ceph'a ly
stroph'u lus
stru'ma
stru'mi form
stru mi'tis
strych'nine
stupe
stu''pe fa'cient
stu''pe fac'tion

stu''pe ma'ni a
stu pid'i ty
stu'por
Sturge-Weber dis ease'
stut'ter er
stut'ter ing
sty'let
sty''lo glos'sus
sty''lo hy'oid
sty''lo man dib'u lar
sty''lo mas'toid
sty''lo pha ryn'ge us
sty'lus
sty''ma to'sis
styp'tic
sub''ab dom'i nal
sub''a cro'mi al
sub''a cute'
sub al''i men ta'tion
sub an''co ne'us
sub''a or'tic
sub ap'i cal
sub''ap o neu rot'ic
sub a'que ous
sub''a rach'noid
sub''a re'o lar
sub''as trin'gent
sub au'ral
sub''au ric'u lar
sub brach''y ce phal'ic
sub''cal ca're ous
sub''cal lo'sal
sub cap'su lar
sub chon'dral
sub chron'ic
sub cla'vi an
sub cla'vi us
sub clin'i cal
sub''col lat'er al

sub″con junc ti′val
sub con′scious
sub con′scious ness
sub″con tin′u ous
sub cor′a coid
sub cor′ti cal
sub cos′tal
sub″cos tal′gi a
sub crep′i tant
sub″crep i ta′tion
sub cul′ture
sub″cu ta′ne ous
sub″cu tic′u lar
sub cu′tis
sub″de lir′i um
sub del′toid
sub den′tal
sub der′mic
sub″di a phrag mat′ic
sub″di vi′ded
sub dol″i cho ce phal′ic
sub duct′
sub du′ral
sub″e pen″dy mo′ma
sub″epi the′li al
sub fas′cial
sub ga′le al
sub gle′noid
sub″glos si′tis
sub″grun da′tion
su bic″u lum
sub″in fec′tion
sub″in vo lu′tion
sub ja′cent
sub jec′tive
sub jec′to scope
sub la′tion
sub le′thal
sub′li mate

sub″li ma′tion
sub lime′
sub lim′i nal
sub li′mis
sub lin′gual
sub″lin gui′tis
sub″lux a′tion
sub″mal le′o lar
sub″man dib′u lar
sub′ma rine
sub max″il lar i′tis
sub max′il lar″y
sub men′tal
sub mes″a ti ce phal′ic
sub″mi cro scop′ic
sub mor′phous
sub″mu co′sa
sub nor′mal
sub″nor mal′i ty
sub no″to chor′dal
sub nu′cle us
sub″nu tri′tion
sub″oc cip′i tal
sub″o per′cu lum
sub or″di na′tion
sub pap′u lar
sub par″a lyt′ic
sub″per i os′te al
sub″per i to ne′al
sub phren′ic
sub″pla cen′ta
sub″pla cen′tal
sub pu′bic
sub″sar to′ri al
sub scap′u lar
sub″scap u la′ris
sub″sen sa′tion
sub se′rous
sub sib′i lant

sub si'dence
sub sig'moid
sub sist'ence
sub spi'nous
sub'stage''
sub'stance
sub ster'nal
sub''sti tu''tion
sub'sti tu''tive
sub'strate
sub sul'to ry
sub sul'tus
sub ta'lar
sub''ten to'ri al
sub''te tan'ic
sub thal'a mus
sub thy'roid ism
sub to'tal
sub tro''chan ter'ic
sub trop'i cal
sub u'ber es
sub un'gual
sub vir'ile
sub''vo lu'tion
Su'ca ryl
suc''ce da'ne ous
suc''ce dan'eum
suc cif'er ous
suc'ci nate
suc cin'ic ac'id
suc''cin yl sul''fa thi'a zole
suc''cor rhe'a
suc'cu bus
suc'cu lent
suc cur'sal
suc'cus
suc cus'sion
suck'le
suck'ling

su'crose
suc'tion
suc to'ri al
su da'men
Su dan'
su da'tion
su''da to'ri a
su''da to'ri um
su''do mo'tor
su''do re'sis
su''dor if'er ous
su''dor if'ic
su''dor i ker''a to'sis
su''dor ip'a rous
su'et
suf'fo cate
suf''fo ca'tion
suf fu'sion
sug gest''i bil'i ty
sug gest'i ble
sug ges'tion ist
sug''gil la'tion
su'i cide
sul'cus
sul''fa di'a zine
sul'fa drugs
sul''fa guan'i dine
sul''fa mer'a zine
sul''fa meth'a zine
sul''fa mez'a thine
Sul''fa my'lon
sul''fa nil'a mide
sul''fa pyr'a zine
sul''fa pyr'i dine
sulf ars''phen a mine'
Sul''fa sux'i dine
sul'fate
Sul''fa thal'i dine
sul''fa thi'a zole

sulf"he mo glo'bin
sulf he"mo glo"bi ne'mi a
sulf"hy'dryl
sul'fide
sul'fite
sul fon'a mide
sul'fone
sul'fo nyl
sul"fo nyl u re'a
sul'fur
sul fu'ric ac'id
sul'fu rous
Sulkowitch re a'gent
sum ma'tion
su"per ab duc'tion
su"per a cid'i ty
su"per ac tiv'i ty
su"per a cute'
su"per al"i men ta'tion
su"per cer"e bel'lar
su"per cil'i um
su"per di crot'ic
su"per dis ten'tion
su"per e'go
su"per e vac"u a'tion
su"per ex"ci ta'tion
su"per ex ten'sion
su"per fe"cun da'tion
su"per fe ta'tion
su"per fi'cial
su"per im"preg na'tion
su"per in fec'tion
su pe'ri or
su pe"ri or'i ty
su"per lac ta'tion
su"per le'thal
su"per mo'ron
su"per na'tant
su"per nu'mer ar"y

su"per pig"men ta'tion
su"per sat'u rate
su"per se cre'tion
su"per sen'si tive
su"per sen"si ti za'tion
su"per son'ic
su"per spi na'tus
su"per ve nos'i ty
su"per ven'tion
su'pi nate
su"pi na'tion
su'pi na"tor
su pine'
sup"pe da'ne ous
sup"ple men'tal
sup pos'i to"ry
sup pres'sion
sup'pu rant
sup'pu ra'tion
sup'pu ra"tive
su"pra cho'roid
su"pra cla vic'u lar
su"pra con'dy lar
su"pra con'dy lism
su"pra cos ta'lis
su"pra gle'noid
su"pra glot'tic
su"pra hy'oid
su"pra lim'i nal
su"pra mas'toid
su"pra oc clu'sion
su"pra om"pha lo dym'i a
su"pra or'bit al
su"pra pa tel'lar
su"pra pu'bic
su"pra re'nal
su"pra re"nal ec'to my
su"pra ren'al in
su"pra re"nal op'a thy

su"pra scap'u lar
su"pra scle'ral
su"pra sel'lar
su"pra spi na'tus
su"pra spi'nous
su"pra ster'nal
su"pra ton'sil lar
su"pra troch'le ar
su"pra ver'gence
su"pra vi'tal
su'ra
sur"al i men ta'tion
surd'i ty
sur"ex ci ta'tion
sur'face
sur fac'tants
sur'geon
sur'ger y
sur'gi cal
sur'ro gate
sur"sum duc'tion
sur"sum ver'gence
sur"sum ver'sion
sur vi'vor ship
sus cep"ti bil'i ty
sus cep'ti ble
sus"cep tiv'i ty
sus'ci tate
sus pen'sion
sus pen'soid
sus"pen so'ri um
sus pen'so ry
sus"pi ra'tion
sus"ten tac'u lum
su"sur ra'tion
su sur'rus
su tu'ra
su'tur al
su'ture

sweat
swel'ling
sy co'ma
sy co'sis
Sydenham's cho re'a
syl lab'ic
syl'la bus
syl lep"si ol'o gy
syl lep'sis
syl vat'ic plague
sym bal'lo phone
sym"bi o'sis
sym"bi ot'ic
sym bleph'a ron
sym bleph"a ro'sis
sym bo'li a
sym"bol i za'tion
Syme's am"pu ta'tion
sy me'li a
sym met'ric
sym'me try
sym"pa ral'y sis
sym"pa thec'to my
sym path"e o neu ri'tis
sym"pa thet'ic
sym"pa thet"i co mi met'ic
sym"pa thet"i co ton'ic
sym"pa thet'o blast
sym path"i co blas to'ma
sym path"i co neu ri'tis
sym path"i cop'a thy
sym path"i co to'ni a
sym path'i co trip"sy
sym path"i co trop'ic
sym path'i cus
sym'pa thism
sym'pa thi"zer
sym path'o blast
sym path"o chro'maf fin

sym path''o go'ni a
sym path''o lyt'ic
sym path''o mi met'ic
sym'pa thy
sym pex'i on
sym phal'an gism
sym''phy o ceph'a lus
sym''phy si ec'to my
sym phys'i on
sym''phy si or'rha phy
sym phys'i o tome''
sym''phy si ot'o my
sym'phy sis
sym''phy so ske'li a
sym'plasm
sym po'di a
symp'tom
symp''to mat'ic
symp''tom a tol'o gy
symp to'sis
sym'pus
syn''ac to'sis
syn''a del'phus
syn al'gi a
syn''an as''to mo'sis
sy nan'che
syn an'the ma
syn'apse
syn ap''to lem'ma
syn''ar thro phy'sis
syn''ar thro'sis
syn can'thus
syn ceph'a lus
syn chi'li a
syn''chon dro'sis
syn''chon drot'o my
syn'chro nism
syn'chy sis
Syn cil'lin

syn'cli tism
syn'clo nus
syn'co pal
syn'co pe
syn cyt'i al
syn cyt'i um
syn dac'tyl ism
syn dac'ty lus
syn dac'ty ly
syn'de sis
syn des''med to'pi a
syn''des mi'tis
syn des''mo cho'ri al
syn des''mo di as'ta sis
syn des'mo pex''y
syn''des mor'rha phy
syn''des mo'sis
syn''des mot'o my
syn'drome
syn ech'i a
syn ech'o tome
syn''ech ot'o my
syn''en ceph'a lo cele
syn er'e sis
syn''er get'ic
syn'er gism
syn'er gy
syn''es the'si a
syn''es the''si al'gi a
syn''gen e'si o plas''ty
Syn'ka min
Syn'ka vite
syn''ki ne'si a
syn oph'rys
syn''oph thal'mi a
syn''oph thal'mus
syn or'chid ism
syn os'che os
syn os'te o phyte''

syn'os tosed
syn''os to'sis
syn o'ti a
syn o'tus
syn''o vec'to my
syn o'vi a
syn o'vi al
syn o''vi o'ma
syn o'vi um
syn''o vi'tis
syn'ta sis
syn tax'is
syn'the sis
syn thet'ic
syn to'ci non
syn ton'ic
syn'tro phus
syn''u lo'sis
syn''u lot'ic
syph''il e'mi a
syph'i lid
syph''il i on'thus
syph'i lis
syph''i lit'ic
syph'i lo derm
syph'i loid
syph''i lol'o gist

syph''i lol'o gy
syph''i lo'ma
syph''i lo ma'ni a
syph''i lo nych'i a
syph''i lop'a thy
syph'i lo phobe''
syph''i lo pho'bi a
syph''i lo phy'ma
syph''i lo ther'a py
sy rig''mo pho'ni a
sy rig'mus
syr''ing ad''e no'ma
syr''ing ad''e no'sus
syr'inge
sy rin''go bul'bi a
sy rin''go car''ci no'ma
sy rin'go cele
sy rin''go cyst'ad e no'ma
sy rin''go cys to'ma
syr''in go'ma
sy rin''go my e'li a
sy rin''go my'e lo cele''
sys so'ma
sys so'mus
sys'to le
sys tol'ic
sys trem'ma

T

tab''a co'sis
tab'a gism
Ta ban'i dae
ta bel'la
ta'bes dor sal'is
ta bet'ic
ta bet'i form
ta''bo pa ral'y sis
tab'u lar

tache
ta chet'ic
ta chis'to scope
tach'o gram
ta chog'ra phy
tach''y aux e'sis
tach''y car'di a
tach''y car'di ac
tach'y graph

271

ta chyg'ra phy
tach"y i a'tri a
tach"y lo'gi a
ta chym'e ter
tach"y pha'gi a
tach"y phy lax'i a
tach"yp ne'a
tach"y rhyth'mi a
tach"y sys'to le
tac'tile
tae'di um vi'tae
Tae'ni a
Tae'ni a sag i na'ta
Tae'ni a so'li um
tae'ni a cide"
tae'ni a fuge"
tae ni'a sis
tae'ni form
tae"ni o pho'bi a
tag'ma
taint
ta lal'gi a
talc
tal'i pes
tal"i pom'a nus
tal'low
ta"lo na vic'u lar
ta'lus
tam'bour
Tam'pax
tam'pon
tam"pon ade'
tam'pon ing
tan'nic ac'id
tan'nin
tan'ta lum
tan'trum
Tap'a zole
ta pe'tum

tape'worm
tap"i no ceph'a ly
tap"i o'ca
ta'pir oid
ta"pote"ment'
tar'ant ism
ta ran'tu la
ta ras'sis
ta rax'is
tare
tars ad"e ni'tis
tars al'gi a
tars ec'to my
tar si'tis
tar"so chei'lo plas"ty
tar"so ma la'ci a
tar"so met"a tar'sal
tar"so phy'ma
tar'so plas"ty
tar"sop to'si a
tar sor'rha phy
tar sot'o my
tar'sus
tar'tar
taste
tat too'ing
tau'rine
Taussig, Helen B.
tau"to me'ni al
tau tom'er al
tax'is
tax on'o my
tears
tech ni'cian
tech nique'
tec"to ceph'a ly
tec to'ri al
tec"to spi'nal
tec'tum

te′di ous
Teflon
teg′men
teg men′tal
teg men′tum
tei chop′si a
te′la
tel al′gi a
tel an″gi ec′ta sis
tel an″gi ec tat′ic
tel an″gi ec to′des
tel an″gi i′tis
tel an″gi o′ma
tel an′gi on
tel an″gi o′sis
tel″e car′di o gram″
tel″e car′di o phone″
tel″e cep′tor
tel″e di″as tol′ic
tel″e flu″or os′co py
tel leg′o ny
tel″e ki ne′sis
tel″e lec″tro car′di o gram″
tel″e lec″tro ther″a peu′tics
tel″en ceph′a lon
tel″e ol′o gy
tel″e op′si a
tel″e o roent′gen o gram″
te lep′a thy
tel″e ra″di og′ra phy
tel″e roent″gen og′ra phy
tel″e ster″e o roent″gen
  og′ra phy
tel″es the′si a
tel″e sys tol′ic
tel″e ther′a py
tel′o coele
tel″o den′dron
tel″og no′sis

tel″o lec′i thal
tel″o lem′ma
tel′o phase
tel″o syn ap′sis
Tem a′ril
tem′per ance
tem′per a ture
tem′po ral
tem′po ral″is su″per fi ci al′is
tem″po ri za′tion
tem″po ro man dib′u lar
tem″po ro-oc cip′i tal
tem″po ro pa ri′e tal
tem″po ro pon′tile
tem′u lence
te na′cious
te nac′i ty
te nac′u lum
ten″di ni′tis
ten′din o plas″ty
ten′di nous
ten dol′y sis
ten″do mu′cin
ten′don
ten″do vag″i ni′tis
te nec′to my
te nes′mus
ten i′o la
ten″o de′sis
ten″o dyn′i a
ten″o fi′bril
ten″o my′o plas″ty
ten″o my ot′o my
ten″o nec′to my
ten″on i′tis
ten″o nom′e ter
te non″to my′o plas″ty
te non″to my ot′o my
ten′o phyte

273

ten'o plas"ty
ten or'rha phy
ten"os to'sis
ten"o syn"o vec'to my
ten"o syn"o vi'tis
ten'o tome
te not'o my
ten"o vag"i ni'tis
ten'sile
ten"si om'e ter
ten'sion
ten'si ty
ten'sive
ten'sor
ten'sure
ten'ta tive
ten tig'i nous
ten to'ri um
ten'u ate
ten u'i ty
ten'u ous
teph"ro my"e li'tis
tep'id
ter"a mor'phous
te'ras
ter'a tism
ter"a to car"ci no'ma
ter"a tog'e ny
ter'a toid
ter"a tol'o gy
ter"a to'ma
ter"a to pho'bi a
ter"a to'sis
ter"a to zo o sper'mi a
ter"e bra che'sis
te'res
ter'mi nal
ter"mi nol'o gy
ter'na ry

ter'pin hy'drate
Ter"ra my'cin
ter'tian
ter'ti ar ism
ter'ti ar"y
ter tip'a ra
tes'ti cle
tes tic'u lar
tes'tis
tes tos'te rone
tet'a nal
te tan'i form
tet"a nig'e nous
tet"a nil'la
tet'a nism
tet"a ni za'tion
tet'a node
tet'a noid
tet"a no ly'sin
tet"a no ly'sis
tet"a nom'e ter
tet"a no mo'tor
tet"a no pho'bi a
tet"a no spas'min
tet'a nus
tet'a ny
te tar"ta no'pi a
te tar'to cone
te tar"to co'nid
tet"ra bra'chi us
tet"ra chei'rus
tet"ra cy'cline
Te'tra cyn
tet"ra dac'tyl
tet"ra eth'yl
tet"ra gen'ic
te trag'e nous
te'tral o gy of Fallot
tet"ra mas'ti a

tet″ra mas′ti gote
tet″ra ma′zi a
te tram′er ism
tet″ra nop′si a
tet″ra ploid
tet′ra pus
te tras′ce lus
tet″ra so′mic
tet″ra sti chi′a sis
tex′ti form
tex″to blas′tic
tex′ture
tha lam′ic
thal″a mo cor′ti cal
thal″a mo len tic′u lar
thal″a mo mam′mil lar″y
thal″a mo teg men′tal
thal″a mot′o my
thal′a mus
tha las se′mi a
tha las″so pho′bi a
tha las″so ther′a py
thal′li um
thal″lo tox″i co′sis
tha mu′ri a
than″a to bi″o log′ic
than″a to gno mon′ic
than″a tog′ra phy
than′a toid
than″a tol′o gy
than″a to ma′ni a
than″a to pho′bi a
than′a top sy
than′a tos
thau′ma trope
the′ca
the ci′tis
the′co dont
the co′ma

the″co steg no′sis
the′e lin
the lal′gi a
the lar′che
the las′is
the″la zi′a sis
the′le plas″ty
the li′tis
the′li um
the lon′cus
the″lo phleb″o stem′ma
the″lor rha′gi a
the′lo thism
thel″y ot′o ky
the′nar
the″o ma′ni a
the″o pho′bi a
the″o phyl′line
the″o ple′gi a
the″o ret′i cal
the′o ry
ther″a peu′tic
ther′a pist
ther′a py
ther″en ceph′a lous
The″ri di′i dae
the″ri od′ic
the″ri o′ma
the″ri o mim′ic ry
ther′mal
ther″mal ge′si a
ther″ma tol′o gy
therm″es the′si a
therm″es the″si om′e ter
ther′mic
ther′mite
ther″mo an″al ge′si a
ther″mo an″es the′si a
ther″mo cau′ter y

275

ther″mo chem′is try
ther″mo chro′ism
ther″mo co ag″u la′tion
ther′mo cou″ple
ther″mo du′ric
ther″mo dy nam′ics
ther″mo ex ci′to ry
ther″mo gen′ic
ther mog′e nous
ther″mo hy″per al ge′si a
ther″mo hy″per es the′si a
ther″mo hy″pes the′si a
ther″mo in hib′i to″ry
ther″mo la′bile
ther mol′y sis
ther mom′e ter
ther″mo met′ric
ther mom′e try
ther″mo neu ro′sis
ther moph′a gy
ther′mo phile
ther″mo phil′ic
ther″mo pho′bi a
ther′mo phore
ther′mo phyl′ic
ther′mo pile
ther″mo ple′gi a
ther″mo pol″yp ne′a
ther″mo reg″u la′tion
ther′mo scope
ther″mo sta′ble
ther′mo stat
ther″mo ste re′sis
ther″mo sys tal′tic
ther″mo tax′is
ther″mo ther′a py
ther″mo to nom′e ter
ther″mo tox′in
ther″mo tra″che ot′o my

ther mot′ro pism
the′ro morph
the″ro mor′phi a
the sau″ris mo′sis
the′sis
thi′a mine
thigh
thi″o cy′a nate
thi′o nine
thi″o phil′ic
thi″o sul′fate
thi″o u′ra cil
thi″o u re′a
tho″ra cec′to my
tho″ra cen te′sis
tho rac′ic
tho″ra co a ceph′a lus
tho″ra co a cro′mi al
tho″ra co ce los′chi sis
tho″ra co cyl lo′sis
tho″ra co cyr to′sis
tho″ra co dyn′i a
tho″ra co gas″tro did′y mus
tho″ra co gas tros′chi sis
tho″ra co lap″a rot′o my
tho″ra co lum′bar
tho″ra com′e lus
tho″ra cop′a gus
tho″ra co par″a ceph′a lus
tho′ra co plas″ty
tho″ra cos′chi sis
tho ra′co scope
tho″ra cos′co py
tho″ra cos′to my
tho″ra cot′o my
tho″ra del′phus
tho′rax
Tho′ra zine
tho′ri um

Thornton, M.L.
Tho'ro trast
thre'o nine
threp sol'o gy
thresh'oid
thrill
thrix an''nu la'ta
throm'base
throm''bas the'ni a
throm bec'to my
throm'bin
throm''bo an''gi i'tis
throm''bo ar''te ri'tis
throm'bo blast
throm boc'la sis
throm'bo cyte
throm''bo cy the'mi a
throm''bo cy'to crit
throm''bo cy''to ly'sin
throm''bo cy''to path'i a
throm''bo cy''to pe'ni a
throm''bo cy''to pe'nic
throm''bo cy to'sis
throm''bo em''bo li'sm
throm''bo em''bo li za'tion
throm''bo en''dar ter ec'to my
throm''bo en''do car di'tis
throm''bo gen'ic
throm''bo kin'ase
throm''bo lym''phan gi'tis
throm bol'y sis
throm bop'a thy
throm''bo pe'ni a
throm''bo phil'i a
throm''bo phle bi'tis
throm''bo plas'tic
throm''bo plas'tin
throm''bo plas tin'o gen
throm''bo plas''tin o pe'ni a

throm''bo poi e'sis
throm'bose
throm'bosed
throm bo'sis
throm''bo sta'sis
throm bot'ic
throm'bo zym
throm'bus
thrush
thumb
thyme
thy mec'to my
thy''mer ga'si a
thy'mic
thy'mi on
thy mi'tis
thy'mo cyte
thy''mo ke'sis
thy'mol
thy mo'ma
thy''mo no'ic
thy mop'a thy
thy'mo pex''y
thy''mo priv'ic
thy'mus
thy''re o gen'ic
thy''ro ad''e ni'tis
thy''ro ar''y te'noid
thy''ro car'di ac
thy'ro cele
thy''ro chon drot'o my
thy''ro cri cot'o my
thy''ro ep''i glot'tic
thy rog'en ous
thy''ro glob'u lin
thy''ro glos'sal
thy''ro hy'al
thy''ro hy'oid
thy'roid

thy"roid ec'to my
thy'roid ism
thy"roid i'tis
thy"roid i za'tion
thy"roid ot'o my
thy roid"o tox'in
thy"ro par"a thy"roid
  ec'to my
thy"ro phar yn ge'us
thy"ro pri'val
thy"ro pri'vus
thy"ro pro'te in
thy"rop to'sis
thy ro'sis
thy"ro ther'a py
thy rot'o my
thy"ro tox'ic
thy"ro tox"i co'sis
thy"ro tox'in
thy"ro tro'pic
thy rot'ro pin
thy rox'in
tib'i a
tib'i al
tib"i al'gi a
tib"i a'lis
tib"i o fib'u lar
tic
tic dou"lou reux'
tick'ling
tic tol'o gy
ti'groid
tim'bre
tinc'ture
tine test
tin'e a
tin ni'tus
ti"queur'
tis'sue

ti ta'ni um
ti'ter
tit"il la'tion
ti tra'tion
tit"u ba'tion
toad'head"
to coph'er ol
to'cus
tok"o dy"na mom'e ter
tok'o graph
to kog'ra phy
tok"o ma'ni a
to kom'e try
tok"o pho'bi a
tol'er ance
tol'er ant
tol'u lene
to lu'i dine
Tomes's fi'bers
to'mo gram
to"na pha'si a
tongue
tongue'tie
to nic'i ty
ton"i co clon'ic
ton"i tro pho'bi a
to"no fi'brils
to'no gram
to'no graph
to nom'e ter
to'no plasts
to nos"cil log'ra phy
to'no scope
ton'sil
ton'sil lar
ton"sil lec'tome
ton"sil lec'to my
ton"sil li'tis
ton sil'lo lith

ton sil'lo tome
ton''sil lot'o my
ton sil''lo ty'phoid
ton''sil sec'tor
ton'sure
to'nus
top''ag no'sis
to pal'gi a
to pec'to my
top''es the'si a
to pha'ceous
to'phus
top''o an''es the'si a
top''og nos'tic
to pog'ra phy
top ol'o gy
top''o nar co'sis
top''o neu ro'sis
top''o pho'bi a
top'o phone
Torek's op''er a'tion
tor'mi na
tor'mi nal
tor pes'cence
tor'pid
tor'por
torque
tor''si om'e ter
tor'sion
tor'sive
tor''si ver'sion
tor'so
tor''soc clu'sion
tor''ti col'lar
tor''ti col'lis
tor'tu ous
Tor'u la
tor''u lo'sis
tor'u lus

to'rus
to tip'o tence
tour'ni quet
tox'o phene
tox e'mi a
tox e'mic
tox'ic
tox'i cant
tox'i cide
tox ic'i ty
tox''i co den'drol
tox''i co der'ma
tox''i co der''ma ti'tis
tox''i co der''ma to'sis
tox''i co gen'ic
tox'i coid
tox''i col'o gist
tox''i col'o gy
tox''i co ma'ni a
tox''i co path'ic
tox''i co pho'bi a
tox''i co'sis
tox if'er ous
tox''i ge nic'i ty
tox ig'e nous
tox'in
tox''in fec'tion
tox in'i cide
tox''i ther'a py
tox''i tu ber'cu lide
tox'oid
tox'o phil
tox'o phore
Tox''o plas'ma
tox''o plas'min
tox''o plas mo'sis
tra bec'u la
tra'cer
tra'che a

tra"che a ec'ta sy
tra"che al'gi a
tra"che i'tis
trach"e lag'ra
trach"e lec'to my
trach"e le"ma to'ma
trach"e lis'mus
trach"e li'tis
trach"e lo cyl lo'sis
trach"e lo dyn'i a
trach"e lo ky pho'sis
tra"che lo mas'toid
trach"e lo par"a si'tus
trach"e lo pex'i a
trach"e lo plas'ty
trach"e lor'rha phy
trach"e lor rhec'tes
trach"e los'chi sis
trach"e lo syr"in gor'rha phy
trach"e lot'o my
tra"che o blen"nor rhe'a
tra"che o bron'chi al
tra"che o bron chi'tis
tra"che o bron chos'co py
tra'che o cele
tra"che o e"soph a ge'al
tra"che o fis'sure
tra"che o la ryn'ge al
tra"che o lar"yn got'o my
tra"che oph'o ny
tra'che o plas"ty
tra"che o py o'sis
tra"che or rha'gi a
tra"che or'rha phy
tra"che os'chi sis
tra"che os'co py
tra"che o ste no'sis
tra"che os'to my
tra'che o tome

tra"che ot'o mist
tra"che ot'o mize
tra"che ot'o my
tra"chi el co'sis
tra"chi el'cus
tra cho'ma
tra"chy o nych'i a
tra"chy pho'ni a
tract
trac'tion
trac tot'o my
trac'tus
tra'gi
tra'gi cus
trag"o mas chal'i a
tra'gus
trait
trance
tran'quil iz"er
trans am'i nase
trans au'di ent
trans ca'lent
trans cav'i tar"y
trans con'dy lar
trans"de am"i na'tion
trans duc'tion
tran sec'tion
trans fer'ence
trans fer'rin
trans fix'ion
trans"fo ra'tion
trans'for a"tor
trans"for ma'tion
trans form'er
trans fuse'
trans fu'sion
tran'sient
trans il'i ac
trans"il lu"mi na'tion

tran sis'tor
tran si'tion al
trans lu'cent
trans lu'cid
trans"mi gra'tion
trans mis"si bil'i ty
trans mis'sion
trans mit'tance
trans'o nance
trans par'ent
tran spi'ra ble
tran"spi ra'tion
trans'plant
trans"plan ta'tion
trans pose'
trans"po si'tion
trans sa'cral
trans"sub stan"ti a'tion
tran'su date
tran"su da'tion
trans"u re'thral
trans vag'i nal
trans"ver sa'lis
trans verse'
trans"ver sec'to my
trans ver'sus
trans ves'ti tism
tra pe'zi um
tra pe'zi us
trap'e zoid
trau'ma
trau mat'ic
trau'ma tism
trau'ma tize
trau"ma tol'o gy
trau"ma top'a thy
trau"ma top ne'a
trau"ma to'sis
trav'ail

treat
tre'a
Trem"a to'da
trem'bles
trem'o gram
trem'o graph
tre"mo la'bile
trem'o lo
tre"mo pho'bi a
trem'or
trem"o sta'ble
trem"u la'tion
trem'u lous
Trendelenburg po sit'ion
trep"a nize
tre pan'ing
tre phine'
tre phin'ing
trep'i dant
trep"i da'ti o
trep"i da'tion
Trep"o ne'ma
trep"o ne"ma to'sis
trep"o ne mi'a sis
trep"o ne"mi cid'al
trep op'ne a
tri"acet yl ole an"do my'cin
tri'ad
tri age'
tri"a kai"de ka pho'bi a
tri'an"gle
Tri at'o ma
trib'ade
tri bra'chi us
tri cel'lu lar
tri ceph'a lus
tri'ceps
trich"an gi ec ta'si a
trich"a tro'phi a

trich″es the′si a
trich i′a sis
Tri chi′na
Trich″i nel′la
trich″i no pho′bi a
trich″i no′sis
trich i′tis
tri chlo″ro a ce′tic
tri chlo″ro eth′yl ene
trich″o be′zoar
trich″o car′di a
trich″o clas ma′ni a
trich″o cryp to′sis
trich′o cyst
trich″o ep″i the″li o′ma
trich″o es the′si a
trich″o es the″si om′e ter
trich′o gen
trich″o glos′si a
trich″o hy′a lin
trich′oid
trich′o lith
trich″o lo′gi a
trich ol′o gy
trich o′ma
tri cho″ma de′sis
trich o′ma tose
trich″o ma to′sis
trich′ome
trich″o mo′na cide
trich″o mo′nad
Trich″o mo′nas
Trich″o my ce′tes
trich″o my co′sis
trich″o no′sis
trich″o path″a pho′bi a
trich op′a thy
trich oph′a gy
trich″o pho′bi a

trich″o phy′ta
trich″o phy′tid
trich″o phy′tin
trich″o phy″to be′zoar
Trich″o phy′ton
trich″o phy to′sis
trich″or rhe′a
trich″or rhex′is
trich″or rhex″o ma′ni a
trich o′sis
Trich″o spo′ron
trich″o spo ro′sis
trich″o sta′sis spin″u lo′sa
trich″o stron″gy li′a sis
Trich″o stron′gy lus
trich″o til″lo ma′ni a
tri chot′o my
trich″o zo′a
tri′chro ism
tri′chro mat
tri″chro mat′ic
tri″chro ma top′si a
tri chro′mic
trich″u ri′a sis
Trich u′ris
Trich u′ris trich′i u ra
tri′cro tism
tri cus′pid
tri dac′tyl
tri′dent
tri den′tate
tri der′mic
Tri′di one
trid′y mus
tri eth″yl a mine′
tri fa′cial
tri′fid
tri fo″li o′sis
tri″fur ca′tion

tri gas'tric
tri gas'tri cus
tri gem'i nal
tri gem'i nus
tri gem'i ny
tri gen'ic
tri'gone
tri'go nid
tri"go ni'tis
trig"o no ceph'a lus
trig"o no ceph'a ly
tri go'num
Tri lene
tri lo'bate
tri loc'u lar
tri man'u al
tri men'su al
tri mes'ter
tri"o ceph'a lus
tri"oph thal'mos
tri"o pod'y mus
tri or'chid
tri or'chis
tri'o tus
trip'a ra
tri"pha lan'gi al
tri phas'ic
tri ple'gi a
trip'let
trip"lo blas'tic
tri ploi'dy
trip"lo ko'ri a
trip lo'pi a
tri pro'so pus
trip'sis
tri que'trum
tri sac'cha ride
tris'mus
tri so'mus

tri'so my
tris"ti chi'a sis
tris"ti ma'ni a
tris'tis
trit"an o'pi a
trit'u rate
tro'car
tro chan'ter
tro'che
troch'le a
troch'le ar
troch"le a'ris
troch"o car'di a
troch"o ceph'a lus
troch"o gin'gly mus
tro'choid
Trom bic'u la
trom bic"u lo'sis
trom"o ma'ni a
tro pe'sis
tro"phe de'ma
troph'e sy
troph'ic
tro phic'i ty
troph'ism
tro'pho blast
tro'pho cyte
tro'pho derm
tro"pho dy nam'ics
tro"pho neu ro'sis
tro phop'a thy
tro"pho spon'gi um
tro"pho tax'is
tro"pho ther'a py
tro"pho trop'ic
tro phot'ro pism
tro"pho zo'ite
tro'pism
tro pom'e ter

tro′po sphere
Trousseau's sign
trun′cat ed
trun′cus
truss
tryp′a nide
Tryp″a no so′ma
try pan′o some
tryp″a no so mi′a sis
try pan′o so mide″
tryp ars′a mide
tryp′sin
tryp sin′o gen
tryp′tase
tryp′to phan
tset′se fly
tsut″su ga mush′i fe′ver
tu′bage
tu′bal
tu bec′to my
tu′ber
tu′ber cle
tu ber′cu lar
tu ber′cu la″ted
tu ber″cu la′tion
tu ber′cu lid
tu ber′cu lin
tu ber″cu lo der′ma
tu ber″cu lo fi′broid
tu ber′cu loid
tu ber″cu lo′ma
tu ber″cu lo pho′bi a
tu ber″cu lo sil″i co′sis
tu ber″cu lo′sis
tu ber′cu lous
tu ber′cu lum
tu″ber os′i tas
tu″ber os′i ty
tu′ber ous

tu″bo ab dom′i nal
tu″bo ad nex′o pex″y
tu″bo cu ra′re
tu″bo lig″a men′tous
tu″bo-o va″ri ot′o my
tu″bo per″i to ne′al
tu″bo plas′ty
tu″bo u′ter ine
tu″bo vag′i nal
tu′bu lar
tu′bule
tu″bu li za′tion
tu″bu lo al ve′o lar
tu″bu lo cyst″
tu′bu lus
tu′bus
Tu′i nal
tu″la re′mi a
tu″me fa′cient
tu″me fac′tion
tu′me fy
tu men′ti a
tu mes′cent
tu′mid
tu mid′i ty
tu′mor
tu″mor i gen′ic
tu′mor ous
tu mul′tus
Tun′ga
tun gi′a sis
tung′sten
tu′ni ca
tun′nel
tur′bid
tur″bi dim′e ter
tur′bi nate
tur′bi na″ted
tur″bi nec′to my

tur'bi no tome''
tur''bi not'o my
tur ges'cence
tur ges'cent
tur'gid
tur'gor
tur'pen tine
tur''ri ceph'a ly
tus'sal
tus'sis
tus'sive
tweez'ers
twitch'ing
tyl'i on
ty lo'ma
ty lo'sis
ty''lo ste re'sis
tym''pa nec'to my
tym pan'ic
tym'pa nism
tym''pa ni'tes
tym''pa nit'ic
tym''pa ni'tis
tym''pa no mas'toid
tym''pa no mas''toid i'tis
tym''pa no plas'ty
tym''pa no'sis
tym''pa no sta pe'di al
tym''pa no sym''pa thec'to my
tym''pa not'o my

tym'pa nous
tym'pa num
tym'pa ny
typh''lec ta'si a
typh lec'to my
typh len''ter i'tis
typh li'tis
typh''lo di''cli di'tis
typh''lo em''py e'ma
typh'loid
typh''lo lex'i a
typh''lo li thi'a sis
typh''lo meg'a ly
typh''lo pto'sis
typh lo'sis
typh'lo spasm
typh''lo ste no'sis
typh los'to my
ty''pho bac'te rin
ty'phoid
ty''pho ma'ni a
ty''pho pneu mo'ni a
ty'phus
typ'i cal
ty'po scope
tyr'an nism
ty rem'e sis
ty'roid
ty'ro sin ase
ty'ro sine

U

ud'der
u lag''a nac'te sis
u''la tro'phi a
ul'cer
ul'cer ate
ul''cer a'tion

ul'cer a''tive
ul''cer o mem'bra nous
ul'cus
u''le gy'ri a
u ler''y the'ma
u let'ic

u li′tis
ul′na
ul′nar
ul no car′pe us
u loc′a ce
u″lo der″ma ti′tis
u″lo glos si′tis
u′loid
u″lor rha′gi a
u lo′sis
u lot′ic
u lot′o my
ul″ti mo gen′i ture
ul″tra brach″y ce phal′ic
ul″tra cen′tri fuge
ul″tra fil′ter
ul″tra fil tra′tion
ul″tra mi′cro scope
ul″tra phag″o cy to′sis
ul″tra red′
ul″tra son′ic
ul″tra son′o gram
ul″tra son′o scope
ul″tra struc′ture
ul″tra vi′rus
ul″tra vi′o let
um′ber
um″bi lec′to my
um bil′i cal
um bil′i cate
um bil″i ca′tion
um bil′i cus
um′bo
un′ci form
un′ci nate
un″ci pi″si for′mis
un con′scious
unc′tion
unc′tu ous

un′cus
un dec″y len′ic ac′id
un dine′
un′du lant
un″du la′tion
un′du la to″ry
un guen′tum
un′guis
un′gu la
un′gu late
u″ni ar tic′u lar
u″ni cam′er al
u″ni cel′lu lar
u″ni cen′tral
u″ni cor′nous
u″ni cus′pid
u″ni fa mil′i al
u″ni fi′lar
u″ni grav′i da
u″ni lat′er al
u″ni lo′bar
u″ni loc′u lar
u″ni nu′cle ar
u″ni oc′u lar
u″ni o′val
u″ni ov′u lar
u nip′a ra
u″ni par′i ens
u nip′a rous
u″ni po′lar
u″ni sex′u al
u′ni tar″y
u″ni va′lent
un or′gan ized
un sat′u ra″ted
un sex′
un stri′a ted
un well′
u ra′chal

u ra′chus
u″ra cra′si a
u ra′ni um
u″ra no col″o bo′ma
u′ra no plas″ty
u′ra no ple′gi a
u″ra nor′rha phy
u″ra nos′chi sis
u″ra no staph′y lo plas″ty
u″ra no staph″y lor′rha phy
u″ra ro′ma
u′rate
u″ra tu′ri a
u re′a
u″re am′e ter
u″re am′e try
u″re de′ma
u re′mi a
u re′mic
u re″si es the′si a
u re′ter
u re″ter ec′ta sis
u re″ter ec′to my
u re″ter i′tis
u re′ter o cele
u re″ter o ce lec′to my
u re″ter o co los′to my
u re″ter o cys′tic
u re″ter o cys tos′to my
u re″ter o en ter′ic
u re″ter o en″ter os′to my
u re″ter og′ra phy
u re″ter o hem″i ne
   phrec′to my
u re″ter o hy″dro ne phro′sis
u re″ter o-in tes′ti nal
u re′ter o lith
u re″ter o li thi′a sis
u re″ter o li thot′o my

u re″ter ol′y sis
u re″ter o ne″o cys tos′to my
u re″ter o ne″o py″e los′to my
u re″ter o ne phrec′to my
u re″ter o pel′vic
u re″ter o pel′vi o plas″ty
u re′ter o plas″ty
u re″ter o py″e log′ra phy
u re″ter o py″e lo ne os′to my
u re″ter o py″e lo ne phri′tis
u re″ter o py″e lo ne
   phros′to my
u re″ter o py′e lo plas″ty
u re″ter o py″e los′to my
u re″ter or rha′gi a
u re″ter or′rha phy
u re″ter o sig″moid os′to my
u re″ter os′to my
u re″ter ot′o my
u re″ter o u re′ter al
u re″ter o u re″ter os′to my
u re″ter o u′ter ine
u re″ter o vag′i nal
u re″ter o ves′i cal
u′re thane
u re′thra
u re′thral
u″re threc′to my
u″re thri′tis
u re″thro bulb′ar
u re′thro cele
u re″thro cys ti′tis
u re′thro gram
u re′thro graph
u″re throg′ra phy
u″re throm′e ter
u re″thro phy′ma
u re′thro plas″ty
u re″thro pro stat′ic

u″re thror′rha phy
u re″thror rhe′a
u re′thro scope
u″re thros′co py
u re′thro spasm
u re″thro ste no′sis
u″re thros′to my
u re′thro tome
u″re throt′o my
u re″thro tri″go ni′tis
u re″thro vag′i nal
ur′gen cy
ur″hi dro′sis
u′ric
u′ri nal
u″ri nal′y sis
u″ri na′ry
u′ri nate
u″ri na′tion
u′rine
u″ri nif′er ous
u″ri nif′ic
u″ri nip′a rous
u″ri no cry os′co py
u″ri no gen′i tal
u″ri nog′e nous
u″ri nol′o gy
u″ri no′ma
u″ri nom′e ter
u′′ri nom′e try
u″ri no scop′ic
u′ri nose
u″ri sol′vent
u ri′tis
ur′ning
u″ro ac″i dim′e ter
u″ro bi′lin
u″ro bi″li ne′mi a
u″ro bi″lin ic′ter us

u″ro bi lin′o gen
u″ro bi″li nu′ri a
u roch′e ras
u″ro che′si a
u′ro chrome
u″ro chro′mo gen
u″ro clep′si a
u″ro cris′i a
u″ro cy an′o gen
u″ro cy″a no′sis
u″ro gen′i tal
u rog′e nous
u′ro gram
u rog′ra phy
u′ro lith
u″ro li thi′a sis
u″ro li thol′o gy
u″ro lith ot′o my
u rol′o gist
u rol′o gy
u rom′e lus
u″ro nos′co py
u rop′a thy
u″ro por′phy rin
u″ro por″phy rin′o gen
u″ror rha′gi a
u ros′che sis
u ros′co py
u″ro sep′sis
u ro tro′pin
u″ro tox′ic
ur″ti ca′ri a
ur′ti cate
ur″ti ca′tion
u″ter ine
u″ter is′mus
u″ter i′tis
u″ter o ab dom′i nal
u″ter o cer′vi cal

u″ter o col′ic
u″ter o ges ta′tion
u″ter og′ra phy
u″ter o in tes′ti nal
u″ter o ma′ni a
u″ter om′e ter
u″ter o-o va′ri an
u″ter o pa ri′e tal
u″ter o pel′vic
u″ter o pla cen′tal
u′ter o plas″ty
u″ter o rec′tal
u″ter o sa′cral
u″ter o sal″pin gog′ra phy
u′ter o scope″
u″ter o ton′ic
u″ter o trac′tor
u″ter o tu′bal
u″ter o vag′i nal

u″ter o ven′tral
u″ter o ves′i cal
u′ter us
u′tri cle
u tric″u li′tis
u tric″u lo sac′cu lar
u′ve a
u″ve i′tis
u″ve o pa rot′id
u′vi o lize″
u″vi o re sist′ant
u′vu la
u′vu lae
u″vu lec′to my
u″vu li′tis
u″vu lop to′sis
u′vu lo tome
u″vu lot′o my

V

vac′ci na ble
vac′ci nal
vac′ci nate
vac″ci na′tion
vac′cine
vac cin′i a
vac cin′i form
vac cin″i o′la
vac′ci noid
vac″ci no pho′bi a
vac′ci no style″
vac″ci no ther′a py
vac′u o lar
vac′u o late
vac′u o la″ted
vac″u o la′tion
vac′u ole

vac′u ome
vac′u um
va′gal
va gi′na
vag′i nal
vag″i nec′to my
vag″i nic′o line
vag″i nif′er ous
vag″i nis′mus
vag″i ni′tis
vag′i no cele
vag″i no dyn′i a
vag″i no fix a′tion
vag″i no my co′sis
vag′i no plas″ty
vag′i no scope
vag″i nos′co py

vag"i not'o my
va gi'tus
va got'o mized
va got'o my
va"go to'ni a
va"go trop'ic
va'gus
va'lence
val"e tu"di na'ri an ism
val'gus
val'ine
val lec'u la
Valsalva's test
valve
val vot'o my
val'vu la
val'vu lar
val"vu li'tis
val'vu lo tome
val"vu lot'o my
vam'pire
vam'pir ism
van"co my'cin
va nil'la
va"po cau"ter i za'tion
va"por i za'tion
va"ri a bil'i ty
va'ri ant
var"i ca'tion
var"i cec'to my
var"i cel'la
var"i cel la'tion
var"i cel'li form
var"i cel'loid
var'i ces
va ric'i form
var"i co bleph'a ron
var'i co cele"
var"i co ce lec'to my

var"i cog'ra phy
var'i coid
var"i co phle bi'tis
var'i cose
var"i co'sis
var"i cos'i ty
var"i cot'o my
va ric'u la
Var'i dase
va'ri form
va ri'o la
va ri'o lar
var'i o late
var"i o'li form
var'i o loid
var'ix
va'rus
vas
vas'cu lar
vas"cu lar i za'tion
vas"cu li'tis
vas def'e rans
vas ec'to my
vas"i fac'tion
vas i'tis
vas"o con stric'tion
vas"o con stric'tive
vas"o con stric'tor
vas"o de pres'sor
vas"o dil"a ta'tion
vas"o di la'tor
vas"o ep"i did"y mos'to my
vas"o for ma'tion
va"so gen'ic
va sog'ra phy
vas"o in hib'i tor
vas"o li ga'tion
vas"o mo'tion
vas"o mo'tor

vas″o neu ro′sis
vas″o-or″chid os′to my
vas″o pa ral′y sis
vas″o pa re′sis
vas″o pres′sor
va″so pres′sin
vas″o re″lax a′tion
vas or′rha phy
vas″o sec′tion
vas′o spasm
vas″o stim′u lant
vas os′to my
vas ot′o my
vas″o ton′ic
vas″o to′nin
vas″o troph′ic
vas″o va′gal
vas″o vas os′to my
vas″o ve sic″u lec′to my
vas′tus
Vater, am pul′la of
vec′tion
vec′tis
vec′tor
vec″tor car′di o gram″
vec″tor car′di o graph
ve′hi cle
vein
ve la′men
vel″a men′tum
vel′li cate
vel″li ca′tion
ve′lum
ve′na ca′va
ve na′tion
ven ec′to my
ven″e nif′er ous
ve ne′re al
ve ne″re ol′o gy

ve ne″re o pho′bi a
ven′er y
ven″e sec′tion
ven″e su′ture
ven″i punc′ture
ve noc′ly sis
ve″no con stric′tion
ve′no gram
ven og′ra phy
ven′om
ven″o mo sal′i var″y
ve″no mo′tor
ve″no per″i to ne os′to my
ve″no pres′sor
ve″no scle ro′sis
ve nos′i ty
ve″no sta′sis
ve″no throm bot′ic
ve not′o my
ve′nous
ve″no ve nos′to my
vent′er
ven′ti late
ven″ti la′tion
ven″ti lom′e ter
ven′tral
ven′tri cle
ven tric′u lar
ven tric″u li′tis
ven tric″u lo cis″ter nos′to my
ven tric″u lo cor dec′to my
ven tric′u lo gram″
ven tric″u log′ra phy
ven tric″u lo mas″toid
  os′to my
ven tric″u lom′e try
ven tric″u lo punc′ture
ven tric′u lo scope″
ven tric″u los′co py

ven tric″u los′to my
ven tric″u lo sub″a rach′noid
ven tric′u lus
ven″tri duc′tion
ven tril′o quism
ven″tri me′sal
ven″tro fix a′tion
ven″tro hys′ter o pex″y
ven″tro lat′er al
ven″tro me′di an
ven tros′co py
ven′trose
ven tros′i ty
ven″tro sus pen′sion
ven″tro ves″i co fix a′tion
ven tu′ri me″ter
ven′ule
ve ra′trum vi′ri de
ver big″er a′tion
ver′gen ces
ver″mi ci′dal
ver′mi cide
ver mic′u lar
ver mic′u late
ver mic″u la′tion
ver mic′u lose
ver′mi form
ver′mi fuge
ver″mi lin′gual
ver′min
ver″mi na′tion
ver′min ous
ver″mi pho′bi a
ver′mis
ver′nal
ver′nix ca″se o′sa
ver ru′ca
ver ru′ci form
ver′ru coid

ver′ru cose
ver′si col″or
ver′sion
ver′te bra
ver″te brar te′ri al
Ver″te bra′ta
ver′te brate
ver″te brec′to my
ver″te bro di dym′i a
ver′tex
ver′ti cal
ver′ti cil
ver tig′i nous
ver′ti go
ver″u mon″ta ni′tis
ver″u mon ta′num
ve sa′ni a
ves′i ca
ves′i cal
ves′i cant
ves″i ca′tion
ves′i ca to″ry
ves′i cle
ves″i co pro stat′ic
ves″i cot′o my
ves″i co u′ter ine
ve sic′u la
ve sic′u lar
ve sic′u lase
ve sic″u la′tion
ve sic″u lec′to my
ve sic″u li′tis
ve sic″u lo bul′lous
ve sic′u lo gram″
ve sic″u log′ra phy
ve sic″u lo pap′u lar
ve sic″u lo pus′tu lar
ve sic″u lot′o my
ves′sel

ves ti′bu lar
ves′ti bule
ves tib″u lot′o my
ves′tige
ves tig′i um
ves″ti men′tum mor′tis
ve′ta
vet″er i na′ri an
vet′er i nar″y
vi′a ble
vi′al
vi bra′tion
vi′bra to″ry
Vib′ri o
vi bris′sa
vi brom′e ter
vi car′i ous
vid″e og no′sis
vib″il am′bu lism″
vig′i lance
vil li′tis
vil″lo si′tis
vil′lous
vil′lus
vil″lus ec′to my
vin′cu lum
Vi′ne thene
vi′nyl
Vi o′form
vi″o la′tion
vi′per
vir′al
Virchow, Rudolf L.K.
vi re′mi a
vir′gin
vir′gin al
vir gin′i ty
vir′ile
vir″i les′cence

vir′i lism
vi ril′i ty
vi′ri ons
vi rip′o tent
vi rol′o gist
vi rol′o gy
vir′u lence
vir″u lif′er ous
vi′rus
vi′rus cytes″
vis′ce ra
vis′ce ral
vis″cer al′gi a
vis″cer o in hib′i to″ry
vis″cer o meg′a ly
vis″cer op to′sis
vis″cer o sen′so ry
vis′cer o tome
vis″cer ot′o my
vis″cer o to′ni a
vis″cer o troph′ic
vis′cid
vis″co li″zer
vis″co sim′e ter
vis cos′i ty
vis′cous
vis′cus
vis′i ble
vi′sion
vis″u al i za′tion
vis″u o au′di to″ry
vis″u og no′sis
vis″u om′e ter
vis″u o psy′chic
vis″u o sen′so ry
vi′sus
vi′tal
vi′tal ism
vi tal′i ty

Vi'tal ize
vi tal'li um
vi'tals
vi'ta min
vi'ta zyme"
vit'el lar"y
vi tel'li cle
vi tel'lin
vi tel"lo lu'te in
vi tel"lo mes"en ter'ic
vi tel"lo ru'bin
vi tel'us
vi"ti a'tion
vit"i lig'i nes
vit"i li'go
vi til'i goid
vit're in
vit"re o den'tin
vit're ous
vi tres'cence
vit're um
vi tri'na
vit'ri ol
vit ri'tis
vit"ro den'tin
vit"ro pres'sion
vit'rum
viv"i dif fu'sion
viv"i fi ca'tion
vi vip'a rous
viv"i sec'tion
viv"i sec'tion ist
viv'i sec"tor
vo'cal
vo ca'lis
void

vo'la
vol'a tile
vo le'mic
Volkmann's con trac'ture
Vollmer patch test
vol sel'la
volt
volt'age
volt'a gram"
vol tam'e ter
volt'am"me ter
volt'-am'pere
volt'me"ter
vol'ume
vol'u met'ric
vol'vu lus
vo'mer
vom"er o na'sal
vom'it
vom'i to"ry
vom"i tu ri'tion
vom'i tus
vo ra'cious
Vorhees
vor'tex
vor'ti cose
vox
vo"yeur'
vu"e rom'e ter
vul'can ize
vul'ner a ble
vul'ner ar"y
vul'va
vul vec'to my
vul vi'tis
vul"vo vag"i ni'tis

W

wad'ding
wad'dle
waist
wake'ful ness
Wangensteen's suc'tion
wart
Wassermann's test
wa'ter-brax"y
Waterhouse-Friderichsen
 syn'drome
watt
watt'age
watt'me"ter
Wechsler-Bellevue test
wedge
weep'ing
Weidel re ac'tion
weight
Weil's dis ease'
wen
Wenckebach's phe nom'e non
wheal

wheeze
whey
whip'lash"
whip'worm
whit'low
whoop'ing cough
Widal test
Wilms tu'mor
wind'-bro"ken
wind'gall"
wind'lass
wind'stroke"
Wintrobe meth'od
Wirsung's duct
WISC
with'ers
womb
wound
wrin'kles
wrist
wry'neck"
Wuch"er er'i a

X

xan"the las'ma
xan'thic
xan'thine
xan"thi nu'ri a
xan"tho chroi'a
xan"tho chro mat'ic
xan"tho chro ma to'sis
xan"tho chro'mi a
xan"tho chro'mic
xan thoch'ro ous
xan'tho cyte
xan"tho der'ma

xan'tho dont
xan"tho gran"u lo"ma to'sis
xan tho'ma
xan tho mat'ic
xan tho"ma to'sis
xan thom'a tous
xan'tho phane
xan'tho phore
xan thop'si a
xan thop'sin
xan thop"sy dra'ci a
xan"thor rhe'a

xan″tho sar co′ma
xan tho′sis
xen″o me′ni a
xen″o pho′bi a
xen″oph thal′mi a
xe″no plas′ty
xe ran′tic
xe″ro der′ma
xe″ro me′ni a
xe″ro myc te′ri a
xer on′o sus
xe″ro pha′gi a
xe″roph thal′mi a
xe″ro ra″di og′ra phy
xe ro′sis
xe″ro sto′mi a

xe′ro tes
xe rot′ic
xe″ro trip′sis
xiph″i ster′num
xiph″o cos′tal
xiph od′y mus
xiph″o dyn′i a
xiph′oid
xiph″oid i′tis
xi phop′a gus
X poly so′my
xy′lene
xy′len ol
xy′lol
xy′ro spasm
xys′ma
xys′ter

Y

yawn
yaws

yeast
Y-plasty
yt′tri um

Z

zar an′than
Zeller's test
Zeph′i ran chlo′ride
Ziehl-Neelsen stain
Zika vi′rus
zinc
zo′na
zon″es the′si a
zo nif′u gal
zo nip′e tal
zon′ule
zon″u li′tis
zon″u lot′o my

zo″o er as′ti a
zo og′o ny
zo′o graft
zo″o lag′ni a
zo ol′o gist
zo″o no′sis
zo″o par′a site
zo oph′a gous
zo oph′i lism
zo″o pho′bi a
zo′o plas″ty
zo op′si a
zos′ter

zos ter'i form
zy"ga poph'y sis
zyg'i on
zy"go dac'ty ly
zy go'ma
zy"go mat'ic
zy"go mat"i co fa'cial

zy"go mat"i co tem'po ral
zy"go mat'i cus
zy"go max"il la're
zy'go spore
zy'gote
zy mo'sis
zy mot'ic

SECTION III
PHONETICALLY SPELLED WORD LIST
Selected Medical Words

AS PHONETICALLY SPELLED	AS CORRECTLY SPELLED
ack'nee	acne
ack"row me gal'ic	acromegalic
ack row my'sin	Achromycin
ack'tar	Acthar
ack"ti no migh ko'sis	actinomycosis
a cue'i ty	acuity
a fan'i sis	aphanisis
a fay'je ah	aphagia
a fay'ke ah	aphakia
a fay'zhuh	aphasia
a fee'me ah	aphemia
a fo'nee uh	aphonia
a fon'ic	aphonic
a'fose	aphose
a fray'zhuh	aphrasia
af"ro diz'ee ack	aphrodisiac
af"ro diz'ee uh	aphrodisia
af'tha	aphtha
af tho'sis	aphthosis
af'thus	aphthous
ah'foze	aphose
ah koosh'munt	accouchement
ahr jirr'ee uh	argyria
ahr kay'ick	archaic
ahrs fen'uh meen	arsphenamine
air"en tur eck tay zhuh	aerenterectasia
air o'bik	aerobic
air'o fil"	aerophil
air'o form"	aeriform
air'o lin	Aerolin
air'o seel"	aerocele
air'o sol"	aerosol
a kay'shuh	acacia

AS PHONETICALLY SPELLED	AS CORRECTLY SPELLED
a kigh'lee uh	achylia
A kil'eez	Achilles
al"i fat'ick	aliphatic
al"kuh lee'mee uh	alkalemia
al"o pee'shee uh	alopecia
a men'shee uh	amentia
am fet'uh meen	amphetamine
am"fe the'a ter	amphitheater
am"fi blas'tic	amphiblastic
am"fo gel'	Amphojel
am for'ick	amphoric
am"fo sill'in	amphocillin
am"fo ter'ick	amphoteric
am'i lace	amylase
am'i loyd	amyloid
am'i tol	Amytal
a mor'fick	amorphic
a mor'fus	amorphous
an"gee or'uh fee	angiorrhaphy
ang"kil ohz'is	ankylosis
an"jee o ko lye'tis	angicholitis
an"o for'ee uh	anophoria
an"o nick'ee uh	anonychia
an"te hee"mo fil'ick	antihemophilic
an"ti fag o sit'ick	antiphagocytic
an"ti hem"o roy'dal	antihemorrhoidal
an"ti lit'ick	antilytic
an"ti pye ret'ick	antipyretic
an"ti ra kit'ick	antirachitic
an"ti spy"ro kee'tic	antispirochetic
an"ti tigh'foyd	antityphoid
an'uh fayz	anaphase
an"uh fuh lax'is	anaphylaxis
an'u rizm	aneurysm
a pof'i seal	apophyseal
a pof'i sis	apophysis

AS PHONETICALLY SPELLED	AS CORRECTLY SPELLED
ap"o mor'feen	apomorphine
ap tigh'uh liz um	aptyalism
a rack"nigh'tis	arachnitis
a rack'noyd	arachnoid
Argile Robertson	Argyll Robertson
ar"i epi"glot'ick	aryepiglottic
a reno"blast toe'muh	arrhenoblastoma
a ri"no'ma	arrhenoma
ar'i tee"noyd	arytenoid
a rith'me ah	arrhythmia
ar'kus	arcus
a sef'uh ly	acephaly
as fik'se ah	asphyxia
as fik'se ant	asphyxiate
a sigh'lum	asylum
a sigh'teez	ascites
ass"i do'sis	acidosis
ass'i nigh	acini
ass"i tab'yoo lum	acetabulum
ass'i tate	acetate
ass"i til sal i sil'ick	acetylsalicylic
ass"i tone	acetone
a'tro fe	atrophy
aus kul'tah tor"y	auscultatory
aw"toe fo'bi a	autophobia
aw"toe li'tick	autolytic
aw tol'i sis	autolysis
Ay ee'deez	Aëdes
ay jy'ree uh	agyria
ay ko"lee uh	acholia
ay sigh"uh not'ick	acyanotic
ay sim'i tree	asymmetry
ay thi"re o'sis	athyreosis
ay thy'mick	athymic
az'muh	asthma
az mat'ic	asthmatic

AS PHONETICALLY SPELLED	AS CORRECTLY SPELLED
bay′so fil	basophil
Beck′s sar′coyd	Boeck's sarcoid
bew′bon ick	bubonic
blef″a ror′ah fe	blepharorrhaphy
blef′a ron	blephoron
blef′a ro pla sty	blepharoplasty
blef″a ro plee′gee a	blepharoplegia
blef″a rop′toe sis	blepharoptosis
blef″a ro spa′zm	blepharospasm
blef″a rot′o me	blepharotomy
blen″o re′ah	blenorrhea
brang′kee ul	branchial
bray″kee al	brachial
bray″kee ce fal′ic	brachycephalic
bray″kee ot′o me	brachiotomy
bray′kee um	brachium
brong′kee ol	bronchiole
brong′kigh	bronchi
brong″ko gen′ick	bronchogenic
brong kog′gra fe	bronchography
brong″ko nu mo′ne ah	bronchopneumonia
brong″ko ploor′ul	bronchopleural
brong″ko seel′	bronchocele
brong′kus	bronchus
bron kigh′tis	bronchitis
broo ee′	bruit
brooz′	bruise
buck″o fa rin′jul	buccopharyngeal
buck′o lay′bi al	buccolabial
buy rine′ee uh	birhinia
ca kec′tic	cachectic
care″ee ol′e sis	karyolysis
care″ee o rek′sis	karyorrhexis
care′ee o type″	karyotype
care′ee o fayj″	karyophage

AS PHONETICALLY SPELLED	AS CORRECTLY SPELLED
caw'duh	cauda
cawl	caul
caw'ter ize	cauterize
Chain stokes	Cheyne stokes
clam'i do spore"	chlamydospore
cly"do mass'toyd	cleidomastoid
cly"do stur'nal	cleidosternal
co'cane	cocaine
cock'lee uh	cochlea
cock'sicks	coccyx
Coksacki vi'rus	Coxsackie
co"le cys'tic	cholecystic
co'lic	cholic
Con test	Kahn test
Coplik's spots	Koplik's spots
craw ro'sis	kraurosis
crow'mo some	chromosome
crow"mo so'mal	chromosomal
deh bree'	debris
deng'ghee	dengue
de send'enz	descendens
de sid'u ah	decidua
de sid'u us	deciduous
dess'i bel	decibel
di af"y seal'	diaphyseal
die'uh foe re'sis	diaphoresis
di fo'ne uh	diphonia
dif the're ah	diphtheria
dif'the royd	diphtheroid
dine	dyne
dis ar'thre ah	dysarthria
dis"ar thro'sis	dysarthrosis
dis'en ter"e	dysentery
dis fay'je ah	dysphagia
dis fay'zhuh	dysphasia
dis funk'shun	dysfunction

AS PHONETICALLY SPELLED	AS CORRECTLY SPELLED
dis'ki nee'ze ah	dyskinesia
dis kon''dro pla'zhuh	dyschondroplasia
dis ko'ree ah	dyscoria
dis play'zhuh	dysplasia
disp nee'ah	dyspnea
dis rith'mee uh	dysrythmia
dis toe'ne ah	dystonia
dis toe'se ah	dystocia
dis'tro fe	dystrophy
dis''uh koo'zhuh	dysacousia
dis u're ah	dysuria
doosh	douche
dur'mis	dermis
dur'moyd	dermoid
dur''muh toe'sis	dermatosis
dur''muh ti'tis	dermatitis
dye nam'ick	dynamic
dye'uh fram	diaphragm
dye''uh ree'a	diarrhea
eck''o la'le ah	echolalia
eck'zi muh	eczema
ed'i pal	oedipal
ee''lew rop'sis	aeluropsis
ee kol'o je	ecology
eh fed'rin	ephedrine
eh rith'ro cite	erythrocyte
eh rith''ro po ee' sis	erythropoiesis
eh rith''ro sigh toe'sis	erythrocytosis
ek lamp'se ah	eclampsia
ek tah'pic	ectopic
ek'to derm	ectoderm
ek tro'pe on	ectropion
E kye''no kok'us	Echinococcus
el''e fan tye'ah sis	elephantiasis
em''fi see'muh	emphysema
em''pye ee'muh	empyema

AS PHONETICALLY SPELLED	AS CORRECTLY SPELLED
en''kon dro'muh	enchondroma
en'sef a li''tic	encephalytic
en sef''ah log'rah fe	encephalography
en sef'ah lo gram	encephalogram
en sef''ah lop'ah the	encephalopathy
en''sef ah lye'tis	encephalitis
en sist'ed	encysted
en'zime	enzyme
e pif'i sis	epiphysis
e pif'o rah	epiphora
er''i thee'mah	erythema
er''i them'ah tus	erythematous
er ith'royd	erythroid
Esh''ur eek'ee uh	Escherichia
e sof'ah gus	esophagus
e sof''ah je'al	esophageal
e sof''ah jye'tis	esophagitis
es''o fo're ah	esophoria
ess''car	eschar
ess'truss	oestrus
eth'il	ethyl
eth'i leen''	ethylene
eye'kon	icon
eye'kor	ichor
eye'let	islet
eye o''do fil'e yuh	iodophilia
eye''so fo'ri a	isophoria
eye''so ko'ri a	isocoria
eye''so kro mat'ick	isochromatic
fag o sigh'toe blast	phagocytoblast
fag''o sigh toe'sis	phagocytosis
fag'o site	phagocyte
fahr'mi sist	pharmacist
fahr''muh ko pee'uh	pharmacopeia
fahr''muh sue'tick	pharmaceutic
fair'inks	pharynx

304

AS PHONETICALLY SPELLED	AS CORRECTLY SPELLED
fal'ic	phallic
fal'lus	phallus
Falow	Fallot
Fanensteel's in ci'sion	Pfannenstiel's incision
fan'tum	phantom
Fa'ren hite	Fahrenheit
fa ring'go scope	pharyngoscope
fa ring'go spaz"um	pharyngospasm
far ing jiz'mus	pharyngismus
fa rin"go nay'sal	pharyngonasal
fa ring"o pal'a teen	pharyngopalatine
far"in got'o me	pharyngotomy
far"in jeck'to me	pharyngectomy
far"in jye'tis	pharyngitis
fash'ee uh	fascia
fa sigh'tis	phacitis
fat no re'ah	phatnorrhea
fay kol'e sis	phacolysis
fay"ko muh toe'sis	phacomatosis
fay'ko scope	phacoscope
fay'ko sist	phacocyst
fay'koyd	phacoid
fay'langks	phalanx
fay lan'jeez	phalanges
fay"lan jye'tis	phalangitis
Fayling's re a'gent	Fehling's reagent
faze	phase
fee"no bahr'bi tol	phenobarbital
fee'nol	phenol
fee'no lat ed	phenolated
fee'no type	phenotype
fe nas'i ⁺in	phenacetin
fen'il kee"to nu'ri a	phenylketonuria
Figh"ko my see'teez	Phycomycetes
figh ma toe'sis	phymatosis
figh mo'sis	phimosis
figh'tase	phytase

AS PHONETICALLY SPELLED	AS CORRECTLY SPELLED
figh'tin	phytin
figh''to bee'zor	phytobezoar
fish'er	fissure
fiz''i a'tricks	physiatrics
fizz''ee o lodj'ick	physiologic
fizz''ee ol'o jee	physiology
fleb eck'to me	phlebectomy
fle'bo lith	phlebolith
fleb'o plas''te	phleboplasty
fleb os'tas sis	phlebostasis
fleb'o tome	phlebotome
Fleb ot'o mus	Phlebotomus
fleb bot'o me	phlebotomy
fle bye'tis	phlebitis
fleg ma'tick	phlegmatic
flem	phlegm
flik ten'yool	phlyctenule
flik ten'yool ur	phlyctenular
fo'bi a	phobia
fo''ko mee'li uh	phocomelia
fo nay'shun	phonation
fo net'ick	phonetic
fo'niks	phonics
fo nop'si uh	phonopsia
fos'fate	phosphate
fos for'ick	phosphoric
fo'tizm	photism
fo''to fo'bi uh	photophobia
fo tom'e ter	photometer
fo''to migh'kro graf	photomicrograph
fren''eh cot'o mee	phrenicotomy
fren'ick	phrenic
fren o kol'ick	phrenocolic
fren ol'o je	phrenology
Froid, S.	Freud, S.
Fry test	Frei test
fye'brus	fibrous

AS PHONETICALLY SPELLED	AS CORRECTLY SPELLED
Gheem'suh	Giemsa
ghil'o teen	guillotine
gin'i koyd	gynecoid
glaw ko'mah	glaucoma
gliss'ur ide	glyceride
gliss'ur il	glyceryl
gliss'ur in	glycerin
glye'ko jen	glycogen
glye"ko jen'e sis	glycogenesis
glye"ko jen'ick	glycogenic
glye kol'i sis	glycolysis
glye'ko side	glycoside
glye"ko su're ah	glycosuria
glye see'mee uh"	glycemia
glye'seen	glycine
Goan	Ghon
goo"bur nack'u lum	gubernaculum
grye po'sis	gryposis
guy"ni kol'o jee	gynecology
guy"ni kol'o jist	gynecologist
Guy so'muh	Geisoma
gwy'ack	guaiac
heem	heme
hee"mo fill'e ack	hemophiliac
hee"mo fill'ee uh	hemophilia
hee'mo lize	hemolyze
hee"mo new"mo thor'acks	hemopneumothorax
He mof'i lus	Hemophilus
he mop'ti sis	hemoptysis
hem'o ridj	hemorrhage
hem'o royd	hemorrhoid
het'er fo ne ah	heterophonia
het'er o fil	heterophil
hi'ah lin	hyalin
hi'ah loyd	hyaloid
hi'al u ron'i dase	hyaluronidase

AS PHONETICALLY SPELLED	AS CORRECTLY SPELLED
hi'brid	hybrid
hi dan'toin	hydantoin
hi dat'id	hydatid
hi'dra gog	hydragogue
hi'drate	hydrate
hi dro fil	hydrophil
hi''dro fo'bi a	hydrophobia
hi''dro noo''mo tho'racks	hydropneumothorax
hi'drops	hydrops
hi'dro seel	hydrocele
hi''dro se fal'ick	hydrocephalic
hi''dro sef'uh lus	hydrocephalus
hi'druh zeen	hydrazine
hi'fa	hypha
hi fee'mee uh	hyphemia
hi gro'mah	hygroma
hi'jeen	hygiene
hi'men	hymen
hi'oid	hyoid
hi''pah ku'ze ah	hypacusia
hip no'sis	hypnosis
hip'no tize	hypnotize
hi''per ee'mi a	hyperemia
hi''po cal ee'mee uh	hypokaliemia
hi''po far'inx	hypopharynx
hi''pof'i sis	hypophysis
hi''po fon'ia	hypophonia
hi''po for'ia	hypophoria
hi''po gly see'mee uh	hypoglycemia
hi''po klor high'dree uh	hypochlorhydria
hi''po kon'dree ack	hypochondriac
hi''po kon'dree uh	hypochondria
hi''po kon'dree um	hypochondrium
hi''po nath'us	hypognathous
hi''pur cal ee'mee uh	hyperkalemia
hi pur faj'ee uh	hyperphagia
hi''pur gly see'mee uh	hyperglycemia

AS PHONETICALLY SPELLED	AS CORRECTLY SPELLED
hi"pur kigh'lee uh	hyperchylia
hi"pur koe'lee uh	hypercholia
hi"pur o nick'ee uh	hyperonychia
hi"pur pye ee'zhuh	hyperpiesia
hi"pur pye reck'see uh	hyperpyrexia
hi"pur tri ko'sis	hypertrichosis
hi pur'tro fe	hypertrophy
hiss tear'ia	hysteria
hiss"tur ec'to me	hysterectomy
hiss"tur or'rafy	hysterorrhapy
hoop'ing cough	whooping cough
Hoosay	Houssay
ick ter'ick	icteric
ick'ter us	icterus
ick'thee o'sis	ichthyosis
ick"thee oyd	ichthyoid
ick'tul	ictal
ick'tus	ictus
il"e or'ah fe	ileorrhaphy
ill'eh um	ileum
ill'eh um	ilium (bone)
in"o kon dry'tis	inochondritis
in'sest	incest
in sigh'zor	incisor
in size'd	incised
in"tur ass'i nus	interacinous
in"tur kon'drul	interchondral
in"tur kon'du lur	intercondylar
ip'i kack	ipecac
irr"i do ko"royd i'tis	iridochoroiditis
irr"i do recks'is	iridorhexis
irr"i do sigh klye'tis	iridocyclitis
irr"i do sigh kleck'to mee	iridocyclectomy
is ku're ah	ischuria
iss kee'mee ah	ischemia
iss"kee o bul bo'sus	ischiobulbosus

AS PHONETICALLY SPELLED	AS CORRECTLY SPELLED
iss"kee o pew'bis	ischiopubis
iss"kee o reck'tul	ischiorectal
iss'kee um	ischium
iss'mus	isthmus
jawn'dis	jaundice
jin"i kol'o jee	gynecology
jin"i kol'o jist	gynecologist
jin'i koyd	gynecoid
jin'ji vah	gingiva
jin"ji vek'to me	gingivectomy
jin"ji vye'tis	gingivitis
jin'o plas"te	gynoplasty
juck"sta po zish'un	juxtaposition
jye'rus	gyrus
ka cof'o ny	cacophony
kahl'ick	colic
kahr"dee o new mat'ick	cardiopneumatic
kahr"po fa lan'je al	carpophalangeal
kah tahr'	catarrh
kah tahr'ul	catarrhal
ka keck'see uh	cachexia
ka'se us	caseous
kar"si no'mah	carcinoma
kay'licks	calyx
kay'seck	Casek
Keeahri's net'work	Chiari's network
kee'late	chelate
kee'loyd	keloid
kee'lo plas"ty	cheiloplasty
kee mo'sis	chemosis
kee"mo tak'sis	chemotaxis
kigh az'muh	chiasma
kigh fo'sis	kyphosis
kigh ligh'tis	cheilitis
kigh lo'sis	cheilosis

AS PHONETICALLY SPELLED	AS CORRECTLY SPELLED
kigh"lo tho'racks	chylothorax
kigh'mo graf	kymograph
kigh"mo trip'sin	chymotrypsin
kile	chyle
klav'i kul	clavicle
klo az'muh	chloasma
klo"ro my see'tin	Chloromycetin
kly"do mas'toyd	cleidomastoid
kly'noyd	clinoid
ko ag'yoo late	coagulate
Koksacki vi'rus	Coxsackie virus
ko led'o kus	choledochus
ko'leen	choline
Kolee's frac'ture	Colles's fracture
ko les'ter ol	cholesterol
ko"le li thigh'ah sis	cholelithiasis
kol"i sis tek'to me	cholecystectomy
kol"i sis ti'tis	cholecystitis
kol"i sis'to gram	cholecystogram
ko'lon	colon
ko los'to me	colostomy
ko los'trum	colostrum
kom'uh	coma
kom'uh toce	comatose
kon"di lo'mah	condyloma
kon"dro kos'tal	chondrocostal
kon dro'mah	chondroma
kon'droyd	chondroid
kon'drul	chondral
kon dry'tis	chondritis
koo'muh rin	coumarin
Koos mahl's res"pi ra'tion	Kussmaul's respiration
kor'duh	chorda
ko ree'i form	choreiform
ko ree'uh	chorea
kor'ne ah	cornea
ko'roid	choroid

AS PHONETICALLY SPELLED	AS CORRECTLY SPELLED
kor′pus ul	corpuscle
korr′o nerr″ee	coronary
kouch′ing	couching
krep′i tant	crepitant
kript	crypt
kro′mo fobe	chromophobe
kro′mate	chromate
krome	chrome
kron′ick	chronic
kroop	croup
kro nis′i te	chronicity
kur nick′tuh rus	kernicterus
Kweckenstedt′s sign	Queckenstedt′s sign
kwin′i deen	quinidine
kwin′zee	quinsey
kwod″ri plee′juh	quadriplegia
kwod′ri seps	quadriceps
kwor′en teen	quarantine
kwor′tan	quartan
kwye′nine	quinine
lab′i rinth	labyrinth
lack′ri mul	lacrimal
lack′tate	lactate
lack′tick	lactic
lack′tos	lactose
lar″ing go far′inks	laryngopharynx
lar″ing gol′o gy	laryngology
lar″ing go scope′	laryngoscope
lar″in jeck′to mee	laryngectomy
lar″in ji′tis	laryngitis
lar″in jiz′mus	laryngismus
lar′inks	larynx
lass′uh rate	lacerate
Layehneck′ cir rho′sis	Laennec′s cirrhosis
Leesh may′nee uh	Leishmania
leesh″mun eye′uh sis	leishmaniasis

AS PHONETICALLY SPELLED	AS CORRECTLY SPELLED
Leffler's syn'drome	Loeffler's syndrome
lew'eez	lues
lew kee'mee ah	leukemia
lew kee'moyd	leukemoid
lew"ko durma'	leukoderma
lew ko'muh	leukoma
lew"ko pee'ne ah	leukopenia
lew"ko pee'nic	leukopenic
lew"ko ree'ah	leukorrhea
lew'ko site	leukocyte
lew"ko si toe'sis	leukocytosis
lew'pus	lupus
lew'te al	luteal
limf	lymph
lim fad"eh nop'ah the	lymphadenopathy
lim fad"en ni'tis	lymphadenitis
lim fan"je o'mah	lymphangioma
lim"fan ji'tis	lymphangitis
lim foj'en us	lymphogenous
lim fo'mah	lymphoma
lim"fo sar ko'mah	lymphosarcoma
lim'fo site	lymphocyte
li'sis	lysis
lo"kee o ree'uh	lochiorrhea
lo'kee uh	lochia
lo'shee o	lotio
lo'sigh	loci
lye'kin	lichen
lye kun"if i kay'shun	lichenification
lye"o my o'ma	leiomyoma
ma lay'shee uh	malacia
Mantoo test	Mantoux test
mass'er rate"	macerate
mame	maim
meel'yoo	milieu
me nar'kee	menarche

AS PHONETICALLY SPELLED	AS CORRECTLY SPELLED
me seng'ko muh	mesenchyma
mess'eng kyme	mesenchyme
mew'koyd	mucoid
mew ko'zuh	mucosa
mew'kus	mucous
micks'oyd	myxoid
micks o'muh	myxoma
mid ri'a sis	midriasis
migh at'ro fe	myatrophy
migh cot'ick	mycotic
migh"eh ligh'tis	myelitis
migh'eh lin	myelin
migh'eh lin ayt"ed	myelinated
migh"ek'to me	myectomy
migh"e lo po ee'sis	myelopoiesis
migh'koyd	mycoid
migh kol'o je	mycology
migh ko'sis	mycosis
migh o clo'ne ah	myoclonia
migh'oyd	myoid
migh o'ma	myoma
migh o'ma tus	myomatous
migh"o meck'to me	myomectomy
migh"o me try'tis	myometritis
migh'ope	myope
migh o'pee uh	myopia
migh o'pick	myopic
migh orr'uh fee	myorrhaphy
migh"o si'tis	myositis
migh ot'o me	myotomy
migh o ton'ick	myotonic
migh se toe'ma	mycetoma
mi"ring got'to me	myringotomy
mi ring'o plast te	myringoplasty
mirr"in jy'tis	myringitis
mix'oyd	myxoid
mix o'ma	myxoma

314

AS PHONETICALLY SPELLED	AS CORRECTLY SPELLED
mon o rine'ick	monorhinic
mon o ti'ke al	monoptychial
moo'lahjh	moulage
mor fe'ah	morphea
mor'feen	morphine
mor''fo jen'eh sis	morphogenesis
mor fol'o je	morphology
mor'guh	morgue
my'krobe	microbe
naf'thuh	naphtha
naf'thu leen	naphthalene
Nah thos'to mah	Gnathostoma
nat	gnat
nath'ick	gnathic
na'tho plas''te	gnathoplasty
naw'zee uh	nausea
nayth'ee on	gnathion
nee fral'juh	nephralgia
nee frek'to me	nephrectomy
nee fro'muh	nephroma
nee fro'sis	nephrosis
nee frot'o me	nephrotomy
nee''mass thee'ne uh	mnemasthenia
nee''mo dur'me uh	mnemodermia
nee mon'icks	mnemonics
neh'frick	nephric
neh fry'tis	nephritis
new'klee ate''ed	nucleated
new'klee eye	nuclei
new klee'o lus''	nucleolus
new'klee ur	nuclear
new'kle us	nucleus
new mat'ick	pneumatic
new''mat o seal'	pneumatocele
new''mo cock'al	pneumococcal
new''mo cock see'mee uh	pneumococcemia

315

AS PHONETICALLY SPELLED	AS CORRECTLY SPELLED
new"mo cock'us	pneumococcus
new"mo en sef'a lo gram	pheumoencephalogram
new'mo graf	pneumograph
new"mo hee"mo thor'acks	pneumohemothorax
new"mo mee dee uhs tine'um	pneumomediastinum
new"mo neck'to mee	pneumonectomy
new mon'ick	pneumonic
new"mo nigh'tis	pneumonitis
new mo'ni uh	pneumonia
new"mo per"i card'i um	pneumopericardium
new"mo per'i to ne um	pneumoperitoneum
new"mo tho'racks	pneumothorax
new"muh toe'sis	pneumatosis
new rite'is	neuritis
new"ro jen'ick	neurogenic
new ro'ma	neuroma
new'ron	neuron
new ro'sis	neurosis
new'ral	neural
new'tron	neutron
nick tal'je uh	nyctalgia
nigh seer'ee uh	neisseria
nigh stag'mus	nystagmus
nimf	nymph
nim"foe may'ne ack	nymphomaniac
nos'tick	gnostic
o ee"de o migh ko'sis	oidiomycosis
Oee'de um	Oidium
off thal'mee uh	ophthalmia
off thal'mick	ophthalmic
off"thal mo din'e ah	ophthalmodynia
off"thal mol'o jist	ophthalmologist
off thal'mo scope	ophthalmoscope
off thal mos'co pe	ophthalmoscopy
o fi'as is	ophiasis
ok'u lar	ocular

AS PHONETICALLY SPELLED	AS CORRECTLY SPELLED
ok"u lo mo'tur	oculomotor
ome	ohm
om fal'ick	omphalic
om"fal i'tis	omphalitis
om"fal o mez"en ter'ick	omphalomesenteric
om"fa lot'me	omphalotomy
om fal'o seel	omphalocele
Ong"ko sur'ca	Onchocerca
o nick'ee uh"	onychia
o nik i'tis	onychitis
o nik"ko din'e ah	onychodynia
o nik o'mah	onychoma
on"i ko migh ko'sis	onychomycosis
on ik o'sis	onychosis
on ik'sis	onyxis
on kol'o gy	oncology
o"off"or or'af ee	oophorrhaphy
o"o foe reck'to me	oophorectomy
o"o foe ro hiss"tyr eck'to me	oophorohystercetomy
o"o foe ro pex se	oophoropexy
or"kee eck'to me	orchiectomy
or"kee o peck'see	orchiopexy
or kigh'tis	orchitis
o"to rea'ah	otorrhea
Oxner, Alton	Ochsner, Alton
pack"e durm'a tus	pachydermatous
pack e ji're ah	pachygyria
pack"e kro mat'ick	pachychromatic
pack"i men"in jy'tis	pachymeningitis
pack"i men'inks	pachymenix
pan"flee bi'tis	panphlebitis
pan"his tur eck'to me	panhysterectomy
par"o nick'ee uh	paranychia
pew'bur ty	puberty
pew'biz	pubis
pur'pur uh	puerpera

AS PHONETICALLY SPELLED	AS CORRECTLY SPELLED
pur'pur ul	puerperal
pick'no lep"se	pyknolepsy
Pirkay test	Pirquet test
ploo'rah	pleura
ploo'ri se	pleurisy
ploo"ro din'ee yuh	pleurodynia
pro"fi lack'tick	prophylactic
pro'fayz	prophase
pro"fi lacks'is	prophylaxis
rab"do migh o'muh	rhabdomyoma
rab"do migh"o sar co'muh	rhabdomyosarcoma
raf a'ne ah	raphania
rag'uh deez	rhagades
ra kit'ick	rachitic
ray'fee	raphe
ra"kee o din'ee ah	rachiodynia
ra"kee op'a the	rachiopathy
ra"kee o ple'je ah	rachioplegia
ray'cus	rhacous
ray'ki om'e ter	rachiometer
ray'ki o tome"	rachiotome
ray"ki ot'o me	rachiotomy
ray'kis	rachis
Re'delz stru'ma	Riedel's struma
ree'o base	rheobase
ree"o card"i og'ra fe	rheocardiography
ree'o cord	rheochord
ree ol'o ge	rheology
ree om'e ter	rheometer
ree'o stat	rheostat
ree"o tack'sis	rheotaxes
ree'o tome	rheotome
ree'o trope	rheotrope
reg'mah	rhegma
rent'ghin	roentgen
rent"ghin og'ra fe	roentgenography

AS PHONETICALLY SPELLED	AS CORRECTLY SPELLED
rent'ghin o gram"	roentgenogram
rent'ghin ol'o je	roentgenology
rent"ghin ol'o jist	roentgenologist
reo'stat	rheostat
rew ma tal'je ah	rheumatalgia
rew ma'tick	rheumatic
rew'ma tizm	rheumatism
rew'ma toyd	rheumatoid
rex'is	rhexis
righ'neck	wryneck
righ nigh'tis	rhinitis
Ri'terz syn'drome	Reiter's syndrome
ri'thum	rhythm
rit"i doe plas'te	rhytidoplasty
rit i doe'sis	rhytidosis
ro dop'sin	rhodopsin
rom'boyd	rhomboid
rong'cus	rhonchus
Roos	Rhus
rowl	rale
rye'nal	rhinal
rye nal'jee ah	rhinalgia
rye"no an try'tis	rhinoantritis
rye"no figh'muh	rhinophyma
rye"no foe'ne ah	rhinophonia
rye'no lith	rhinolith
rye nol'o jist	rhinologist
rye"no plas'te	rhinoplasty
rye nop'uth ee	rhinopathy
rye"nor ray'je ah	rhinorrhagia
rye no ree'uh	rhinorrhea
rye nor'uh fee	rhinorrhaphy
rye'ne scope	rhinoscope
rye"no sef'a le	rhinocephaly
rye"no sef'a lus	rhinocephalus
Rye"no spor rid'i um	Rhinosporidium
rye not'o me	rhinotomy

AS PHONETICALLY SPELLED	AS CORRECTLY SPELLED
rye′zome	rhizome
rye zot′o me	rhizotomy
sack′uh rin	saccharin
sac′uh ryde	saccharide
sack′yoo lar	saccular
saf′eh nus	saphenous
sam o′muh	psammoma
see′kum	cecum
see′lee ack	celiac
sef′ah lad	cephalad
se fal′gic	cephalgic
sef′al hee″muh toe′muh	cephalhematoma
sef′al in	cephalin
se fal′ick	cephalic
sef″a lo′ma	cephaloma
sel	cell
sel″u li′tis	cellulitis
ser″e bel′ar	cerebellar
ser″e bel′lum	cerebellum
ser′e bral	cerebral
se roo′men	cerumen
ser′vicks	cervix
ser″vi sy′tis	cervicitis
sfee′ne on	sphenion
sfee″no eth′moyd	sphenoethmoid
sfee″no max′i lar ee	sphenomaxillary
sfee″no pal′uh teen	sphenopalatine
sfee″ne pe tro′sal	sphenopetrosal
sfee″no tree′ze ah	sphenotresia
sfee no′tribe	sphenotribe
sfee′noyd	sphenoid
sfee″noyd i′tis	sphenoiditis
sfeer′o site	spherocyte
sfeer′oyd	spheroid
sfeer′ule	spherule
sfig mo′graf	sphygmograph

AS PHONETICALLY SPELLED	AS CORRECTLY SPELLED
sfig'moyd	sphygmoid
sfig''mo ma nom'e ter	sphygmomanometer
sfing'go my'eh lin	sphyngomyelin
sfink''ter al'je ah	sphincteralgia
sfink''ter i'tis	sphincteritis
sfink''ter ot'o me	sphincterotomy
sfink'tur	sphincter
shang'ker	chancre
Shick test	Schick test
Shil'derz dis ease'	Schilder's disease
shis''to so mye'a sis	schistosomiasis
shwon o'muh	schwanoma
sib'a lum	scybalum
Sidinham's cho re'a	Sydenham's chorea
sif'i lid	syphilid
sif''i lit'ick	syphilitic
sif il o'mah	syphiloma
sif'i loyd	syphiloid
sif''i lo ther'a pe	syphilotherapy
sif'i lus	syphilis
sigh at'ick	sciatic
sigh at'i kuh	sciatica
sigh''kass thee'ne uh	psychasthenia
sigh'kee	psyche
sigh''kee at'rick	psychiatric
sigh'kick	psychic
sigh''ko an al'i sis	psychoanalysis
sigh''ko dye nam'icks	psychodynamics
sigh kol'o gee	psychology
sigh kol'o jist	psychologist
sigh''ko me'trics	psychometrics
sigh''ko mo'tor	paychomotor
sigh''ko new ro'sis	psychoneurosis
sigh''ko new rot'ick	psychoneurotic
sigh'ko path	psychopath
sigh ko'sis	psychosis

AS PHONETICALLY SPELLED	AS CORRECTLY SPELLED
sigh"ko so ma'tick	psychosomatic
sigh'nate	cynate
sigh tite'is	scytitis
sigh tol'ogy	cytology
sik'ah triks	cicatrix
si kigh'uh tree	psychiatry
si kigh'uh trist	psychiatrist
sil'a bus	syllabus
sil'e air"ee	ciliary
sil'e ate"ed	ciliated
sil'ee ah	cilia
sim blef'uh ron	symblepharon
sim"bi o'sis	symbiosis
sim e'le ah	symelia
Sime's am"pu ta'tion	Syme's amputation
sim'fi sis	symphysis
sim fiz'ee o tome"	symphisiatome
sim'i try	symmetry
sim"pa theh'tick	sympathetic
sim"pa thek'to me	sympathectomy
sim path"e kop'a the	sympathicopathy
sim path"e o nu ri'tis	sympathoneuritis
sim"pa thet"i ko mi met'ick	sympatheticomimetic
sim path"o lit'ick	sympatholytic
sim path"o mi met'ick	sympathomimetic
simp'tom	symptom
sin'aps	synapse
sin"ar thro'sis	synarthrosis
sin dack'til ee	syndactyly
sin'drome	syndrome
sing'ko pee	syncope
sing"kon dro'sis	synchondrosis
sink'a men	Synkamin
sin'ka vite	Synkavite
sin'ko py	syncopy
sin"os toe'sis	synostosis
si no"vee o'muh	synovioma

AS PHONETICALLY SPELLED	AS CORRECTLY SPELLED
si no′vee ah	synovia
sin″o vy′tis	synovitis
sin sill′in	Synicillin
sin thet′ick	synthetic
sint′ti gram	scintigram
sin′ur jiz um	synergism
si″ring go′ma	syringoma
si ring″go migh ee′lee ah	syringomyelia
si ring″go seel′	syringocele
si ring″o sist toe′mah	syringocystoma
si′rinj	syringe
si row′sis	cirrhosis
sist	cyst
sis′tick	cystic
sis′to lee	cystole
sis tol′ick	cystolic
sis′to seel	cystocele
sis′to scope	cystoscope
sis tos′ko pe	cystoscopy
sis′turn	cistern
sis tur′nah	cisterna
sit″a ko′sis	psittacosis
Skanzoni′s ma neu′ver	Scanzoni's maneuver
skee′mo graf	schemograph
skil′izm	scillism
skirr′oyd	scirrhoid
skirr′us	scirrhous or scirrhus
skiz″o fren′ick	schizophrenic
skiz″o fren′i ah	schizophrenia
skiz og′o ne	schizogony
skiz″o may′ni ah	schizomania
skiz′oyd	schizoid
skle″ro ma la′she ah	scleromalacia
skle ro nik′e ah	scleronychia
skle ro′sis	sclerosis
sklerr eck′to me	sclerectomy
sklerr ee′muh	sclerema

AS PHONETICALLY SPELLED	AS CORRECTLY SPELLED
sklerr eye'tis	scleritis
sklerr o'muh	scleroma
sklerr''ro durm'ah	scleroderma
skle'ruh	sclera
skli rot'ick	sclerotic
skli roze'	sclerose
sko''lee o'sis	scoliosis
sko'lex	scolex
sko toe'muh	scotoma
skra'fu luh	scrofula
sku'ba di'ving	scuba diving
skur'vee	scurvy
sor''ee at'ick	psoriatic
so''rye ass'i form	psoriasiform
so rye'uh sis	psoriasis
so'us	psoas
spy'ro keet	spirochete
staf''i lo cock'al	staphylococcal
staf''i lo cock see'me uh	staphylococcemia
staf''i lo cock'us	staphylococcus
staf'i loma	staphyloma
stip'tick	styptic
strick'nin	strychnine
sty'lit	stylet
sty''lo high'oyd	stylohyoid
sty'lus	stylus
sue''dar thro'sis	pseudarthrosis
sue''do an jye'nuh	pseudoangina
sue''du bul'bar	pseudobulbar
sue''do hee''mo fill'ee ah	pseudohemophilia
sue''do high pur'tro fee	pseudohypertrophy
sue''do hur maf'ro dite	pseudohermaphrodite
sue''do mem'brane	pseudomembrane
sue''do mo'nus	pseudomonas
sue''do mew'sin	pseudomucin
sue''do pa ree'sis	pseudoparesis
sue''do par ral'e sis	pseudoparalysis

AS PHONETICALLY SPELLED	AS CORRECTLY SPELLED
sue"do po'dee um	pseudopodium
sue"do sigh ee'sis	pseudocyesis
sue"do sist'	pseudocyst
sue"do tay'beez	pseudotabes
sue"do tie'foyd	pseudotyphoid
sub fren'ick	subphrenic
su'krose	sucrose
sul'fur	sulphur
supra high'oyd	suprahyoid
sur"kum sizh'un	circumcision
tack'ee card'i uh	tachycardia
tack"ip nee'uh	tachypnea
tahr'mick	ptarmic
taw'reen	taurine
tee'nee uh	taenia
tee'nee uh fuj"	taenifuge
Teet'see fly	Tsetse fly
teh ridj'ee um	pterygium
tel'o faze	telophase
terr'ee on	pterion
terr'i goyd	pterygoid
thigh'mawl	thymol
thigh meck'to mee	thymectomy
thigh'mick	thymic
thigh mo'muh	thymoma
thigh'mus	thymus
thigh my'tis	thymitis
thigh rock'sin	thyroxin
thigh"ro gen'ick	thyrogenic
thigh"ro gloss'ul	thyroglossal
thigh"ro high'oyd	thyrohyoid
thigh ro'sis	thyrosis
thigh"ro trope'in	thyrotropin
thigh'royd	thyroid
thigh"royd eck'to mee	thyroidectomy
thigh"royd i'tis	thyroiditis
tie lo'sis	ptilosis

AS PHONETICALLY SPELLED	AS CORRECTLY SPELLED
tif leck'to mee	typhlectomy
tif lye'tis	typhlitis
tif los'to mee	tiphlostomy
ti'foyd	typhoid
ti'fus	typhus
tim'pa nee	tympany
tim pan'ick	tympanic
tim''pan it'ick	tympanitic
tim'pan um	tympanum
ti'ro seen	tyrosine
toe'sis	ptosis
track'i lor'ud fee	trachelorrhaphy
track''i lot'o mee	trachelotomy
track''i lye'tis	trachelitis
tra ko'muh	trachoma
traw mat'ick	traumatic
traw'muh	trauma
traw'muh tize	traumatize
tray''kee i'tis	tracheitis
tray'kee o brong'kee ul	tracheobronchial
tray''kee o brong kigh'tis	tracheobronchitis
tray''kee o lar in'jul	tracheolaryngeal
tray''kee o ste no'sis	tracheostenosis
tray''kee os'tomy	tracheostomy
tray''kee ot'o mee	tracheotomy
tray'kee uh	trachea
tree ahj'	triage
tre fine'	trephine
Trick''i nel'uh	Trichinella
trick''i no'sis	trichinosis
trick''ko bee'zoar	trichobezoar
tric'ko lith	tricholith
Trick''o migh ko'sis	Trichomycosis
Trick''o mo'nas	Trichomonas
Trick yoo'ris	Trichuris
tri kigh'nuh	trichina
Tri kof'e tin	Tricophyton

AS PHONETICALLY SPELLED	AS CORRECTLY SPELLED
trip'sin	trypsin
tro can'tur	trochanter
trock'lee uh	trochlea
trock'lee ur	trochlear
tro'fick	trophic
tro'fizm	trophism
tro'fo blast	trophoblast
tro"fo zo'ite	trophozoite
tro'kee	troche
try cot'o mee	trichotomy
try fay'zick	triphasic
turn'eh kit	tourniquet
tye'al in	ptyalin
tye al'o gog	ptyalogogue
tye'sis	ptysis
u'fo ni a	euphonia
u'fo ri a	euphoria
u jen'ics	eugenics
u ko'le ah	eucholia
u mor'fic	eumorphic
u'nuck	enuch
u ray'cus	urachus
u"thah nay'ze ah	euthanasia
vack'seen	vaccine
vack sin'ee uh	vaccinia
vack'sin oyd	vaccinoid
vair'icks	varix
vane	vein
veck'tor	vector
vur'gin	virgin
waw bain	ouabain
zan'theen	xanthine
zan"thi laz'muh	xanthelasma

AS PHONETICALLY SPELLED	AS CORRECTLY SPELLED
zan"tho crow'mee uh	xanthochromia
zan tho"ma toe'sis	xanthomatosis
zan tho'ma tus	xanthomatous
zan tho'muh	xanthoma
zan tho'sis	xanthosis
zeer"o dur'muh	xeroderma
zeer"of thal'mee uh	xerophthalmia
zef'e ran	Zephiran
zer an'tic	zerantic
ae ro'sis	xerosis
ze rot'ick	xerotic
zi'goma	zygoma
zif'oyd	xiphoid
zi'gee on	zygion
zi'goat	zygote
zi go mat'ick	zygomatic
zi'leen	xylene
zi'lol	xylol

SECTION IV
ALPHABETICAL LIST OF:

Arteries
Veins
Muscles
Diseases
Syndromes
Commonly Performed Tests
Surgical Incisions
Dental Surfaces
Descriptive Positions, i.e., Anatomical

Arteries

Aberrant
Acetabular
Acromial
Acromiothoracic
Alveolar
Angular
Antral
Aorta
Appendicular
Arciform
Arcuate (foot, kidney)
Auditory
Aruicular
Axillary
Azygos (of vagina)

Basilar
Brachial
Bronchial
Buccal
Buccinator

Calcaneal
Calcarine
Caroticotympanic
Carotid
Carpal
Cavernous
Celiac
Central (of retina)
Cerebellar
Cerebral
Cervical
Choroid
Ciliary
Circumflex
Clitoral

Colic
Collateral
Communicating
Conjunctival
Coronary
Costocervical
Cremasteric
Cricothyroid
Crural
Cystic

Deferential
Dental
Digital (fingers, toes)
Diploic
Dorsalis pedis

Epigastric
Episcleral
Esophageal
Ethmoidal

Facial
Femoral
Frontal

Gastric
Gastroduodenal
Gastroepiploic
Genicular
Gluteal

Hallucis
Helicine
Hemorrhoidal
Hepatic
Humeral

Hypogastric
Hypophyseal

Ileal
Ileocolic
Iliac
Iliolumber
Infraorbital
Innominate
Intercostal
Interlobar (of kidney)
Interosseous
Intestinal

Jejunal

Labial
Lacrimal
Laryngeal
Lenticulostriate
Lienal
Lingual
Lumbar

Malleolar
Mammary
Masseteric
Mastoid
Maxillary
Median (hand, spinal cord)
Mediastinal
Meningeal
Mental
Mesenteric
Metacarpal
Metatarsal
Musculophrenic

Nasal

Nasopalatine
Neubauer's
Nutrient (femur, fibula,
    tibia, humerus)

Obturator
Occipital
Ophthalmic
Ovarian

Palatine
Palmar
Palpebral
Pancreatica
Pancreaticoduodenal
Penis
Perforating (of thigh)
Pericardiacophrenic
Perineal
Peroneal
Pharyngeal
Phrenic
Plantar
Pontine
Popliteal
Preventricular
Princeps cervicis
Princeps hallucis
Princeps pollicis
Profunda brachia
Profunda femoris
Profunda linguae
Pterygoid canal, Artery of
Pudendal
Pulmonary
Pyloric

Radial
Ranine

Recurrent (tibial, ulnar, radial)
Renal

Sacral
Saphenous
Scapular circumflex
Scapular transverse
Sciatic
Scrotal
Septal, posterior (nose)
Sigmoid
Spermatic
Sphenopalatine
Spinal
Spiral
Splenic
Stapedial
Sternocleidomastoid
Stylomastoid
Subclavian
Subcostal
Sublingual
Submental
Subscapular
Supraorbital
Suprarenal
Suprascapular
Sural

Tarsal
Temporal
Terminal

Testicular
Thoracic
Thoracoacromial
Thoracodorsal
Thymic
Thyrocervical trunk
Thyroid
Tibial
Tonsilar
Trabecular
Transverse (facial, neck,
    perineal, scapular)
Tympanic

Ulnar
Umbilical
Urethral
Uterine

Vaginal
Vasa Brevia
Vertebral
Vesical
Vidian
Volar (digital, radial)

Wilkie's (supraduodenal)
Willis, circle of

Zinn's
Zygomatico-orbital

Veins

Accesory, cephalic
Accessory. hemiazygos
Accessory, saphenous
Angular
Anterior auricular
Anterior bronchiole
Anterior coronary
Anterior facial
Anterior jugular
Anterior mediastinal
Anterior parotid
Anterior tibial
Anterior vertebral
Articular (knee, mandible)
Ascending lumbar
Axillary
Azygos

Basilic
Basivertebral
Branchial
Bronchial

Cephalic
Cerebellar
Cerebral
Choroid
Colic
Comitans (lateralis, medialis)
Coronary
Costoaxillary
Cystic

Deep cervical
Deep circumflex iliac
Deep iliac circumflex
Deferentiales

Dental
Digital
Diploic
Dorsal digital (hand, foot)
Dorsal metacarpal
Dorsal metatarsal
Dorsal (of penis)
Ductus venosus
Duodenal

Emissary
Esophageal
External iliac
External jugular
External nasal
External pudic

Femoral
Femoropopliteal
Frontal

Galen
Gastroepipoloic
Gluteal
Great saphenous

Hemiazygos
Hepatic
Hypogastric

Ileocolic
Iliolumbar
Inferior epigastric
Inferior gluteal
Inferior mesenteric
Inferior ophthalmic
Inferior palpebral

Inferior petrosal sinus
Inferior phrenic
Inferior thyroid
Inferior vena cava
Innominate
Intercapitular
Intercostal
Internal auditory
Internal circumflex
Internal iliac
Internal jugular
Internal mammary
Internal maxillary
Internal pudendal
Internal pudic
Internal vertebral
Intervertebral

Jugular

Labial
Lateral circumflex femoral
Lateral plantar
Lateral sacral
Lienal (splenic)
Lingual
Lumbar

Marginal right
Median
Median antebrachial
Median temporal
Meningeal
Metacarpal
Middle cardiac
Middle colic
Middle hemorrhoidal
Middle sacral
Musculophrenic

Nasofrontal

Obturator
Occipital
Ophthalmic
Orbital
Ovarian

Palatine
Palmar
Pancreatic
Pancreaticoduodenal
Paraumbilical
Pericardial
Peroneal
Pharyngeal
Plantar
Popliteal
Portal
Posterior auricular
Posterior bronchiole
Posterior facial
Posterior mediastinal
Posterior parotid
Posterior scrotal
Posterior tibial
Prostatic
Pubic
Pudendal
Pyloric

Radial
Renal

Short gastric
Short saphenous
Sigmoid
Spermatic
Sphenoparietal

Splenic
Stylomastoid
Subclavian
Supraorbital
Suprarenal

Temporal, superficial
Testicular
Thoracic
Thoracoepigastric
Transverse cervical

Transverse facial
Transverse scapular

Ulnar
Urethral
Uterine
Uterovaginal

Vaginal
Vertebral
Vesicular
Volar

Muscles

Abductor digiti minimi
(foot, hand)
Abductor hallucis
Abductor pollicis (brevis,
longus)
Accelerator urinae
Accessorius
Adductor brevis
Adductor hallucis
Adductor hallucis transversus
Adductor longus
Adductor magnus
Adductor minimus
Adductor pollicis
Agitator caudae
Anconeus
Antitragicus
Arrectores pilorum
Articularis genus
Aryepiglottic
Arytenoepiglotticus
Arytenoid (oblique, transverse)
Attollens aurem
Attrahens aurem
Auricularis anterior
Auricularis superior
Auricularis posterior
Azygos uvulae

Biceps brachii
Biceps femoris
Biventer cervicis
Brachialis
Brachioradialis
Broncho-oesophageus
Buccinator
Buccopharyngeus

Bulbocavernosus

Caninus
Cephalopharyngeus
Ceratocricoideus
Ceratopharyngeus
Cervicalis ascendens
Chondroglossus
Chondropharyngeus
Ciliary
Coccygeus
Complexus
Compressor naris
Compressor urethrae
Compressor vaginae
Constrictor of pharynx
(inferior, middle, superior)
Coracobrachialis
Corrugator cutis ani
Corrugator supercilii
Costalis
Costocervicalis
Costocoracoideus
Cremaster
Cricoarytenoid (lateral,
posterior)
Cricopharyngeus
Cricothyroid
Crureus

Dartos
Deltoid
Depressor alae nasi
Depressor anguli oris
Depressor epiglottidis
Depressor labii inferioris
Depressor septi

Depressor urethrae
Detrusor urinae
Diaphragm
Digastric
Dilator naris
Dilator pupillae

Ejaculator seminis
Epicranius
Erector clitoridis
Erector penis
Erector pili
Extensor brevis digitorum
Extensor brevis pollicis
Extensor carpi radialis
brevis
Extensor carpi radialis
longus
Extensor carpi ulnaris
Extensor coccygis
Extensor digiti quinti
proprius
Extensor digitorum brevis
Extensor digitorum longus
Extensor hallucis brevis
Extensor hallucis longus
Extensor indicis proprius
Extensor ossis metacarpi
pollicis
Extensor pollicis brevis
Extensor pollicis longus

Flexor brevis hallucis
Flexor carpi radialis
Flexor carpi ulnaris
Flexor digiti quinti brevis
Flexor digitorum brevis
Flexor digitorum longus
Flexot digitorum profundus

Flexor digitorum sublimis
Flexor hallucis brevis
Flexor hallucis longus
Flexor sublimis digitorum
Frontalis

Gastrocnemius
Gemellus (inferior, superior)
Genioglossus
Geniohyoid
Glossopalatinus
Glossopharyngeus
Glutens maximus
Gluteus medius
Gluteus minimus
Gracilis

Helicis major
Helicis minor
Hyoglossus
Hypopharyngeus

Iliacus
Iliococcygeus
Iliocostalis cervicis
Iliocostalis dorsi
Iliocostalis lumborum
Iliocostocervicalis
Iliopsoas
Infracostals
Infraspinatus
Intercostal (external,
internal)
Interossei, dorsal (of
hand, foot)
Interossei, plantar
Interossei, volar
Interspinalis
Intertransversarii

Ischiocavernosus
Ischiofemoralis

Latissimus dorsi
Levator anguli oris
Levator ani
Levator costae
Levator glandulae
  thyroideae
Levator labii inferior
Levator labii superior
Levator labii superioris
  alaeque nasi
Levator menti
Levator palati
Levator palpebrae
  superioris
Levator prostatae
Levator scapulae
Levator veli palatini
Levatores costarum
Longissimus capitis
Longissimus cervicalis
Longissimus dorsi
Longissimus thoracis
Londitudinalis dorsi
Longitudinalis inferior
Longitudinalis superior
Longus capitis
Longus colli
Lumbricals (toes, fingers)

Masseter
Mentalis
Multifidus
Mylohyoid
Mylopharyngeal

Nasalis

Obliquus abdominis
  externus
Obliquus abdominis
  internus
Obliquus auriculae
Obliquus capitis
  inferior
Obliquus capitis superior
Obliquus oculi inferior
Obliquus oculi superior
Obturator externus
Obturator interus
Occipitalis
Occipitofrontalis
Omohyoid
Opponens digiti quinti
  (hand, foot)
Opponens pollicis
Orbicularis oculi
Orbicularis oris
Orbicularis palpebrarum
Orbitalis

Palatoglossus
Palatopharyngeus
Palatosalpingeus
Palmaris brevis
Palmaris longus
Pectinatus
Pectineus
Pectoralis major
Pectoralis minor
Peroneus accessorius
Peroneus brevis
Peroneus tertius
Pharyngopalatinus
Piriformis
Plantaris
Platysma

Popliteus
Procerus
Pronator pedis
Pronator quadratus
Pronator teres
Psoas major
Psoas minor
Pterygoideus externus
Pterygoideus internus
Pterygopharyngeus
Pubocavernosus
Pubococcygeus
Puboprostaticus
Puborectalis
Pubovesicalis
Pyramidalis abdominis
Pyramidalis auriculae
Pyramidalis nasi
Pyriformis

Quadratus femoris
Quadratus labii inferioris
Quadratus labii superioris
Quadratus lumborum
Quadratus plantae
Quadriceps femoris

Rectococcygeus
Rectus abdominis
Rectus capitis anterior
Rectus capitis anticus
    major
Rectus capitis anticus
    minor
Rectus capitis lateralis
Rectus capitis posterior major
Rectus capitis posterior minor
Rectus femoris
Rectus oculi inferior

Rectus oculi internus
Rectus oculi lateralis
Rectus oculi medialis
Rectus oculi superior
Retrahens aurem
Rhomboideus major
Rhomboideus minor
Risorius
Rotatores

Sacrococcygeus
Sacrolumbalis
Sacrospinalis
Salpingopharyngeus
Sartorius
Scalenus anterior
Scalenus medius
Scalenus posterior
Semimembranosus
Semispinalis capitis
Semispinalis cervicis
Semispinalis dorsi
Semitendinosus
Serratus anterior
Serratus posterior inferior
Serratus posterior superior
Soleus
Sphincter ani externus
Sphincter ani internus
Sphincter oris
Sphincter pupillae
Sphincter urethrae membranaceae
Sphincter vaginae
Sphincter vesicae
Spinalis capitis
Spinalis cervicis
Spinalis dorsi
Spinalis thoracis
Splenius cervicis

Splenius colli
Stapedius
Sternalis
Sternoclavicularis
Sternocleidomastoid
Sternocostalis
Sternohyoid
Sternothyroid
Styloauricularis
Styloglossus
Stylohyoid
Stylolarngeus
Stylopharyngeus
Subanconeus
Subclavius
Subcostals
Subcrureus
Subscapularis
Supinator
Supinator longus
Supinator radii brevis
Supraspinalis
Supraspinatus

Tarsalis (inferior, superior)
Temporal
Tensor fasciae latae
Tensor palati
Tensor tarsi
Tensor tympani
Tensor vaginae femoris
Tensor veli palatini
Teres major
Teres minor
Thyroarytenoid
Thyroepiglottic

Thyrohyoid
Thropharyngeus
Tibialis (interior, posterior)
Tibiofascialis anterior
Trachelomastoid
Tragicus
Transversalis colli
Transverospinalis
Transversus abdominis
Transversus auriculae
Transversus linguae
Transversus menti
Transversus nuchae
Transversus pedis
Transversus perinei profundus
Transversus perinei superficialis
Transversus thoracis
Trapezius
Triangularis
Triangularis labii (inferior,
    superior)
Triangularis sterni
Triceps brachii
Triceps surae
Trochlearis

Uvulae

Vastus externus
Vastus intermedius
Vastus internus
Vastus lateralis
Vastus medialis
Ventricularis
Verticalis linguae
Vocalis

Zygomatic

ABC hemolytic
Acosta's
Adams-Stokes
adaptation
Addison's
Adenocystic
air sac
Albers-Schönberg
Albert's
Albright's
Alexander's
alkali
alligator skin
Alper's
Alzeimer's
amyloid
Ander's
anserine
Aran-Duchenne
arc-welder's
attic
Aujeszky's
Australian X
autoimmune
aviator's
Ayerza's

Babinski-Froehlich
bagasse
Bamberger-Marie
Bang's
Bannister's
Banti's
Barcoo
Barlow's
Basedow's
Batten-Mayou's

Bazin's
Behcet's
Bekhterev's
Bell's
Bernhardt's
Besnier-Boeck-Schaumann
Biermer's
Bornholm
Bouillaud's
Bourneville's
Bowen's
Bright's
Brill's
Brill-Symmers
Buaki
Buerger's
Buschke's
Busquet's
Busse-Buschke's

caisson
California
Calvé's
Carrión's
Castellani's
cat-scratch
celiac
Chargas'
Charcot-Marie-Tooth
Chauffard-Still's
Chiari's
Christian-Weber
Christmas
cobalt deficiency
collagen
communicable
Concato's

congenital
congenital polycystic
constitutional
contagious
Cooley's
Coxsackie
Cruveilhier's
Cushing's
cutaneous caisson
cystic d. of breast
cystine
cytomegalic inclusion

Darier's
Darling's
David's
de Beurmann-Gougerot
deficiency
degenerative
degenerative joint
demyelinating
Dercum's
DiGuglielmo's
Duchenne-Aran
Duhring's
Durand-Nicolas-Favre
Durand's

Eale's
Ebstein's
Economo's
Eddowe's
endemic
Engelmann's
Engel-Recklinghausen's
epidemic
Erb-Charcot

Favre

Fete-Riga's
fibrocytic
Flajani's
Fordyce's
Fox-Fordyce
Freiberg's
Frei's
Friedreich's
functional

Gaisböck's
Gamna's
Gaucher's
Gee-Herter
Gee's
Gee-Thayson
Gilchrist's
glycogen storage
Gougerot's
Graefe's
Grave's
Guillain-Barré
Gull and Sutton's

Habermann's
Hailey-Hailey
Hammond's
Hand-Schüller-Christian
Hanot's
Hansen's
Hashimoto's
Haxthausen's
Heberden's
Hebra's
Heine-Medin
hemorrhagic
hemorrhagic d. of the newborn
hereditary
Heubner-Herter

Hippel-Lindau
Hirschsprung's
Hodgkin's
Holla
Hopf's
Huntington's
Hurler's
hyaline membrane
hypertensive vascular

idiopathic
inclusion
intercurrent

Jaffé-Lichtenstein
Johne's
Jüngling's

Kahler's
Kaiserstuhl
Kakke
Kaposi's
Kienböck's
Kimmelstiel-Wilson
Köhler's
König's
Kufs'
Kümmel's

Larsen-Johansson
Legg-Calvé-Perthes
Leiner's
Léri's
Letterer-Siwe
Lewandowsky's
Libman-Sacks
Lindau's
lipoid storage
Little's

Lobstein's
loco
Looser-Milkman's
Lutembacher's

Majocchi
malignant
Marie's
Mediterranean
Ménière's
milkman's
Mitchell's
Moeller-Barlow
Monge's
Morquio-Brailsford
mosaic

Newcastle
Niemann-Pick

Ollier's
organic
Osgood-Schlatter
Osler-Rendu-Weber
Osler-Vaquez
Owren's

Paget's
Paget's of nipple
pandemic
pararheumatic
parasitic
Parkinson's
Parry's
Pel-Ebstein's
periodic
periodontal
Peyronie's
Pfeiffer's

Phoca's
Pick's
Pictow
Pinkus'
Plummer's
pneumatic hammer
policeman's
Pollitzer's
polyhedral
Pompe's
Poncet's
porcupine
Posada-Wernicke's
Potain's
Pott's
Poulet's
Preiser's
Pringle's
Profichet's
Puente's
pullorum
Purtscher's
pyramidal

Quervain's
Quincke's
Quinquand's

Raugier's
Rayer's
Raynaud's
Recklinghausen's
Recklinghausen-Applebaum
Reclus'
Reed-Hodgkin
Refsum's
Reichmann's
Reiter's
Rendu-Osler-Weber

Renikhet
rheumatic heart
rheumatoid
Ribas-Torres
Riedel's
Riga's
Riga-Fede
Riggs'
Ritter's
Rivolta's
Robinson's
Robles'
Roger's
Rokitansky's
Romberg's
Rose
Rosenbach's
Roth's
Roth-Bernhardt
Roussy-Lévy's
Rowland's
Rummo's
Runneberg's
Rust's
Ruysch's

Sachs'
sacroiliac
St. Agatha's
St. Aignon's
St. Aman's
St. Anthony's
St. Appolonia's
St. Avertin's
St. Avidus'
St. Blasius'
St. Clair's
St. Dymphna's
St. Erasmus'

St. Fiacre's
St. Francis'
St. Gervasius'
St. Gete's
St. Giles'
St. Gotthard's tunnel
St. Hubert's
St. Job's
St. Main's
St. Mathurin's
St. Modestus'
St. Roch's
St. Sement's
St. Valentine's
St. Zachary's
salivary gland
San Joaquin Valley
Sander's
sartian
Saunders'
Savill's
Schamberg's
Schanz's
Schaumann's
Scheuermann's
Schilder's
Schimmelbusch's
Schlatter's
Schmorl's
Scholz's
Schönlein's
Schönlein-Henoch
Schottmüller's
Schriddes'
Schroeder's
Schüller's
Schüller-Christian
Schultz's
Secretan's

Senear-Usher
senecio
septic
serum
Sever's
Shishito
shuttlemaker's
silage
silo-filler's
Simmonds'
Simons'
Sjogren's
Skevas-Zerfus
Smith's
Spencer's
Spielmeyer-Stock
Spielmeyer-Vogt
sponge-divers'
sporadic
Stargardt's
Steinert's
Sterbe
sterility
Sternberg's
Stieda's
Still's
Stiller's
Stokes'
Stokes-Adams
Stokvis'
Strachan's
Strümpell's
Strümpel-Leichtenstern
Strümpell-Marie
Stuhmer's
Sturge's
Sturge-Weber-Dimitri
Stuttgart
subacute

subchronic
Sudeck's
Sutton's
Sutton and Gull's
Swediaur's
Swift's
Swift-Feer
Sylvest
Symmers'

Taenzer's
Talfan
Talma's
Tangier
tarabagan
tartaric
Tay's
Tay-Sachs
Taylor's
Teschen
Theiler's
Thomsen's
Thomson's
Thornwaldt's
Tietze's
Tillaux's
Tomaselli's
Tourette's
Traum's
Trevor's
Trousseau's
tsetse fly
tsutsugamushi
Tyzzer's

Underwood's
Unna's
Unverricht's

Urback-Oppenheim
Urbach-Wiethe's

vagabonds'
vagrants'
Valee's
Valsuani's
Vaquez'
Vaquez-Osler
veldt
venereal
Verneuil's
Verse's
Vidal's
Vincent's
Virchow's
Vogt's
Vogt-Spielmeyer
Volkmann's
Voltolini's
von Economo's
von Gierke's
von Hippel's
von Jaksch's
von Recklinghausen's
von Willebrand's

Wagner's
Waldenstrom's
Wardrop's
Wartenberg's
Wassilieff's
Weber's
Weber-Christian
Weber-Dimitri
Wegner's
Weil's
Weingartner's
Weir Mitchell's

Wenckebach's
Werdnig-Hoffmann
Werlhof's
Werner-His
Werner-Schultz
Wernicke's
Westberg's
Westphal-Strümpell
Whipple's
White's
Whitmore's
Whytts'
Widal-Abrami
Wilks'

Willis'
Wilson's
Wilson-Brocq
Winckel's
Windscheid's
Winkelman's
winter vomiting
Winton
Woillez's

Zagari's
Zahorsky's
Ziehen-Oppenheim
zymotic

Syndromes

Abercrombie's
Achard-Thiers
Adair-Dighton
Adams-Stokes
addisonian
Adie's
adiposogenital
adrenogenital
Albright's
Albright-McCune-Sternberg's
Aldrich's
amnestic
amyostatic
Andersen's
Angelucci's
anginal
anginose
anterior cornual
Apert's
Arnold's nerve reflex
Arnold-Chiari
Ascher's
asphyctic
auriculotemporal
Avellis's
Ayerza's

Babinski's
Babinski-Frolich
Babinski-Nageotte
Babinski-Vacquez
Banti's
Bard-Pic
Bardet-Biedl
Barré-Guillain
Bassen-Kornzweig
Beau's

Behcet's
Benedikt
Bernard's
Bernard-Horner
Bernard-Sergent
Bernhardt-Roth
Bernheim's
Bertolotti's
Bianchi's
Biedl's
Biemond's
Binney-Bow
Blatin's
Blum's
Bonnevie-Ullrich
Bonnier's
Bouillaud's
Bouveret's
Brenneman
Briquet's
Brissaud-Marie
Brissaud-Sicard
Bristow's
Brock's
Brown-Sequard
Brugsch's
Brun's
bundle of Kent
Burnett's
Bywater's

callosal
Capgras's
capsulothalamic
carotid sinus
carpal tunnel
cavernous sinus

centroposterior
cerebellar
cervical
cervical rib
cervicobrachial
Cestan's
Cestan-Chenais
Cestan-Raymond
Charcot-Weiss-Barber
Chargot's
Charlin's
Chauffards's
Chauffard-Still
Chiari's
Chiari-Arnold
Chiari-Frommel
chiasma
chiasmatic
chorea
Christian's
Citelli's
Clarke-Hadfield
Claude's
Claude-Bernard-Horner
Clough and Richter's
Collet's
Collet-Sicard
cor pulmonale
corpus striatum
Costen's
costoclavicular
Cotard's
Courvoisier-Terrier
Crigler-Najjar
Cruveilhier-Baumgarten
cubital tunnel
Cushing's
Cyriax's

Da Costa's
Danlos'
defibrination
Dejerine's
Dejerine-Roussy
de Toni-Fanconi
Dighton-Adair
Di Guglielmo
Doan and Wiesman's
Down's
Dresbach's
Duane's
Dubin-Johnson
Dubin-Sprinz
Dubreuil-Chambardel
Duchenne's
Duchenne-Erb
dumping
Duplay's
Dupre's
dysglandular
dystrophia-dystocia

Eddowes'
Ehlers-Danlos
Eisenmenger's
Ellis-van Creveld
encephalotrigeminal vascular
epiphysial
Epstein's
Erb's

Faber's
Fabry's
Fallot's
Fanconi
Felty's
Fitz's

Syndromes

Forssman carotid
Foster Kennedy's
Foville's
Frey's
Friedmann's vasomotor
Frolich's
Froin's

Gailliard's
Gaisbock's
Ganser's
gastrocardiac
Gee-Herter-Heubner
Gelineau's
general adaptation
Gerhardt's
Gerlier's
Gerstmann's
globus pallidus
Goplan's
Gougerot's
Gouley's
Gower's
Gradenigo's
Graham-Little
Gronblad-Strandberg
Guillain-Barré
Gunn's

Hadfield-Clark
Hallervorden-Spatz
Hamman's
Hamman-Rich
Hand's
Hand-Schuller
hand-shoulder
Hanot's
Hanot-Chauffard

Hare's
Harris'
Hassin's
Hayem-Widal
hemiparaplegic
hemohistioblastic
hemopleuropneumonic
hemorrhagic fever
Hench-Rosenberg
hepatorenal
Heyd's
Hines-Bannick
Hoffmann-Werdnig
Holmes-Adie
Homen's
Horner's
Horner-Bernard
Horton's
humoral
Hunt's
Hunt's striatal
Hunterian glossitis
Hurler's
Hutchinson's
Hutchinson-Gilford
hyaline membrane
hypercalcemia
hyperophthalmopathic
hypophyseal

Jackson's
Jacquet's
jejunal
jugular foramen

Karroo
Kartagener's
Kast's

Kennedy's
Kimmelstiel-Wilson
Kleine-Levin
Klinefelter's
Klippel-Feil
Klumpke-Dejerine
Kocher's
Konig's
Korsakoff's

Landry's
Lasegue's
Laubry-Soule
Launois'
Laurence-Biedl
Laurence-Moon-Biefl
Lawen-Roth
Leredde's
Leriche
Lermoyez's
Leschke
Levi's
Levy-Roussy
Lhermitte and McAlpine
Libman-Sacks
Lichtheim's
Lightwood's
loculation
Loffler's
Lowe's
Lutembacher's
lymphoproliferative

McArdle
Mackenzie's
Maffucci's
malabsorption
Malin's
Maranon's

Marchiafava-Micheli
Marcus Gunn
Marfan's
Marie's
Marie-Robinson
Meigs'
Ménière's
mesodermal
metameric
middle radicular
Mikulicz's
Milian's
milkman's
Millard-Gubler
Minkowski-Chauffard
Mobius
Monakow's
Moore's
Morel's
Morgagni's
Morgagni-Stewart-Morel
Morquio's
Morton's
Morvan's
Mosse's
Munchausen's
Murchison-Sanderson
myasthenia gravis
myeloproliferative

Naffziger's
nephrotic
neurocutaneous
nitritoids
Nonne's
Nonne-Milroy-Meige
Nothnagel's

oculocerebrorenal

Syndromes

Oglivie's
orodigitofacial
orofacial-digital
Ostrum-Furst

paleostriatal
pallidal
pallidomesencephalic
Pancoast's
pancreaticohepatic
paralysis agitans
paratrigeminal
Parinaud's
Parke's
Parkinson's
parkinsonian
Paterson's
Patton's
Pellazzi's
Pepper
pericolic-membrane
Peutz
Peutz-Jeghers
phrenogastric
physiopathic
Picchini's
Pick's
pickwickian
Pierre Robin
pineal
Pins'
pituitary
Plummer-Vinson
pluriglandular
polyglandular
pontine
postcommissurotomy
posterolateral
postgastrectomy

postirradiation
postpericardiotomy
Potain's
Pozzi's
premotor
Profichet's
Putnam Dana

radicular
Raymond-Cestan's
Refsum's
Reichmann's
Reiter's
Renon-Delille
retroparotid space
Riley's
rolandic vein
Romberg-Paessler
Rosenbach's
Roth's
Rothmund's
Roussy-Levy
Rust's

Sawii
scalenus
scalenus anticus
scapulocostal
Schanz's
Schaumann's
Schmidt's
Schonlein-Henoch
Schroeder's
Schuller's
Schuller-Christian
Schultz
segmentary
Selye
Senear-Usher

Sezary
Sezary reticulosis
Sheehan's
Sicard's
Siemens'
Silverskiold's
Silverstrini-Corda
Simmonds'
Sjogren's
Sluser's
Spens's
Spurway
Stein-Leventhal
Stevens-Johnson
Stewart-Morel
Still-Chauffard
Stokes's
Stokes-Adams
striatal
Stryker-Halbeisen
Sturge's
Sturge-Kalischer-Weber
Sturge-Weber
subclavian steal
Sudeck-Leriche
superaspinatus

Tapia's
Taussig-Bing
tegmental
temporomandibular joint
Terry's
testicular feminization
thalamic
Thibierge-Weissenbach

Thiele
thromboembolic
Tietze's
Timme's
Toland's
Tomaselli's
Treacher-Collins
Troisier's
Turner's

vago-accessory
van der Hoeve's
vascular
Vernet's
Villaret's
Vogt's
Vogt-Koyanagi
Volkmann's
von Welty's

Wallenberg's
Waterhouse-Friderichsen
Weber
Weber-Dubler
Weingarten's
Werdnig-Hoffmann
Werner's
Wernicke's
Widal
Wilson's
Wolff-Parkinson-White
Wright's

Young's

Zollinger-Ellison

Commonly Performed Tests

Abderhalden's
Abelin's
Abrams'
acetanilid
acetic acid
aceto-acetic acid
acetone
acetonitril
Achard and Castaigne's
acidity reduction
acidosis
Acree-Rosenheim
acrolein
Adamkiewicz's
Adam's
Addis'
Adler's
Admiralty
adrenalin
agglutination
Agostini's
Aiello's
Albarran's
albumin
aldehyde
Aldrich-McClure
Alfraise's
alizarin
alkali
alkaloid
Allen's
Allen-Doisy
Allesandri-Guaceni
Almen's
aloin
Alper's
alpha

alphanaphthol
Althausen
Amann's
amidopyrine
amino-acid nitrogen
aminopyrine
ammonia
ammonium sulfate
amylase
amyl nitrite
amylopsin
Andersch and Gibson
Anderson's
Anderson and Goldberger's
Andre's
Andreasch's
Andrewe's
Anstie's
antiformin
antimony
antipyrine
antithrombin
antitrypsin
Antonucci
anvil
apomorphine
aptitude
Arakawa's
Archetti's
Arloing-Courmont
Arnold's
Aron's
arsenic
arsphenamine
Aschheim-Zondek
Aschner-Danini
Ascoli's

Atkinson and Kendall's
atropine
Auricchio and Chieffi's
autohemolysis
auto-urine
Axenfeld's
Ayer's
Ayer-Tobey
A-Z
azorubin

Babcock's
Babinski
Babinski-Weil
Bachman
Bachmeier's
bactericidal
bacteriolytic
Baeyer's
BAJ
Baldwin's
Balfour's
Bang
Barany's
Barberio's
Bardach's
Bareggi's
Barfoed's
Bargehr
Barral's
Basham's
basophil
Bass-Watkin
Bauer's
Baumann's
Baumann and Goldmann's
Bayer's
Bayrac's
B.C.G.

Bechterew's
Becker's
Bedson's
Behre and Benedict's
Bell's
Bellerby's
Bendien's
Benedict's
Benedict and Denis'
Benedict and Murlin's
bentonite
benzidine
benzidine peroxidase
bensoin
Bercovitz
Berenreuther
Bergmann-Meyer
Berthelot's
Bertoni-Raymondi
Bertrand's
Berzelius's
beta
beta-oxybutyric acid
Bettendorff's
Bettmann's
Bial's
bicarbonate tolerance
bicolor guaiac
bile pigment
bilirubin
Binet's
Binet-Simon
Bing's entotic
Binz's
biological
Birkhaug
Bischoff's
bismuth
bitterlung

biuret
Black's
Blackberg and Wanger's
blanche
Blaxland's
Block-Steiger
blood cholesterol
blood-urea clearance
Bloor's
Bloxam's
Blum's
Blumenau's
Blyth's
Boas'
Bodal's
Boedeker's
Beorner-Luckens
Bohmansson's
Bolen
Boltz's
Bonanno's
Borchardt's
Borden's
Bordet-Gengou
Bordet's
Boston's
Botelho's
Bottger's
Bottu's
Bouchardt's
Bouin and Ancel
Bourdon's
Bourget's
Boveri's
Boyksen's
Bozicevich's
Brahmachari's
Bram's
Brande's

Braun's
Braun-Husler
Bremer's
Brieger's
bromine
bromsulphalein
Brouha
Brown's
brucellin
Brugsch's
Bryce's
Bufano
Burchard-Liebermann
Burger's
Burnam's
Busacca's
Buscaino's
butyric acid
Bychowski's

caffeine
Caillan's
calcium
Callaway's
Calmette's
caloric
Calvert's
Cammidge's
Campani's
Campbell's
camphor
Cantani
capillary resistance
capon comb growth
Cappagnoli's
Capranica's
carbohydrate
carbon monoxide
Carnot's

carotinemia
Carr-Price
Carrez's
Casamajor's
casein
Casilli's
Casoni's intradermal
Castellani's
catoptric
cellulose
cephalin-cholesterol flocculation
Chapman's
Chautard's
Chediak's
Chick-Martin
Chiene's
Chimani-Moos
chloride balance
chlorophyll
cholera red
cholesterol
choline
Chopra's antimony
Chorine's
Chrobak
chromatin
chromic acid
Ciamician and Magnanini's
Cipollina's
citochol
Clark's
Clauberg
Clive's
coagulation
cobra venom
coccidiodin
cockscomb
coffee

Cohen's
Cohn's
coin
colchicin
cold pressor
Cole's
colloidal benzoin
colloidal gold
Comessatti's
complement-fixation
concentration
Congo red
conjugate glycuronates
conjunctival
connective tissue
contact
Contejean
Cooke's
Coombs'
Cope's
Corner-Allen
Costa
Cowie's guaiac
Craft's
Craig's
Cramer's
Crampton's
creatinine
Crismer's
Cronin Lowe
Cuboni's
Cuignet's
Cunisset's
currant
Curschmann
Cutler-Power-Wilder
Cutola
Cutting's

cysteine
cystine
cytosin

Daclin
Dalldorf's
D'Amato's
Daranyi
dark-adaptation
Davy's
Day's
Dedichen's
Deen's
Degener's
Dehio's
dehydrocholate
Dejust's
Delff's
Deniges'
Dennis and Silverman's
Derrien's
desmoid
dextrose
diacetic acid
diacetyl
dialysis
Diamond slide
diastase
diazo
Dick
Dicken's
Dienst
digestive function
digitalin
dilution
dimethylamino-azrobenzene
Dold's
Dolman's

Donaldson's
Donath's
Donath-Landsteiner
Donders'
Donne's
Donogany's
Dorn-Sugarman
double-blind
Dowell
Dragendorff's
Drechsel's
Dreyer's
Duane's
Dugas'
Duke's
Dumontpallier's
Dungern's
Dupont's
Dwight-Frost

Eagle
Ebbighaus'
Eberson's
edestin
Edlefsen's
Ehrard's
Ehrlich's
Ehrmann's
Eijkman's
Einhorn's
Eiselt's
Eitelberg's
Ellermann and Erlandsen's
Elton's ring
Ely's
Emanuel-Cutting
epinephrine
epiphanin

Erdman's
Erichsen
erythrocyte sedimentation
Esbach's
Escherrich's
Escudero's
ether
ethyl acetate
ethyl butyrate
euglobulin lysis
Eustis's
Ewald's
extinction
Exton's
Exton and Rose

Fabre's
Fahraeus'
Falk and Tedesco's
Falls'
Farber's
Faust's
Fearon's
Fehling's
fermentation
ferric chloride
Feulgen's
fibrinogen
Fieux's
Finckh's
Fischer's
Fishberg
Fishberg and Friedfeld
fistula
fixation
Flack
Fleig's
Fleischl's
Fleitmann's

flocculation
Florence
fluorescent treponemal
  antibody-absorption
Flushmann's
Focker's
Folin's
Folin and Denis'
Folin and McEllroy's
Folin and Wu's
formaldehyde
formalin
formol-gel
Fornet-s ring
Foshay's
Foubert's
Fouchet's
Fournier
fragility
Francis'
Frank and Goldberger
Frank and Nothmann's
Frankel's
Franken's
Frei
Fridweichsen's
Friedman's
Friedman-Hamburger
Fröhde's
Frohn's
Frommer's
fructose
Fuchs's
Fuld's
Fuld-Goss
Furbringer's
furfurol

Gairdner's coin

galactose
Gali Mainini
Gallois'
Ganassini's
Gannther's
Gardiner-Brown
Garriga's
Garrod's
Gate and Papacostas'
Gault
Gauran
Gawalowski's
Gay-Force
Gayer
Geissler's
Gelle's
Gentele's
Geraghty's
Gerhardt's
Gerrard's
Ghedini-Weinberg
Gibbon and Landis
Gies'biuret
Glenard's
globulin
glucose
glutoid
Gluzinski's
glycerol
glycerol-cholesterol
glycerophosphate
glycuronates
glyclitryptophan
glyoxylic acid
Gmelin's
Goetsch's
Goldscheider's
gold-sol
Gordon's

Gothlin's
Graefe's
Graham's
Grandeau's
Graupner's
Gregerson and Boas'
Greig
Greppi-Villa
Griess's
Grigg's
Grobly's
Grocco's
Gross'
Gruber's
Gruber-Widal
Grünbaum's
Grünbaum-Widal
Gruskin
guaiac
Gunning's
Gunning-Lieben
Gunzburg's
Guterman
Gutzeit's

Hager's
Haines'
Hallion's
Ham
Hamburger's
Hamel's
Hamilton-Swartz
Hamilton's
Hammarsten's
Hammer's
Hammerschlag's
Hanganatziu-Deicher
Hanger's
Hanke and Koessler's

Harding and Ruttan's
Harrington-Flocks
Harris and Ray
Harrison spot
Harrower's
Hart's
Hassall's
Hawk's
Hay's
Hecht's
Hecht-Weinberg
Hecht-Weinberg-Gradwohl
Heichelheim's
Heller's
hematein
hematoporphyrin
hemin
hemoglobin
hemosiderin
Hench-Aldrich
Henderson's
Henie-Coenen
Hennebert's
Henry's
Henshaw
hepatic function
Hering's
Herman-Perutz
Herring's
Herring-Binet
Herter's
Herz's
Herzberg's
Hess capillary
Heynsius'
Hildebrandt's
Hindenlang's
Hines and Brown
Hinton
hippuric acid

Hirschfeldt's
Hirst
Hirst and Hare
histamine
histidine
Hitzig
Hoffmann's
Hofmann's
Hofmeister's
Hogben
Holmgren's
Holten's
Hopkins' thiophene
Hopkins-Cole
Hoppe-Seyler
hormone
Horsley's
Hotis
Houghton's
Howell's
Huddleson's
Huggins
Huhner
Hunt's
Huppert's
Huppert-Cole
Hurtley's
hydrobilirubin
hydrochloric acid
hydrogen peroxide
hydrophilia skin
hydrostatic
hydroxylamine
hyperemia
hyperpnea
hypochlorite-orcinol
hypoxanthine

icterus index
Ide

Iefimov
Ilimow's
Iloxvay's
Imhof's
imidazole
immunologic pregnancy
indican
indigo carmine
indole
indophenol
inoculation
inosite
intelligence
intracutaneous tuberculin
intradermal salt solution
inulin clearance
iodine
iodipin
iodoform
Ishihara's
Israelson's
Ito-Reenstierna

Jacobsthal's
Jacoby's
Jacquemin's
Jadassohn's
Jadassohn-Bloch
Jaffe's
Jaksch's
Janet's
Jansen's
Javorski's
Jendrasic's
Jenner-Kay
Jenning's
Johnson's
Jolles'
Jones and Cantarow

Jorissen's
Justus'

Kabatschnik's
Kafka's
Kahn
kairin
Kamnitzer's
Kantor and Gies'
Kapeller-Adler
Kaplan's
Kapsinow's
Kashiwado's
Kastle's
Kastle-Meyer
Katayama's
Kathrein
Katzenstein's
Kauffmann's
Keller's ultraviolet
Kelling's
Kelly's
Kendrick's
Kentmann's
Kerner's
Killian's
Kinberg's
Kitzmiller
Kiutsi-Malone
Kjeldahl's
Klausner's
Klein
Klemperer's
Klimow's
Kline
Kline-Young
Knapp's
Kober
Kobert's
Koch's

Koenecke's
Koh's
Kolmer's
Kondo's
Konew's
Knosuloff's
Korotkoff's
Kossel's
Kottmann's
Kowarsky's
Krauss'
Krokiewicz's
Kuhlmann
Kultz's
Kurzrok-Miller
Kustallow's
Kveim

Laborde's
lactose
Ladendorff's
Landau color
Lang's
Lange's
Laughlen
Lautier's
Leach's
Lebbin's
Lechini's
Lee's
Legal's
Leiner's
Le Nobel's
lentochol
Leo's
lepromin
Lesser's
Lesieur-Privey
leucine

Levinson
levulose
Lewis and Pickering
Lichtheim
Lieben's
Lieben-Ralfe
Liebermann's
Liebermann-Burchardt
Liebig's
Ligat's
Lignieres'
Lindemann's
Lindner's
Links'
Linzenmeier's
lipase
Lipps'
Lipschuetz's
litmus mild
liver function
Livierato's
Loewe's
Loewi's
Lombard's
Lowenthal's
Lowy's
Lucke's
Luebert's
Luenbach-Koeppe
luetin
lupus induction
Luttge-Mertz
Luttke's
Lyle and Curtman's
lysis time

McClure-Aldrich
MacDonagh's
Macdonald's

Macht
McKendrick
McKinnin's
Maclagan's
MacLean
MacLean-de Wesselow
MacMunn's
MacQuarrie
MacWilliams
magnesionitric
Magpie's
Malerba's
Malmejde's
Malot's
maltose
Maly's
Mandel's
Manoiloff's
Manson evaluation
Mantoux
Manzullo's
Marechal's
Marechal-Rosin
Marie's three-paper
Markee
Marlow's
Marquardt's
Marquis's
Marris atropine
Marsh's
Marshall's
Maschke's
Masselon
Masset's
Master's
mastic
Matas'
Matefy
Mathews'

Maumene
Mauthner's
Mayer-Tanret
Mayer's
Mayerhofer's
Mazer-Hoffman
Mazzini
Mehu's
Meigs's
Meinicke
melanin
melitin
Meltzer-Lyon
Mendel's
Mendeleeff's
Mendelsohn's
mercury
Mérieux-Baillion
Mester's
methylene blue
methyl-phenyl-hydrazine
Mett's
Meyer's
Michaelides'
Michailow's
microprecipitation
Middlebrook-Dubos
Millard's
Miller-Kurzrok
Millon's
Mills's
miostagmin
Mitscherlich's
Mitsuda-Rost
Mittlemeyer's
Mohr's
Molisch's
Moloney
monosaccharide

Montigne's
Moore's
Morelli's
Moretti's
Moritz
Morner's
Moro's
morphine
Morton's
Moschowitz
Mosenthal's
Moynihan's
mucic acid
mucification
Muck's
Mulder's
Muller's
Muller-Jochmann
Murata
murexide
Murphy's
mucobiologic
mycologic
Myersand Fine
Mylius'

Naffziger's
Nagle's
Nakayama's
Napier's serum
Nasso's
Nathan's
Neisser and Wechsberg's
Nencki's
neosalvarsan
Nessler's
Neubauer and Fischer's
Neufeld's
Neukomm's

neutralization
Newcomer's
Nickerson-Kveim
Nickles'
ninhydrin
Nippe's
nitrate reduction
nitric acid
nitric acid-magnesium sulfate
nitrites
nitrogen partition
nitropropiol
nitroprusside
nitroso-indole-nitrate
Nobel's
Noguchi's
Nonne's
Nonne-Apelt
nonverbal
Norrie' atropine
Nothnagel's
nuclear
nucleus
nucleo-albumin
Nyiri's
Nylander's
nystagmus

Ober's
Obermeyer's
Obermuller's
obturator
occult blood
Oliver's
one-stage prothrombin time
orcinol
organoleptic
orientation
orthotoluidine

osazone
Osgood-Haskins'
osmotic resistance
Osterberg's
Otani's
Ott's
oxyphenylsulfonic acid

Pachon's
Page and van Slyke's
Paget's
palmin
palmitin
pancreatic function
Pandy's
Papanicolaou
para-dimethyl-amino
    benzaldehyde
parallax
Parnum's
partial thromboplastin time
paternity
Patrick's
Patterson's
Paul's
Paul-Bunnell
Paunz'
Pavy's
Peck
Pelouse-Moore
Pels and Macht
pentose
Penzoldt's
Penzoldt-Fischer
peppermint
pepsin
peptone
perchloride
percutaneous tuberculin

Peret's
Peria's
Perls'
permanganate
peroxidase
Perthes'
Peterman's
Petri's
Pettenkofer's
Petzetaki's
phenacetin
phenol
phenolphthalein
phenolsulfonphthalein
phenoltetrachlorophalein
phenylhydrazine
phlorizin
phloroglucin
phosphatase
phosphoric acid
phrenic-pressure
phthalein
phytotoxin
Piazza's
picrotoxin
Pincus
Pintner-Patterson
Piorkowski's
Piria's
Pirquet's
plasmacrit
Plesch's
Plugge's
Poehl's
Pohl's
Politzer's
Pollacci's
Pollatschek-Porges
polyuria

Porges-Meier
Porges-Pollatschek
Porges-Salomon
porphobilinogen
Porter's
Porteus maze
Posner's
potassium iodide
Pratt's
precipitin
precipitation
Pregl's
pregnancy
Prendergast's
presumptive
Preyer's
Proetz
prostigmine
protein
protein tyrosin
proteose
prothrombin
protozoan
psychometric
Purdy's
purine bodies
pyramidon
pyridine
pyrocatechin

quadriceps
Queckenstedt's
quelling
Quick's
quinine
Quinlan's

Raabe's
Rabuteau's

Ralfe's
Ramon flocculation
Randolph's
Rantzman's
Raygat's
Rees's
Reh's
Rehberg's
Rehfuss'
Reichi's
Reid Hunt's
Reinsch's
Remont's
rennin
Renton's
resorcinol
resorcinol-hydrochloric acid
Reuss's
Reynold's
Rh
rhubarb
Rieckenberg's
Riegel's
Riegler's
Rimini's
Ringold
Rinne's
Rivalta's
Roberts'
Roffo's
Roger's
Roger-Josue
Romer's
Ronchese
Rorschach
Rose's
rose bengal
Rose-Waaler
Rosenbach's

Rosenbach-Gmelin
Rosenheim's
Rosenheim-Drummond
Rosenthal's
Rosett's
Rosin's
Ross's
Ross-Jones
Rossel's aloin
Rothera's
Rotter's
Rous's
Roussin's
Rowntree and Geraghty's
Rubin's
Rubino's
Rubner's
Ruge and Phillipp's
Ruhemann's
Rumpel-Leede
Russo's
Ruttan and Hardisty's
Ryan's skin
Rytz

Saathoff's
Sabrazes
saccharimeter
Sachs's
Sachs-Georgi
Sachs-Witebsky
Sachsse's
safranine
Sahli's
Sahli-Nencki
salicylaldehyde
salicylic acid
Salkowski's
Salkowski and Schipper's

salol
Salomon's
salvarsan
Sandrock
Sanford's
santonin
Saundby's
scarification
Schaffer's
Schalfijew's
Scherer's
Schick
Schiff's
Schiller's
Schilling
Schirmer's
Schlessinger's
Schmidt's
Schneider
Schneider's
Schonbein's
Schopfer's
Schroeder's
Schubert-Dannmeyer
Schulte's
Schultz's
Schultz-Charlton
Schultze's
Schultze's indophenol oxydase
Schumm's
Schurmann's
Schwabach
Schwartz's
Schwartz-McNeil
Schwarz's
Scivoletto's
secretin
sedimentation
Seidel's

Seidlitz powder
Selivanoff's
Sellards'
semen
Senn's
senna
sensitized sheep cell
sero-enzyme
serologic
serum neutralization
Sgambati's
shadow
Shaw-Mackenzie
Shear's
sheep cell agglutination
Sicard-Cantelouble
sickling
Siddall
Siebold and Bradbury's
sigma
Simonelli's
Sims'
Sivori and Rebaubi
skatole
Smith's
Snellen's
Snider match
sodium chloride balance
Soldaini's
Solera's
solubility
Sonnenschein's
specific gravity
sphenopalatine
Spiegler's
Spiro's
Staehlin's
Stanford-Binet
steapsin

Stein's
Steinle-Kahlenberg
Stenger
Stern's
Stern's fermentation
Stewart's
Stieglitz
Stock
Stokes's
Stokvis'
Storck's
Strange's
Strassburg's
Straus's biological
Strauss's
Struve's
strychnine
Stypven time
sulfonal
sulfosalicylic acid
sulfur
Sulkowitch's
Sullivan's
Suranyi's
syphilis
Szabo's

Takata-Ara
Taliqvist's
tannic acid
tannin
Tanret's
Tardieu's
Targowla's
taurine
Taylor's
Teichmann's
tellurite
Terman

thalleioquin
thermoprecipitin
thiocyanate
Thomas-Binetti
Thompson's
Thormahlen's
Thorn
thromboplastin generation
Thudichum's
thumb-nail thymol
   turbidity
thyroid
Tidy's
Tizzoni's
Tobey-Ayer
Tollens'
Tollens, Neuberg and
   Schwket's
Topfer's
Torquay's
tourniquet
Trambusti
trapeze
Trendelenburg's
Tretop's
Triboulet's
trichophytin
triketohydrindene
Trommer's
Trousseau's
trypsin
tryptophan
Tschernogowbou's
Tsuchiya's
tuberculin
Tuffier's
Twort
typhoidin
tyrosine

Tyson's
Tzanck

Ucko's
Udranszky's
Uffelmann's
Uhlenhuth's
Ulrich's
Ultzmann's
Umber's
uracil
urea
urease
uric acid
urobilin
urochromogen
urorosein
Urriolla's

Valenta's
Valsalva's
van Deen's
van den Bergh's
van der Velden's
vanillin
Van Slyke
Van Slyke and Cullen's
Vaughn and Novy's
Venning Browne
ventilation
Vernes'
virulence
Visscher-Bowman
Vitali's
vocabulary
Voelcker and Joseph's
Voge's
Vogel and Lee's
Vogus-Proskauer

Volhard's
Vollmer's
von Aldor's
von Dungern's
von Frisch
von Jaksch's
von Maschke's
von Pall's
von Pirquet's
von Recklinghausen's
von Zeynek and Mencki's
Vulpain

Waaler-Rose
Wagner's
Walter's bromide
Wang's
Warren's
Wassermann
Waterhouse pus
Watson-Schwartz
Weber's
Webster's
Weichdrodt's
Weidel's
Weil's
Weinberg's
Weinstein's
Weisman's
Weiss permanganate
Weiss's
Well-Felix
Welland's
Weltmann's serum
Welty's
Wender's
Wenzell's
Weppen's
Wernicke's

Wetzel's
Weyl's
Wheeler and Johnson's
Whipple's
Widal's
Wideroe's
Widmark's
Wilbrand's prism
Wilbur and Addis'
Wildbolz's
Wilkinson and Peter's
Williamson's blood
Wilson's
Winckler
Winslow's
Winternitz's
Wishart
Witz's
Wohlgemuth's
Woldman's
Wolff-Eisner
Wolff-Junghans
Woodbury's
Woods's
Worm-Muller
Wormley's
worsted
Wreden's
Wurster's
Wys's

xanthemia
xanthine
xanthroproteic
Xenopus
xylidine
xylose concentration

Yakinoff's
Yefimov's

Yerkes-Bridges
Young
Yvon's

Zaleski's
Zambrini's
Zangemeister
Zappacosta's
Zeisel's

Zeller's
Zenoni's
Ziechen's
Ziffern's
Zitovitch's
Zondek-Aschheim
Zouchlos'
Zsigmondy's gold number
Zwenger's

Surgical Incisions

Auvray

Banks and Laufman
Bar
Battle
Bergmann
Bevan
buttonhole

celiotomy
circumscribing
confirmatory
crescent
crosshatch
crucial (Cruciate)

Deaver
Dührssen

endaural
exploratory

Fergusson
Fowler

Gatellier

Halsted
Harmon
Heerman
hockey-stick

Kehr

Kocher
Kustner

Lamm
Langenbeck
lateral rectus
Lempert
Longuet

Mackenrodt
Mayo-Robson
McArthur
McBurney
median
Meyer

Ollier

paramedian
Parker
Perthe
Pfannenstiel
Phemister

relief

saber cut
semilunar

Wilde

Visscher

Dental Surfaces

axial	labial
	lingual
basal	
buccal	masticating
	masticatory
distal	mesial
glenoid	occlusal
incisal	subocclusal

Descriptive Positions, i.e., Anatomical

Bonner's
Bozeman's
Brickner's

Casselberry's
centric

dorsal
dorsoanterior
dorsoposterior
dorsosacral

eccentric
Edebohls

Fowler's
frontoanterior
frontoposterior

genucubital

hinge candylar
hinge mandibular
hinge terminal

intercuspal

knee-chest
knee-elbow

lateral recumbent

leapfrog
lithotomy

Mayo Robson's
mentoanterior
mentoposterior
Mercurio's

Noble's

occipitoanterior
occipitoiliac
occipitolevoanterior
occipitolevoposterior
occipitoposterior
occlusal

prone
protrusive

sacroanterior
Scultetus'
semiprone
Simon's
Sims'
supine

Trendelenburg's

Valentine's

Walcher

OFTEN USED WORD ABBREVIATIONS
OFTEN USED PRESCRIPTION ABBREVIATIONS
Abbreviations

A.A.	achievement age
AAL	anterior axillary line
abbr.	abbreviation
a.c.	ante collation or before meals
ACTH	adrenocorticotrophic hormone
a.d.	right ear
ADH	antidiuretic hormone
ad lib	at pleasure
adm.	administration
AEq	age equivalent
AHD	arteriosclerotic heart disease
AID	acute infectious disease
anat.	anatomy
ant.	anterior
ante	before
anti.	antidote
A.P.	anter-posterior or front to back; anterior pituitary gland
A.P.L.	anterior pituitary like
app.	appendix
A.Q.	achievement quotient
Aq.	water
aq. dest.	distilled water
ARD	acute respiratory disease
art.	artery
AS	Anglo-Saxon
ASCVD	arteriosclerotic cardiovascular disease
ASHD	arteriosclerotic heart disease
assn.	association
Asso; Assoc.	associate
AT-10	dihydrotachysterol
at. no.	atomic number
at. wt.	atomic weight
AU	ears (both)
A.V.	arteriovenous; atrioventricular
A-Z	Ascheim-Zondek
bact.	bacteriology

BAL	British Anti-Lewisite
baso.	basophil
BBA	born before arrival
BBT	basal body temperature
bd.	board
B.E.	barium enema
bet.	between
b.i.d.	twice daily
biol.	biology
B.M.R.	basal metabolic rate
BP	blood pressure
br.	branch, branches
brp	bathroom privileges
B.S.	blood sugar
BSP	bromsulphalein
BTU; B.Th.U.	British thermal unit
BUN	blood urea nitrogen
c̄	with
C	carbon
C	centigrade
c; cert; ct	certified
CBC	complete blood count
Ca	calcium
ca	cancer
Cal.	large calorie
cal.	small calorie
caps.	capsules
carbo.	carbohydrates
card; cardiog	cardiography
cardiol	cardiologist, cardiology
c.c.	chief complaint
cc.	cubic centimeter
cent.	centigrade
cf.	compare
cg.	centigram
CHD	congestive heart disease
chem.	chemistry
chm	chairman

Cl	chlorine
cm.	centimeter
CNS	central nervous system
commun	communicable
comp.	composition
cons	consultant, consulting
contra.	contraindication
conv.	convalescent
C. P.	cerebral palsy
cran	cranial
CSF	cerebrospinal fluid
Cu	copper, cuprum
CVA	cerebrovascular accident
CVD	cardiovascular disease
CVRD	cardiovascular renal disease
d.	daily
D.D.S.	dentist
DDT	dichloro-diphenyl-trichloroethane
def.	deficiency
der.	derivative
derm	dermatology
diag	diagnosis
dir	director
dis	disease
DJD	degenerative joint disease
DMSO	dimethyl sulfoxide
DNA	deoxyribonucleic acid
D.O.	Doctor of Osteopathy
DOA	dead on arrival
DPH	Doctor of Public Health
DPT	Diptheria, Pertussis, Tetanus
Dx.	diagnosis
E.	English
(e	alternate word ending
EENT	ear, eye, nose and throat
ECHO	entero-cytopathogenic human orphan virus
EDC	expected date of confinement
EDTA	ethylenediaminetetraacetate

EE	eye and ear
EEE	Encephalitis, Eastern Equine
EEG	electroencephalogram
e.g.	for example
EKG; ECG	electrocardiogram
elect.	electricity
elix	elixir
encephalog	encephalography
endocrin	endocrinology
EOM	extraocular movements
eos.	eosinophils
ESP	extrasensory perception
esp.	especially
ESR	erythrocyte sedimentation rate
etiol.	etiology
ex.	example
ext.	exterior, external
F	Fahrenheit
F.A.	first aid
FAD	flavine-adenine dinucleotide
FDA	Food and Drug Administration
Fe	iron, ferrum
fem.	female, feminine
ff. ind.	fact-finding index
FH	family history
fl	fluid
Fr.	French
frict.	friction
FSH	follicle stimulating hormone
funct.	function
FUO	fever of undetermined origin
FX	fracture
G.	Greek
g; gm	gram
gas-int; G.I.	gastro-intestinal
gastroent; ge	gastroenterology
GB	gall bladder
Ger.	German

Abbreviations

ger	geriatrics
GP	general practice
gr.	grain
grad.	graduate
GTH	gonadotropic hormone
GTT	glucose tolerance test
gtt	one drop
gtts	drops
G-U	genito-urinary
gyn; gyec	gynecology
H	hydrogen
h.	hour
H & E	hematoxylin and eosin
Hb	hemoglobin
HBP	high blood pressure
hematol	hematology
HEW	Health, Education and Welfare
HMO	Health Maintenance Organization
H_2O	water
hosp	hospital
ht.	height
I	iodine
I & O	intake and output
ICM	intercostal margin
ICS	intercostal space
ICSH	interstitial cell-stimulating hormone
i.e.	that is
IM	infectious mononucleosis
I.M.	intramuscular injection
immun	immunology
ind.	indication
Ind Med	industrial medicine
ind sur	industrial surgery
inf.	inferior
Infec. dis.	infectious disease
INH	isoniazid
inst.	institute
int.	intern, internal; interior

int med	internal medicine
IOP	intraocular pressure
IPPB	intermittent positive pressure breathing
I.Q.	intelligence quotient
I.U.	international unit
IV	intravenous
jt.	joint
K	potassium, kalium
kg	kilogram
KUB	kidney, ureter and bladder
KV	kilovolt
KW	kilowatt
L.	Latin
L & A	light and accomodation
L & W	living and well
lab	laboratory
lar; laryng	laryngology
lat.	lateral
lb.	pound
LCM	lymphocytic chorio-meningitis
LE	lupus erythematosus
LH	luteinizing hormone
LL.	late Latin
LLQ	left lower quadrant
L.M.D.	local medical doctor
L.M.P.	last menstrual period
L.O.A.	left occiput anterior
L.O.P.	left occiput posterior
L.S.P.	left sacroposterior
LTH	luteotropic hormone
LVN	licensed vocational nurse
LUQ	left upper quadrant
m.	male
M.Sc.	Master of Science
MA	mental age
malig	malignant
mat	maternity
MC	Medical Corps
mc	millicurie

MCHC	mean corpuscular hemoglobin concentration
mcg	microgram
MCV	mean corpuscular volume
med	medicine, medical
metab.	metabolism
mEq	milliequivalent
Mg	magnesium
mg.	milligram
mgh.	milligram-hour
min	one drop of water
min.	minim
ml.	milliliter
MLD	minimal lethal dose
MM	mucous membrane
mM	millimole
mm.	millimeter
mos.	months.
M.S.L.	midsternal line
Mt	membrane tympana
mu; u	micron
N	nitrogen
N and V	nausea and vomiting
Na	sodium
neur	neurologist, neurology
neuropath	neuropathology
N.F.	National Formulary
NFIP	National Foundation for Infantile Paralysis
NIH	National Institutes of Health
NND	new and nonofficial drugs
N.N.R.	new and nonofficial remedies
NP	nursing procedure
NPH insulin	neutral protamine hegedorn insulin
N.P.N.	nonprotein nitrogen
NS soln.	normal saline solution
nut.	nutrients
NVD	nausea, vomiting and diarrhea; Newcastle virus disease
NYD	not yet diagnosed
O	oxygen

ob; obst	obstetrician, obstetrics
o.d.	right eye
O.Fr.	Old French
o.l.; o.s.	left eye
O.M.	otitis media
OMPA	otitis media, purulent, acute
ONP	operating nursing procedure
OPD	outpatient department
oph; ophth	ophthalmology
opp.	opposite
O.R.	operating room
or; orth	orthopedics; orthopedist
orig.	origin
O.T.	old tuberculin
ot; oto; otol	otolaryngology
o.v.	both eyes
oz.	ounce
p	phosphorus
p.	page
P & A	percussion and auscultation
P.A.	pernicious anemia; professional association
PAL	posterior axillary line
PAS	para-amino salicylic acid
path	pathological; pathologist; pathology
PBI	protein bound iodine
pcu	packed cell volume
PDR	Physician's Desk Reference
ped; pd	pediatrics, pediatrician
periph vas dis	peripheral vascular disease
pert.	pertaining
P-G	post-graduate
PH	Public Health
phar	pharmacology, pharmacy
Ph.G.	graduate pharmacist
phy; phys	physician
phy med	physical medicine
phys	physiology
physiol	physiological; physiologist; physiology
physiother	physiotherapy

pl.	plural
plast sur	plastic surgery
PM & Rehab	physical medicine and rehabilitation
PMI	point of maximum impulse
post.	posterior
PPLO	pleuropneumonia-like organism
pre.	prefix
prenat	prenatal
pro.	protein
proct	proctology; proctologist
prog.	prognosis
prof	professor
PSRO	Professional Standards Regulatory
psy	psychiatrist, psychiatry
psych	psychologist, psychology
PT	physical therapy
pt.	pint
PTA	plasma thromboplastin component
q:	each, every
q.d.	every day
q.h.	every hour
q.i.d.	four times daily
q.s.	as much as suffices
qt.	quart
q.v.	which see
r	roentgen
RBC	red blood cell
RCM	right costal margin
rel.	relating
RES	reticuloendothelial system
RHD	rheumatic heart disease
rheum	rheumatic, rheumatism
RLF	retrolental fibroplasia
RLQ	right lower quadrant
R.N.	registered nurse
RNA	ribonucleic acid
R.O.A.	right occiput anterior
roent	roentgenologist, roentgenology
R.O.P.	right occiput posterior

R.Q.	respiratory quotient
RS	related subjects
R.T.	x-ray technician
R.U.	roentgen unit
RUQ	right upper quadrant
RVH	right ventricular hypertrophy
S	sulfur
s.	left
SBE	sub-acute bacterial endocarditis
SCUBA	self-contained underwater breathing apparatus
S.G.O.	Surgeon General's Office
SGO-T	serum glutamic oxalopyruvic transaminase
sig.	let it be labeled
sing.	singular
soc.	society
sp. gr.	specific gravity
SPCA	serum prothrombin conversion accelerator
ss, ss	half
STS	serologic test for syphilis
sup.	superior
supt.	superintendent
sur; surg	surgeon, surgery
sym	symptoms
symb	symbol
syn	synonym
syph	syphilologist, syphilology
T.	temperature
T & A	tonsillectomy and adenoidectomy
TAT	tetanus antitoxin
TAO	triacetyloleandomycin
Tb; Tbc	tuberculosis
Thor sur	thoracic surgery
tid	thrice daily
TLC	tender loving care
TPR	temperature, pulse and respiration
TSH	thyroid stimulating hormone
UCHD	usual childhood diseases
USA	United States Army
USN	United States Navy

U.S.P.	United States Pharmacopeia
U.S.P.H.S.	United States Public Health Service
URI	upper respiratory infection
v.	volt
VA	Veteran's Administration
Vas Dis	vascular disease
VD	venereal disease
V.D.R.L.	venereal disease research laboratory test
viz.	namely
VOD	vision right eye
VOS	vision left eye
WBC	white blood cell
WEE	Western Equine Encephalitis
WHO	World Health Organization
WN, WD	well nourished, well developed

Prescription Abbreviations

a̅a̅ (ana)	of each (equal parts)
a.c. (ante cibum)	before meals
aq. (aqua)	water
b.i.d. (bis in die)	twice a day
caps. (capsula)	capsule
chart. (chartulae)	papers (powders)
ft. (fiat)	make
h.s. (hora somni)	at bedtime
M. (misce)	mix
m. dict. (modo dictu)	as directed
non rep. (non repetatur)	do not repeat (do not refill)
o.d. (oculus dexter)	right eye
o.s. (oculus sinister)	left eye
p.c. (post cibum)	after meals

p.r.n. (pro re nata	as needed
q.h. (quaque hora)	every hour
q.i.d. (quater in die)	four times a day
q.s. (quantum sufficit)	a sufficient quantity
℞ (recipe)	take (thou) a recipe
sig. (signa)	write on label
stat. (statim)	immediately
t.i.d. (ter in die)	three times a day
ut dict. (ut dictum)	as directed
gr.	grain or grains
gtt. (gutta(e))	drop(s)
m.	minim
3 $\overline{\text{iss}}$	one and one-half drams
3 $\overline{\text{i}}$	one ounce
3 $\overline{\text{ss}}$	one-half ounce
cc.	cubic centimeter
Gm.	gram
mg.	milligram
mcg.	microgram
ml.	milliliter

Reprinted from the twentieth edition of *The Pocketbook of Medical Tables* with the permission of Smith, Kline and French Laboratories.

SECTION VI
COMMONLY PRESCRIBED
PHARMACEUTICALS—GENERIC NAMES

acetaminophen
acetazolamide
acetic acid
acetyl sulfisoxazole
adiphenine hydrochloride
adrenocorticotropic hormone
allantoin
aluminum hydroxide
aminobenzoic acid
aminophylline
aminosalicylic acid
amitriptyline hydrochloride
ammonium chloride
amobarbital
amphetamine
amphotericin
ampicillin
ampicillin trihydrate
amylolytic enzyme
androgen
anthraquinone
antipyrine
ascorbic acid
aspirin
atropine
bacitracin
barbiturate
belladonna
benzocaine
benzoic
benzthiazide
benzyl alcohol
betamethasone
bioflavonoids
bisacodyl
bishydroxy coumarin

brompheniramine maleate
butabarbital
butalbital
butyrophenone
caffeine
calamine
calciferol
calcium carbonate
calcium gluconate
calcium panothenate
candicidin
cantharidin
carbamide
carbenicillin indanyl sodium
carboxymethylcellulose
    sodium
carisoprodol
cascara sagrada
cephalexin monohydrate
cephaloglycin dihydrate
cephaloridine
cephalothin sodium
chloral hydrate
chloramphenicol
chlordantoin
chlordiazepoxide
    hydrochloride
chlorhydroxyquinoline
chlorophyll
chloroquine hydrochloride
chlorothiazide
chlorphenesin carbamate
chlorpheniramine gluconate
chlorpheniramine maleate
chlorpromazine
chlorpropamide

chlorprothixene
chlortetracycline
chlorzoxazone
chorionic gonadotropin
cinoxate
clidinium bromide
chlorzoate dipotassium
codeine phosphate
colchicine
colistimethate sodium
colistin sulfate
cortisone acetate
coumarin
cyanocobalamin
cyclizine
cyclophosphamide
cyproheptadine hydrochloride
danthron
demeclocycline
deoxycorticosterone
desipramine hydrochloride
desoxycorticosterone acetate
desoxyribonuclease
dexamethasone
dexbrompheniramine maleate
dexpanthenol
dextran
dextroamphetamine sulfate
dextromethophran
    hydrobromide
diatrizoate
diazepam
dibucaine hydrochloride
dicyclomine hydrochloride
diethylpropion hydrochloride
diethylstilbestrol
digitalis
digitoxin

dihydromorphione
    hydrochloride
dihydroxy aluminum
    aminoacetate
diiodohydroxyquinoline
dimenhydrinate
dimercaprol
dioctyl
diperodon
diphenhydramine
diphenoxylate hydrochloride
diphenylhydantoin
dipyrone
d-isoephedrine sulfate
doxepin
doxepin hydrochloride
doxycycline
dyphylline
endocrine
entsufon
ephedrine
ergocalciferol
ergonovine maleate
ergot
ergotamine tartrate
erythromycin
estradiol
estrogen
ethaverine hydrochloride
ethinyl estradiol
ethosuximide
ethynodiol diacetate
euprocin hydrochloride
ferrous fumerate
ferrous sulfate
fibrinolysin
fludrocortisone acetate
fluocinolone acetonide

fluorine
fluphenazine
flurandrenolide
flurazepam hydrochloride
folic acid
furazolidone
gentamicin sulfate
glucagon
glutamic acid
glutethimide
glycerin
glycerol guaiacolate
glycopyrrolate
gramicidin
griseofulvin
haloperidol
heparin
hexachlorophene
homatropine methyl
    bromide
hydantoin
hydralazine hydrochloride
hydrochlorothiazide
hydrocodone bitartrate
hydrocortisone
hydroflumethiazide
hydromorphone
hydroquinone
hydroxyamphetamine
    hydrobromide
hydroxychloroquine sulfate
hydroxyzine hydrochloride
hyoscine hydrobromide
hyoscyamine
ichthamol
imipramine hydrochloride
indomethacin
inositol

iodochlorhydroxyquin
iopanoic acid
ipecac
ipodate
isoniazid
isopropamide
isopropyl
isoproterenol
kanamycin sulfate
kaolin
lactobacillus acidophilus
lactobacillus bulgaricus
lantocide C
lanolin
lecithin
levallorphan tartrate
levartenol bitartrate
levodopa
lidocaine
lincomycin hydrochloride
    monohydrate
liotrix
lipolytic
lithium carbonate
luturin
lysine
magnesium carbonate
magnesium hydroxide
magnesium trisilicate
mannitol
mazindol
meclizine hydrochloride
medoxyprogesterone acetate
meglumine diatrizoate
meglumine iodipamide
menthol
meperidine
mephenytoin

mephobarbital
meprobamate
mercaptomerin sodium
mestranol
methacycline hydrochloride
methadone hydrochloride
methamphetamine hydrochloride
methapyrilene
methapyrilene fumerate
methaqualone
metharbital
methdilazine
methenamine
methicillin
methimazole
methiodal sodium
methionine
methocarbamol
methotrexate
methscopolamine
methylcellulose
methyldopa
methylene blue
methylphenidate hydrochloride
methylprednisolone
methylprylon
methylsergide maleate
methyl testosterone
metronidazole
mithramycin
monoamine-oxidase
nafcillin
nalidixic acid
naloxone hydrochloride
naphazoline hydrochloride
neomycin
neostigmine bromide
neostigmine methyl sulfate
niacinamide

nicotinic acid
nifuroxime
nikethamide
nitrofurantoin
nitrofurazone
nitroglycerin
nitromersol
nonoxynol
norethindrone acetate
norethynodrel
norgestrel
nortriptyline hydrochloride
nux vomita
nystatin
opium
orphenadrine citrate
oxacillin sodium
oxazepam
oxycodone
oxymetazoline hydrochloride
oxymetholone
oxyphencyclimine
    hydrochloride
oxyphenonium bromide
oxyquinoline sulfate
oxytetracycline
oxytocin
panthenol
pantothenate calcium
papaverine hydrochloride
para-aminobenzoate
para-aminobenzoic acid
para-aminosalicylic
paraldehyde
paramethadione
paramethasone acetate
paregoric
p-disobutylphenoxypoly-
    ethoxyethanol

pectin
penicillin G, benzathine
penicillin G, dibenzylethyene
   diamine
penicillinase
pentaerythritol tetranitrate
pentzocine hydrochloride
pentobarbital
pentylenetetrazol
pepsin
perphenazine
phenacemide
phenacetin
phenazopyridine
phendimetrazine tartrate
phenethicillin potassium
phenformin
pheniramine maleate
phenmetrazine hydrochloride
phenobarbital
phenol
phenolphthalein
phenothiazine
phenoxybenzamine HC1
phensuximide
phentermine
phentolamine
phenylalanine
phenylbutazone
phenylephrine
phenylmercuric acetate
phenylpropanolamine
phenyltoloxamine citrate
phenyltoloxamine dihydrogen
   citrate
phosphorated carbohydrate
physostigamine
pipenzolate bromide
piperacetazine

piperazine
pitressin tannate
polycarbophil
polyestradiol phosphate
polymixin
polyoxyethylene
potassium guaiacolsulfonate
prednisolone
prednisone
primaquin phosphate
primidone
probenecid
procaine
prochlorperazine
progesterone
promethazine hydrochloride
propranodol
propantheline bromide
propoxyphene napsylate
propylene glycol
propylhexedrine
proteolytic
protoveratrine
protriptyline
pseudoephedrine
psyllium
pyridoxine
pyrilamine
pyrvinium pamoate
quinethazone
quinidine
racephedrine
rauwolfia
reserpin
resorcin
resorcinol
riboflavin
rutin
salicylamide

salicylic acid
scopolamine
secobarbital
selenium sulfate
senna
silicone
simethicone
sodium amytal
sodium ampicillin
sodium butabarbital
sodium cloxacillin
  monohydrate
sodium dehydrocholate
sodium dicloxacillin
  monohydrate
sodium levothyroxine
sodium liothyronine
sodium pentobarbital
sodium secobarbital
sodium sulfacetamide
sodium sulfbromophthalein
sodium thiopental
sodium thiosulfate
sodium warfarin
spectinomycin dihydrochloride
  pentahydrate
streptokinase-streptodornase
sulfacetamide
sulfadiazine
sulfamethazole
sulfamethoxazole
sulfanilamide
sulfathiazole
sulfisoxazole
terpin hydrate
testosterone
tetracaine hydrochloride

tetracycline
tetrahydrozoline
  hydrochloride
theobromine
theophylline
thiamine HC1
thimerosal
thioridazine
thiothixene
thioxanthene
thrombin
thyroid
thyroxine
tolazoline hydrochloride
tolbutamide
tolnoftate
triacetin
triamcinolone
tridihexethyl chloride
trifluoperazine hydrochloride
trihexphenidyl
trimeprazine tartrate
trimethadione
trimethobenzamide hydrochloride
tripelennamine
triprolidine
trisulfapyrimidines
troleandomycin
undecylenate
undecylenic acid
vancomycin
vincristen sulfate
xanthine
xylometazoline hydrochloride
zirconium oxide
zolamine hydrochloride

COMMONLY PRESCRIBED
PHARMACEUTICALS—PROPRIETARY NAMES

Aarane
Achromycin V
Achrostatin V
Actidil
Actifed
Adapin
Adeflor
Adrenosem
Afrin
Aldactazide
Aldactone
Aldomet
Aldoril
Allbee
Ambenyl
Amcill
Amesec
Ampicillin
Amytal
Ananase
Anaspaz
Anavar
Android
Antabuse
Antepar
Antivert
Anusol
Apresoline
Aquasol
Aralen
Aristocort
Artane
Asbron
Ascriptin
Atarax
Atromid

Aventyl
Azo Gantanol
Azo Gantrisin
Azo-mandelamine
Azulfidine
Bactrim
Bamadex
Becofin
Belladenal
Bellergac
Benadryl
Bendectin
Benemid
Benisone
Bentyl
Benylin
Benzedrine
Berocca
Beta-chlor
Betepen
Bontril
Bristacycline
Bristamycin
Bronchobid
Brondecon
Butazolidin
Butibel
Butiserpazide
Butisol
Butiserpine
Butisol
Cafergot
Calcinate
Camalox
Cantil
Cardilate

Cedilanid
Celestone
Celontin
Chloromycetin
Chlor-trimeton
Choledyl
Chymoral
Cleocin
Cogentin
Colace
Colbenemid
Combid
Compazine
Compocillin
Conar
Cordrian
Coricidin
Cortisporin
Coryban
Cotazyn
Coumadin
Crystodygin
Cyclospasmol
Cytomel
Cytoxan
Dalmane
Darvocet
Darvon
Deaner
Decadron
Declomycin
Declostatin
Deltasone
Demazin
Demerol
Demulin
Deprol
Deronil
Desoxyn

Dexamyl
Dexedrine
Diabinese
Dialose
Diamox
Dibenzyline
Dicumarol
Didrex
Digoxin
Dilantin
Dimacol
Dimetane
Dimetapp
Disomer
Disopherol
Diupres
Diuril
Dolene
Donnatol
Donnazyme
Dorbane
Doriden
Dramamine
Drixorial
Dulcolax
Dyazide
Dynapen
Elavil
Elixophyllin
Emperin
Exprazil
E-mycin
Enduron
Enduronyl
Engran
Enovid
Equagesic
Equanil
Erythrocin

Erythromycin
Esidrex
Eskabarb
Eskalith
Eskatrol
Estinyl
Etrafon
Euthroid
Evex
Fastin
Fedrazil
Feminins
Feosol
Ferancee
Fer-in-sol
Fero-folic
Fero-grad
Ferrobid
Filibon
Fiorinal
Flagyl
Forhistal
Formatrix
Fulvicin
Gantanol
Gantrisin
Garamycin
Gaviscon
Gelusil
Gemonil
Geocillin
Gitaligin
Grifulvin
Grisactin
Haladol
Halotestin
Harmonyl
Histabid
Hormonin

Hydergine
Hydrodiuril
Hydromox
Hydropres
Hygroton
Iberet
Iberol
Ilosone
Ilutycin
Imuran
Inderal
Indocin
Intal
Indo-niacin
Ionamin
Isoniazid
Isopto-carpine
Isordil
Isuprel
Kafucin
Kantrex
Kaon
Keflex
Kenalog
K-lyte
Kolantyl
Lanoxin
Larodopa
Lasix
Leukeran
Librax
Libritabs
Librium
Lincocin
Lithane
Loestrin
Lomotil
Maalox
Macrodantin

Mandelamine
Maolate
Marax
Mebaral
Medicone
Medrol
Mellaril
Menest
Meprobomate
Meprospan
Merezine
Mesantoin
Methergine
Meticorten
Mi-cebrin
Midrin
Milpath
Miltown
Minocin
Mintezol
Moderil
Mol-iron
Mudrane
Multicebrin
Mulvidren
Mylanta
Mylicon
Myosoline
Mysteclin-F
Naldecon
Naqua
Naturetin
Navane
Negram
Nembutal
Neobiotic
Neo-decracon
Neopap
Neosporin

Nicotinic acid
Nilstat
Nitroglycerin
Nitrospan
Noctec
Noludar
Norflex
Norgesic
Norinyl
Norlestrin
Norpramin
Novahistine
Ogen
Omnipen
Optilets
Oracon
Oragrafin
Oralen
Oreton
Orinase
Ornacol
Ornade
Ornex
Ortho-novum
Oscal
Ovral
Ovulen
Pabalate
Pamine
Panmycin
Paradione
Parafon
Paredrine
Paregoric
Parest
Pathilon
Pathocil
Pavabid
Pedameth

Pediamycin
Penbritin
Penicillin
Pentids
Penvee
Percodan
Periactin
Peri-colace
Peritrate
Permitil
Pertofrane
Pfizerpen
Phenaphen
Phenergan
Phenobarbital
Phenurone
Placidyl
Polaramine
Polycillin
Polymagma
Pondimin
Povan
Pramilet
Prednisone
Preludin
Premarin
Principen
Priscoline
Pro-banthene
Prolixin
Proloid
Pronestyl
Prostaphlin
Provera
Pyribenzamine
Pyridium
Quaalude
Quibron
Quide

Quinamm
Quinidex
Quinidine sulfate
Raudixin
Rauzide
Regitine
Regroton
Renese
Reserpine
Ritalin
Robaxin
Robinul
Roblate
Rondec
Rondomycin
Salutensin
Sanorex
Sansert
Seconal
Ser-AP-es
Serax
Seromycin
Serpasil
Sinequan
Singlet
Sinubid
Sinutab
Soma
Sparine
Stelazine
Sterazolidin
Stero-darvon
Stresscaps
Stress tabs
Stuartinic
Sudafed
Sumycin
Surbex-T
Synalar

Synalgos
Synthroid
Tacaryl
Tace
Talwin
Tandearil
Tao
Taractan
Tedral
Tegopen
Teldrin
Telepague
Temaril
Tempra
Tenuate
Tepanil
Terramycin
Terrastatin
Tessalon
Tetracycline HCl
Tetracyn
Tetrastatin
Tetrex
Theragran
Thiosulfil
Thorazine
Thyroid
Thyrolar
Tigan
Titralac
Tofranil
Tolinase
Torecan
Tranxene
Trasentine
Triaminic
Triavil

Tridione
Trilafon
Trinsicon
Troph-iron
Trophite
Tuinal
Tussagesic
Tussend
Tuss-ornade
Tylenol
Unipen
Urised
Urispas
Urobiotic
Ursinus
Uticillin
Valisone
Valium
Valmid
Vanobid
Vasodilan
V-cillin
Veetids
Verequad
Versapen
Vibramycin
Vicon
Vidaylin
Vioform
Vistaril
Viterra
Vivactil
Voranil
Wyanaid
Zarontin
Zeste
Zyloprim

SECTION VII

LIST OF RECOGNIZED MEDICAL SPECIALTIES

Allergist—A physician who treats diseases caused by sensitivity to substances found in food, water, air, etc.

Anesthesiologist—A physician specializing in the administration of drugs for the relief of pain and discomfort, usually during operative procedures.

Cardiologist—A physician who diagnoses and treats diseases of the heart and blood vessels.

Dermatologist—A physician who diagnoses and treats disease of the skin and integument.

Endocrinologist—A physician, usually a specialist in internal medicine, who manages problems associated with the endocrine (glandular) system.

Endodontist—One who specializes in the diagnosis and treatment of diseases and injuries of the dental pulp and periapecal tissues of the teeth.

Exodontist—A dentist who extracts teeth.

Gastroenterologist—A physician, usually an internist, who deals with diseases of the stomach, intestine and associated organs.

General Practitioner—A physician who diagnoses and treats general disease of the entire body, usually in all ages.

Geriatrician—A physician who handles medical problems of the elderly.

Gynecologist—A physician specializing in medical and surgical disorders of the female reproductive system.

Industrialist—A physician who specializes in medical problems of industry.

Internist—A physician who specializes in diagnosis and treatment of non-surgical medical diseases.

Neurologist—A physician who diagnoses and treats nonpsychiatric disease of the nervous system.

Obstetrician—A physician who cares for a woman before, during and after childbirth.

Oncologist—A physician who specializes in the diagnosis and treatment of tumors.

Ophthalmologist—A physician who specializes in caring for diseases of the eye.

Oral Surgeon—A dentist who surgically treats natural or traumatic diseases of the mouth and adjacent tissue.

Orthodontist—A dentist trained to treat malformed teeth and oral problems.

Orthopedist—A physician who specializes in disease of the bones, joints, muscles, etc.

Osteopath—One who has been awarded a degree of Doctor of Osteopathy (D.O.). This field encompasses all of medicine with particular emphasis on the manipulation of the skeletal system to treat illness.

Otolaryngologist—A physician specializing in the disorders of the ear, nose and throat.

Pathologist—A physician who specializes in the disorders of diseased tissue or body fluids, usually under laboratory conditions.

Pediatrician—A physician who specializes in the treatment and care of infants, children and adolescents.

Pedodontist—A dentist who specializes in the treatment and prevention of disease of the gums.

Physiatrist—A physician specializing in the rehabilitation of patients following disease, trauma or surgery.

Plastic Surgeon—A physician who specializes in the reconstruction and repair of diseased, damaged or poorly functioning tissue.

Preventive Medicine—A medical specialty practiced by a physician whose main interest is in the prevention of disease and its spread.

List of Recognized Medical Specialties

Proctologist—A physician who treats diseases of the rectum, anus and large intestine.

Psychiatrist—A physician who treats and prevents mental health disorders.

Radiologist—A physician who specializes in the use of radiation to diagnose and/or treat disease.

Surgeon—A physician who operates to cure or prevent disease.

Urologist—A physician who specializes in the treatment of disease of the urogenital system (bladder, kidneys, penis, etc.).

ALASKA

Alaska Health Science Library
P O Box 7-741
Anchorage, AK 99510

ALABAMA

Ralph Brown Draughon Library
Auburn University
Auburn, AL 36830
Tel. (205) 826-5409

Baptist Medical Center Princeton
701 Princeton Ave.
Birmingham, AL 35211
Tel. (205) 785-8031 Ext. 360

Medical Library
Carraway Methodist Medical Center
1615 North 25th Street
Birmingham, AL 35234
Tel. (205) 254-6265

Lister Hill Library of the Health
Sciences
University of Ala. in Birm.
University Station
Birmingham, AL 35294
Tel. (205) 934-5460
Twx. JA-MED-LIB BHM
810-733-3613

Professional Library
USAF Hospital
Building 50
Maxwell AFB, AL 36112
Tel. (205) 265-5621 Ext. 7807

Biomedical Library
University of South Alabama
Mobile, AL 36688
Tel. (205) 460-7043

School of Nursing Library
Troy State University
P O Drawer 588
Montgomery, AL 36101
Tel. (205) 264-3912

Medical Library
V A Hospital
Tuscaloosa, AL 35401
Tel. (205) 553-3760 Ext. 263

Medical Library
Veterans Administration
V A Hospital
Tuskegee, AL 36083
Tel. (205) 727-0550 Ext. 647

Health Science Library
University of Alabama
P.O. Box 2938
University, AL 35486

ARKANSAS

Regional Health Sciences Lib.
Sparks Regional Medical Center
1311 So. I St.
Ft. Smith, AR 72901
Tel. (501) 441-4221
Twx. JA 910-723-7697

Baptist Medical Center Library
9600 W. 12th Street
Little Rock, AR 72201
Tel. (501) 227-2671

Medical Library
Consolidated VA Hospital
300 E. Roosevelt Rd.
Little Rock, AR 72206
Tel. (501) 372-8361 Ext. 294

Library
University of Arkansas Med.Center
P.O. Box 2381
Little Rock, AR 72203
Tel. (501) 664-5000 Ext. 257
Twx. ARU-M-LIB- 910-722-7349

ARIZONA

Medical Library
Arizona State Hospital
2500 East Van Buren
Phoenix, AZ 85008
Tel. (602) 244-1331 Ext. 278

Medical Library
Good Samaritan Hospital
P.O. Box 2989
Phoenix, AZ 85062
Tel. (602) 252-6611 Ext. 3627

Medical Library
Maricopa County General Hospital
2601 E. Roosevelt
Phoenix, AZ 85008
Tel. (602) 267-5197

Maricopa County Med.
Society Library

2025 N. Central Ave.
Phoenix, AZ 85004
Tel. (602) 252-8054
Twx. MCMSL-PHOENIX
109-511-598

Medical Library
St. Joseph's Hospital
P.O. Box 2017
Phoenix, AZ 85001
Tel. (602) 277-6611 Ext. 3362

Arizona Medical Center Library
University of Arizona
Tucson, AZ 85724
Tel. (602) 882-6241
Twx. AZU-M-TUCSON 910-952-1238

CALIFORNIA

Medical Library
La Vina Hospital
for Respiratory Diseases
3900 N. Lincoln
Altadena, CA 91001
Tel. 791-1241 Ext. 219

Medical Library
Tripler Army Medical Center
APO San Francisco, CA 96438

Supply & Services Division
US Army Hospital-Okinawa Japan
APO San Francisco, CA 96331

Professional Library
Atascadero State Hospital
Drawer A

Atascadero, CA 93422
Tel. (805) 466-2200 Ext. 26

Medical Library
Saint Joseph Hospital
501 Buena Vista
Burbank, CA 91503

Medical Library
Peninsula Hospital
1703 El Camino Real
Burlingame, CA 94010
Tel. (415) 697-4061

Medical Library
Fairview State Hospital
2501 Harbor Blvd.
Costa Mesa, CA 92626

Health Sciences Library HSTS
University of California-Davis
Davis, CA 95616
Tel. (916) 752-1162

Medical Library
Rancho Los Amigos Hospital
7601 E. Imperial Hwy.
Downey, CA 90242
Tel. (213) 922-7696

Medical Library
Rio Hondo Memorial Hospital
8300 E. Telegraph Road
Downey, CA 90240
Tel. (213) 861-6761

Piness Medical Library
City of Hope

Duarte, CA 91010
Tel. (213) 359-8111 Ext. 211

Professional Library
Sonoma State Hospital
P.O. Box 1400
Eldridge, CA 95431
Tel. (707) 966-1011

Department of the Army
    Med. Library
U.S. Army Medical Dept. Activity
    MEDDAC Fort Ord
Fort Ord, CA 93941
Tel. (408) 242-3889

Medical Library
Valley Med. Center of Fresno
445 S. Cedar Ave.
Fresno, CA 93702

Medical Library
NAPA State Hospital
Imola, CA 94558
Tel. (707) 226-2011 Ext. 477

Allergan Pharmaceuticals Library
Allergan Pharmaceuticals
2525 Du Pont Drive
Irvine, CA 92664
Tel. (714) 833-8880 Ext. 271

Medical Sciences Library
University of California-Irvine
Irvine, CA 92664
Tel. (714) 833-6651
Twx. AZ 910-595-1510

Hupp Medical Library
Scripps Clinic & Research Fdn.
476 Prospect St.
La Jolla, CA 92037
Tel. (714) 454-6141

Biomedical Library
University of Calif.-San Diego
La Jolla, CA 92037
Tel. (714) 453-2000 Ext. 1979
Twx. CUSD-BIOMED
910-337-1279

Hospital Library
VA Hospital
Livermore, CA 94550
Tel. (415) 447-2560

Vernier Radcliffe Memorial Library
Loma Linda University
Loma Linda, CA 92354
Tel. (714) 796-7311 Ext. 2916
Twx. LLNDAU LIBRARY
910-332-1314

Joseph E. Bellis Medical Library
Bauer Hospital-St. Mary Medical Ctr.
P.O. Box 887
Long Beach, CA 90801
Tel. (213) 435-4441

Medical Library
Long Beach Community Hospital
1720 Termino Ave.
Long Beach, CA 90804
Tel. (213) 597-6655 Ext. 351

Medical Library
Memorial Hospital Medical Center

2801 Atlantic Avenue
Long Beach, CA 90801
Tel. (213) 595-3841

Medical Library
Naval Regional Medical Center
7500 Carson St.
Long Beach, CA 90801
Tel. (213) 421-4741 Ext. 287

Medical Library
Pacific Hospital
2776 Pacific Ave.
Long Beach, CA 90806
Tel. (213) 595-1911 Ext. 291

Medical Library
VA Hospital
5901 E. 7th St.
Long Beach, CA 90804

Medical Library
Children's Hospital of Los Angeles
4650 Sunset Blvd.
Los Angeles, CA 90027
Tel. (213) 663-3341 Ext. 255
Twx. CHLA LSA 910-321-2468

Medical Library
Kaiser Foundation Hospital
4867 Sunset Blvd.
Los Angeles, CA 90027
Tel. (213) 663-8411 Ext. 1340

The Library
Los Angeles City Medical Assn.
634 S. Westlake Ave.
Los Angeles, CA 90057
Tel. (213) 483-4555

Medical Library
Los Angeles Orthopaedic Hospital
2400 Flower St.
Los Angeles, CA 90007
Tel. (213) 747-4481 Ext. 228

Anna Freud Research Library
Reiss-Davis Child Study Center
9760 W. Pico Blvd.
Los Angeles, CA 90035
Tel. (213) 273-0111 Ext. 301

Biomedical Library
University of California
Center for the Health Sciences
Los Angeles, CA 90024
Tel. (213) 825-5781
Twx. CLU-BIOMEDUCLA
910-342-6897

Norris Medical Library
USC School of Medicine
2025 Zonal Avenue
Los Angeles, CA 90033
Tel. (213) 226-2232
Twx. USCNORRISM LSA
910-321-2434

Courville-Abbott Memorial Library
White Memorial Medical Center
1720 Brooklyn Ave.
Los Angeles, CA 90033
Tel. (213) 269-9131 Ext. 215

Medical Library
Merced County General Hospital

P.O. Box 231
Merced, CA 95340
Tel. (209) 723-2861

Medical Library
Alameda Contra Costa Med. Assn.
2850 Vallecito Pl.
Oakland, CA 94606
Tel. (415) 534-8055 Ext. 257

School of Nursing Library
Kaiser Foundation
3451 Piedmont Ave.
Oakland, CA 94611
Tel. (415) 645-6485

Medical Library
Kaiser Foundation Hospital
280 Mac Arthur Blvd. W.
Oakland, CA 94611
Tel. (415) 645-5033

Medical Library
Naval Regional Medical Center
Bldg. 500
Oakland, CA 94627
Tel. (415) 639-2070 Ext. 2031
Twx. NAV HOSP OAK 910-366-7333

Medical Library
Samuel Merritt Hospital
Hawthorne & Webster
Oakland, CA 94609
Tel. (415) 655-4000 Ext. 150

Burlew Medical Library
St. Joseph Hospital
P.O. Box 5627

Orange, CA 92667
Tel. (714) 968-1352

Library
Syntex Corp.
3401 Hillview
Palo Alto, CA 94304
Tel. (415) 327-0110 Ext. 337

Health Science Library
Huntington Memorial Hospital
100 Congress Street
Pasadena, CA 91105
Tel. 796-0371
Twx. NA 910-588-3277

Staff Library
Pacific State Hospital
Box 100
Pomona, CA 91768
Tel. (714) 595-1221

Medical Library
Porterville State Hospital
P.O. Box 2000
Porterville, CA 93257

Paul H. Guttman Library
Sacramento County Med. Society
5380 Elvas Avenue
Sacramento, CA 95819

Thompson Medical Library
Naval Regional Medical Center
Bldg. 8
San Diego, CA 92134
Tel. (714) 233-2367

Rees Stealy Med. Clinic Library
2001 4th Ave.
San Diego, CA 92101
Tel. (714) 234-6216

Medical Library
VA Hospital
San Diego, CA 92161
Tel. (714) 453-7500 Ext. 3421

Schmidt Library
Calif. College of Podiatric Medicine
P.O. Box 7855 Rincon Annex
San Francisco, CA 94120
Tel. (415) 563-3444 Ext. 246-247

Emge Medical Library
Children's Hospital of
San Francisco
P.O. Box 3805
San Francisco, CA 94119
Tel. (415) 387-8700 Ext. 534

Medical Library
Harkness Community Hospital
1400 Fell St.
San Francisco, CA 94117
Tel. (415) 346-8781

Medical Library
Kaiser/Permanente Medical Center
2425 Geary Blvd—P.O. Box 7612
San Francisco, CA 94120
Tel. 929-4101

Medical Library
Rm. 338 Bldg. 1100
Letterman Army Medical Center

Presidio of San Francisco
San Francisco, CA 94129
Tel. (415) 561-2465

Sinai Memorial Library
Mt. Zion Hospital & Med. Center
Box 7921
San Francisco, CA 94120
Tel. (415) 567-6600

Medical Library
St. Mary's Hospital & Medical Center
2200 Hayes Street
San Francisco, CA 94117
Tel. (415) 668-1000 Ext. 319

The Library-Acquisitions Division
Univ. of Calif.-San Francisco
San Francisco, CA 94143
Tel. (415) 666-2334
Twx. NA 910-372-6518

Santa Clara Valley Medical
Center Library
751 S. Bascom Ave.
San Jose, CA 95128
Tel. (408) 293-0262 Ext. 255

San Mateo County
Health & Welfare Library
225 37th Ave.
San Mateo, CA 94403

Medical Library
Marin General Hospital
Box 2129
San Rafael, CA 94902
Tel. 461-0100

Medical Library
Santa Ana Community Hospital
600 E. Washington Ave.
Santa Ana, CA 92701
Tel. (714) 542-6744 Ext. 342

Santa Barbara County Medical
Society Library
300 W. Pueblo St.
Santa Barbara, CA 93105
Tel. (805) 966-7393

Medical Library
Kaiser Foundation Hospital
900 Kiely Blvd.
Santa Clara, CA 95051
Tel. (408) 244-5500 Ext. 296

St. John's Hospital
Kyser Medical Library
1328 22nd St.
Santa Monica, CA 90404
Tel. (213) 829-5111 Ext. 197

Medical Center Library
Santa Monica Hospital
1225 15th St.
Santa Monica, CA 90404
Tel. (213) 451-1511 Ext. 280

Medical Library
Comm. Hospital of Sonoma County
3325 Chanate Rd.
Santa Rosa, CA 95402
Tel. 544-3340

Medical Library
Kaiser/Permanente Medical Center
1200 El Camino Real

South San Francisco, CA 94080
Tel. (415) 876-0408

Lane Medical Library
Stanford Univ. Medical Center
Stanford, CA 94305
Tel. (415) 321-1200 Ext. 5111

Science Library
University of the Pacific
Stockton, CA 95204
Tel. (209) 946-2568

Medical Library
David Grant USAF Hospital
Travis AFB, CA 94535
Tel. (707) 438-3257

Library for Medical & Health
Sciences
Valley Presbyterian Hospital
15107 Vanowen St.
Van Nuys, CA 91405
Tel. (213) 782-6600 Ext. 211

Medical Library
Kaiser Foundation Hospital
1425 South Main Street
Walnut Creek, CA 94596
Tel. 933-3000 Ext. 2567

CANAL ZONE

Samuel Taylor Darling Mem. Library
Box 3
Balboa Heights, CZ 06720
Tel. 052-3927

COLORADO

Webb Memorial Library
Penrose Hospital
2215 N. Cascade Avenue
Colorado Springs, CO 80907
Tel. 475-3227

Denver Medical Society Library
1601 E. 19th Ave.
Denver, CO 80218
Tel. (303) 222-5817

Dept. of Health & Hospital Library
West 8th Ave. & Cherokee St.
Denver, CO 80204
Tel. 893-7422

Medical Technical Library
Fitzsimons Army Medical Center
Denver, CO 80240
Tel. (303) 531-1252 Ext. 30

Medical Technical Library
Fitzsimons General Hospital
Denver, CO 80240
Tel. (303) 366-5311 Ext. 24118

Fort Logan Mental Health Center
3520 W. Oxford Ave.
Denver, CO 80236

Medical Library
General Rose Memorial Hospital
1050 Claremont St.
Denver, CO 80220

Medical Library
Mercy Hospital

1619 Milwaukee St.
Denver, CO 80206
Tel. 388-6288

Medical Library
National Jewish Hospital and
Research Center
3800 E. Colfax Ave.
Denver, CO 80206
Tel. (303) 322-1881 Ext. 340

Memorial Medical Library
St. Anthony's Hospital Systems
4231 West 16th Avenue
Denver, CO 80204
Tel. (303) 825-9011 Ext. 2432

Medical Nursing Library
St. Luke's Hospital
601 E. 19th Ave.
Denver, CO 80203
Tel. (303) 292-0600 Ext. 2460

Charles Denison Memorial Library
University of Colorado Med. Center
4200 E. 9th Avenue
Denver, CO 80220
Tel. (303) 394-7469
Twx. COU-M-DENVER
910-931-2681

Medical Library
VA Hospital
1055 Clermont St.
Denver, CO 80220
Tel. (303) 399-8020 Ext. 351

Medical Library
Swedish Medical Center
501 E. Hampden Ave.
Englewood, CO 80110
Tel. (303) 761-0560 Ext. 259

Medical Library
US Army Hospital
Bldg. 6235
Ft. Carson, CO 80913
Tel. (303) 579-3209

Professional Library
Colorado State Hospital
1600 W. 24th Street
Pueblo, CO 81003
Tel. (502) 117-0267 Ext. 7

US Air Force Academy Library
Medical Library Branch
Air Force Academy
USAF Academy, Co 80840

Medical Library
Lutheran Hospital and
Medical Center
8300 W. 38th Ave.
Wheat Ridge, CO 80033

CONNECTICUT

Medical Library
Bridgeport Hospital
267 Grant St.
Bridgeport, CT 06602
Tel. (203) 334-0131

Medical Library
St. Vincent's Hospital
2820 Main St.
Bridgeport, CT 06606
Tel. (203) 334-1081 Ext. 302

Health Sciences Library
Danbury Hospital
Danbury, CT 06810
Tel. (203) 744-2300 Ext. 279

Lyman Maynard Stowe Library
University of Conn. Health Center
Farmington, CT 06032
Tel. (203) 674-2547
Twx. U-CONN-E/C-LIB
710-423-5521

Fray Carter Library
Greenwich Hospital
Greenwich, CT 06830
Tel. (203) 869-0177

Library Code 04822
NAVSUMEDRSCHLAB
Box 600 Naval Submarine Base
Groton, CT 06340
Tel. (203) 449-3629

Medical Library
Hartford Hospital
80 Seymour St.
Hartford, CT 06115

Hartford Medical Society Library
230 Scarborugh St.
Hartford, CT 06105
Tel. (203) 236-5613

Medical Library
Institute of Living
400 Washington St.

Hartford, CT 06106
Tel. (203) 278-7950 Ext. 412

Medical Library
New Milford Hospital
New Milford, CT 06776

Hallock Medical Library
Connecticut Valley Hospital
P.O. Box 351
Middletown, CT 06457
Tel. (203) 347-5651 Ext. 304

Health Sciences Library
Milford Hospital
2047 Bridgeport Ave.
Milford, CT 06460
Tel. (203) 878-3551

Norwich Hospital Medical Library
P.O. Box 508
Norwich, CT 06360
Tel. (203) 889-7361 Ext. 788

Medical Library
New Britain General Hospital
92 Grand St.
New Britain, CT 06052
Tel. (203) 223-2761 Ext. 280

Yale Medical Library
333 Cedar St.
New Haven, CT 06510
Tel. (203) 436-4784
Twx. YALE-MED-LIB 710-465-1145

St. Raphael Hospital Medical
Library
1450 Chapel St.
New Haven, CT 06511
Tel. (203) 772-3900 Ext. 491

Medical Library
Fairfield Hills State Hospital
Newtown, CT 06470
Tel. (203) 426-2531

Purdue Frederick Co. Medical
Research Library
50 Washington Street
Norwalk, CT 06856
Tel. (203) 853-0123

Wiggans Library
Norwalk Hospital
24 Stevens St.
Norwalk, CT 06856
Tel. (203) 838-3611 Ext. 326

Medical Library
The Stamford Hospital
Shelburne Rd. & W. Broad St.
Stamford, CT 06902
Tel. (203) 327-1234 Ext. 408

Health Science Library
St. Mary's Hospital
56 Franklin St.
Waterbury, CT 06702
Tel. (203) 756-8351

Medical Library
Waterbury Hospital
Robbins St.
Waterbury, CT 06720
Tel. 573-6148

DISTRICT OF COLUMBIA

Library
Armed Forces Institute of
Pathology
6825 16th Street N.W.
Washington, DC 20305

Medical Library
District of Columbia General
Hospital
19th & Massachusetts Ave. S.E.
Washington, DC 20003
Tel. (202) 626-5349

William Mercer Sprigg Mem. Library
Doctors Hospital
1815 Eye Street N.W.
Washington, DC 20006
Tel. (202) 541-1700

Dahlgren Memorial Library
Georgetown Univ. Med. Center
3900 Reservoir Rd. N.W.
Washington, DC 20007
Tel. (202) 625-7578
Twx. DGU-M WSH 710-822-1103

Medical-Dental Library
Howard University
600 W. Street N.W.
Washington, DC 20059

Tel. (202) 636-6433
Twx. HOWARD-U-LIB 710-822-9798

Medical Library
Malcolm Grow USAF Medical Center
Box 2097 Andrews AFB
Washington, DC 20331
Tel. (301) 981-8354

Joint Medical Library
Office of the Surgeon Gen.
USA-USAF
Forrestal Bldg. Rm. 6E040
Washington, DC 20314
Tel. 693-5870

Library
Pan American Sanitary Bureau
525 - 23rd Street N.W.
Washington, DC 20037
Tel. (202) 223-4700

VA Hospital Medical Library
50 Irving St. N.W.
Washington, DC 20422
Tel. (202) 483-6666

Medical Library
Walter Reed Army Medical Center
Bldg. 1-D Rm. C 206
Washington, DC 20012
Tel. (202) 576-3614
Twx. IDS CODE 198

Medical Library Rm. 2A-21
Washington Hospital Center
110 Irving St. N.W.
Washington, DC 20010
Tel. (202) 541-6221

Documentation Center
Washington Technical Institute
4100 Connecticut Ave. N.W.
Washington, DC 20008
Tel. (202) 629-7524

DELAWARE

Medical Library
Beebe Hospital of Sussex County
P.O. Drawer No. 226
Lewes, DE 19958
Tel. (302) 645-6211

Alfred I. Du Pont Institute of the
Nemours Foundation Library
P.O. Box 269
Wilmington, DE 19899
Tel. (302) 655-6386 Ext. 243

Delaware Academy of Medicine,
Inc. Library
Lovering Ave. & Union St.
Wilmington, DE 19806
Tel. (302) 656-1629

Medical Library
VA Center
Wilmington, DE 19805

FLORIDA

Medical Library
Boca Raton Community Hospital
800 Meadows Rd.
Boca Raton, FL 33432
Tel. (305) 395-7100

Medical Library
Bethesda Memorial Hospital
2315 S. Seacrest Blvd.
Boynton Beach, FL 33435

Dr. W.E. Wentzel Library
Manatee Memorial Hospital
206 2nd St. E.
Bradenton, FL 33505
Tel. (813) 746-5111 Ext. 121

Medical Library
Halifax Hospital Medical Center
Clyde Morris Boulevard
Daytona Beach, FL 32014
Tel. 255-0161

Health Center Library
University of Florida
Gainesville, FL 32603
Tel. (904) 392-3051
Twx. U-OF-F-HC-LIBR
810-825-6334

Medical Library Bldg. H-2080
Naval Regional Med. Center
Jacksonville, FL 32211
Tel. (904) 772-3439

Division of Health Library
Florida Dept. of Health and
Rehabilitative Services
P.O. Box 210
Jacksonville, FL 32201
Tel. (904) 354-3961

James L. Borland Medical Library
Jacksonville Hospitals

Educational Program Inc.
555 Bishop Gate Lane
Jacksonville, FL 32204
Tel. (904) 353-8574

Staff Medical Library
Mercy Hospital
3663 South Miami Ave.
Miami, FL 33133
Tel. 854-4400

Library
Papanicolaou Cancer
Research Institute
P.O. Box 23-6188
Miami, FL 33123
Tel. (305) 324-5572

Louis Calder Memorial Library
University of Miami
School of Medicine
P.O. Box 52875 Biscayne Annex
Miami, FL 33152
Tel. (305) 547-6441 Ext. 71-7
Twx. FMUMED LIB 810-848-6392

Medical Library 546/123
Veterans Administration Hospital
1201 N.W. 16th St.
Miami, FL 33125
Tel. (305) 377-2441 Ext. 3461

Medical Library
St. Francis Hospital
Allison Island
Miami Beach, FL 33141
Tel. (305) 866-7741 Ext. 736

Naval Aerospace
Medical Institute - Code 12
Naval Aviation Medical Center
Pensacola, FL 32512
Tel. (904) 452-2256

Medical Library
Memorial Hospital
1901 Arlington Street
Sarasota, FL 33579
Tel. (813) 959-1238

Medical Library
Bayfront Medical Center Inc.
701 Sixth St. S.
St. Petersburg, FL 33701
Tel. (813) 894-1161 Ext. 476

Medical Library
St. Joseph's Hospital
3001 W. Buffalo Ave.
Tampa, FL 33607
Tel. (813) 877-8161

Medical Library
Tampa General Hospital
Tampa, FL 33606
Tel. (813) 253-0711 Ext. 328

Medical Center Library
University of South Florida
4202 Fowler Ave.
Tampa, FL 33620
Tel. (813) 974-2399 Ext. 1-7
Twx. LI TPA 810-876-0829

Richard S. Beinecke Medical Library
Good Samaritan Hospital
P.O. Box 3166
West Palm Beach, FL 33402
Tel. (305) 833-1741 Ext. 246

Medical Staff Library
St. Mary's Hospital
900 49th St.
West Palm Beach, FL 33407

GEORGIA

CDC Library
Center For Disease Control
1600 Clifton Rd. N.E.
Atlanta, GA 30333
Tel. (404) 633-3311 Ext. 3396

Medical Library
Crawford W. Long Memorial Hosp.
35 Linden Ave. N.E.
Atlanta, GA 30308
Tel. (875) 441-1319

A.W. Calhoun Medical Library
Emory University
Woodruff Research Bldg.
Atlanta, GA 30322
Twx. EMORY-MED LIB
810-751-8512

Sheppard W. Foster Library
Emory University School of
Dentistry
1462 Clifton Road N.E.
Atlanta, GA 30322

Library
Georgia Dept. Human Resources
321-H 47 Trinity Ave. S.W.
Atlanta, GA 30334
Tel. (404) 656-4969

Professional Library
Georgia Mental Health Institute

1256 Briarcliff Rd. N.E.
Atlanta, GA 30306
Tel. (404) 873-6661

Medical Library
Georgia Baptist Hospital
300 Boulevard N.E.
Atlanta, GA 30312
Tel. (404) 659-4211 Ext. 2232

Library
Georgia Retardation Center
4770 N. Peachtree Rd.
Atlanta, GA 30341
Tel. (404) 458-5111

H. Custer Naylor Library
Mercer University
Southern School of Pharmacy
345 Boulevard N.E.
Atlanta, GA 30312
Tel. (404) 523-2891

Sauls Memorial Library
Piedmont Hospital
1968 Peachtree Rd. N.W.
Atlanta, GA 30309
Tel. (404) 355-7611 Ext. 305

Russell Bellman Health Sci. Library
St. Joseph's Infirmary
265 Ivy St. N.E.
Atlanta, GA 30303
Tel. (404) 525-4681 Ext. 298

Medical Library
Medical College of Georgia
Augusta, GA 30902
Tel. (404) 724-7111
Twx. MCG-LIB 810-755-4039

University Hospital Medical Library
1350 Walton Way
Augusta, GA 30901
Tel. (404) 724-7171 Ext. 2329

Medical Library
VA Hospital
Augusta, GA 30904
Tel. (404) 733-4471 Ext. 2450680

Simon Schwob Medical Library
Medical Center
710 Center St.
Columbus, GA 31902
Tel. (404) 324-4711

Hospital Professional Library
Martin Army Hospital
Ft. Benning, GA 31905
Tel. 544-1351

Max Mass Library
Medical Center of Central
Georgia
P.O. Box 6000 Hosp. Box 147
Macon, GA 31208
Tel. (912) 742-1122 Ext. 3335

Medical Library
Central State Hospital
Milledgeville, GA 31062
Tel. 453-4483

Doctors Library
Memorial Medical Center
P.O. Box 6688 Station C
Savannah, GA 31405
Tel. 355-3200 Ext. 269

417

Ralph Perkins Memorial Library
John D. Archbold Memorial Hosp.
P.O. Box 1018
Thomasville, GA 31792
Tel. (912) 226-4121 Ext. 166

GUAM

Medical Reference Library
Guam Memorial Hospital
P.O. Box AX
Agana, GU 96910
Tel. 746-9138

HAWAII

Hawaii Medical Library Inc.
1221 Punchbowl St.
Honolulu, HI 96813
Tel. (808) 536-9302

Hastings H. Walker Medical Library
Leahi Hospital
3675 Kilauea Ave.
Honolulu, HI 96816
Tel. 734-0221 Ext. 314

St. Francis Hospital Library
2230 Liliha St.
Honolulu, HI 96817
Tel. 524-2100 Ext. 240

Maui Memorial Hospital Medical
Library
221 Mahalani St.
Wailuku Maui, HI 96793

IOWA

Veterinary Medical Library
Iowa State University
Ames, IA 50010
Tel. (515) 294-2225

Health Science Library
St. Luke's Methodist Hospital
1026 A Avenue N.E.
Cedar Rapids, IA 52402
Tel. (319) 398-7358

Oliver J. Fay Memorial Library
Iowa Methodist Hospital
1200 Pleasant St.
Des Moines, IA 50308
Tel. (515) 283-6490

State Library Commission of Iowa
Medical Dept.
East 12th and Grand Ave.
Des Moines, IA 50319
Tel. (515) 281-5772

University of Iowa Libraries
Serials Dept.
Iowa City, IA 52242
Tel. (319) 353-4137

IDAHO

Science Library
Idaho State University
Pocatello, ID 83201
Tel. (208) 232-8564

ILLINOIS

Medical Staff Library
Northwest Community Hospital
800 W. Central Road
Arlington Heights, IL 60005
Tel. 259-1000 Ext. 228

Library
Mercy Center
1325 N. Highland Avenue
Aurora, IL 60506
Tel. (312) 859-2222

Health Sciences Library
Mennonite Hospital & School of
Nursing
804 N. East St.
Bloomington, IL 61701
Tel. (309) 828-5241

Morris Library-Periodicals
Southern Illinois University
Carbondale, IL 62901
Tel. (618) 453-2700

Library
American College of Surgeons
55 East Erie Street
Chicago, IL 60611
Tel. (312) 664-4050

Bureau of Library Services
American Dental Association
211 E. Chicago Ave.
Chicago, IL 60611
Tel. (312) 944-6730

ASA Bacon Memorial Library
American Hospital Association
840 N. Lake Shore Drive
Chicago, IL 60611
Tel. (312) 645-9530

Archive-Library Department
American Medical Assn.
535 N. Dearborn St.
Chicago, IL 60610
Tel. (312) 751-6013
Twx. MC 910-221-0300

Carl. A. Hedberg Health Sci. Library
Augustana Hosp. & Health
Care Center
411 W. Dickens Ave.
Chicago, IL 60614
Tel. (312) 348-1000

Library
Chicago Col. of Osteopathic
Medicine
5200 S. Ellis Ave.
Chicago, IL 60615
Tel. (312) 363-6800 Ext. 487-8-9

Professional Library
Chicago-Read Mental Health Center
6500 W. Irving Park Rd.
Chicago, IL 60634
Tel. (312) 794-3746

Joseph Brennemann Memorial Lib.
Children's Memorial Hospital
700 W. Fullerton Avenue
Chicago, IL 60614
Tel. (312) 649-4505

Ill. Central Community Hosp. Lib.
5800 Stony Island Ave.

Chicago, IL 60637
Tel. (312) 643-9200

Carl F. Shepard Memorial Library
Illinois College of Optometry
3241 S. Michigan Ave.
Chicago, IL 60616
Tel. (312) 225-1700 Ext. 13

Illinois College of Podiatric
Medicine Library
1001 N. Dearborn St.
Chicago, IL 60610
Tel. (312) 664-3301

Noah Van Cleef Medical
Memorial Library
Illinois Masonic Medical
Center
836 Wellington Avenue
Chicago, IL 60657
Tel. (312) 525-2300 Ext. 328

Professional Library
Illinois State Psychiatric
Institute
1601 W. Taylor Street
Chicago, IL 60612
Tel. (312) 341-8318

Institute for Psychoanalysis
180 N. Michigan Avenue
Chicago, IL 60601
Tel. (312) 726-6300 Ext. 63

Medical Library
Jackson Park Hospital Foundation
7531 Stony Island Avenue
Chicago, IL 60649
Tel. (312) 363-6000 Ext. 516

John Crerar Library
35 West 33rd Street
Chicago, IL 60616
Tel. (312) 225-2526
Twx. JOHN-CRERAR-CG
910-221-5131

Medical Library
Mercy Hospital
Stevenson Expresswy at King Dr.
Chicago, IL 60616
Tel. (312) 842-4700 Ext. 363

Lillian W. Florsheim Mem.
Medical Library
Michael Reese Hospital
29th and Ellis Ave.
Chicago, IL 60616
Tel. (312) 791-2474

School of Nursing Library
Michael Reese Hospital
2816 S. Ellis Ave.
Chicago, IL 60616

Lewison Memorial Library
Mount Sinai Hospital
Medical Center
California Ave. at 15th St.
Chicago, IL 60608
Tel. (312) 542-2056

Archibald Church Medical Library
Northwestern University
303 Chicago Ave.
Chicago, IL 60611
Tel. (312) 649-8133
Twx. JO 910-221-0913

The Dental School Library
Northwestern University
311 E. Chicago
Chicago, IL 60611
Tel. (312) 649-8332

Medical-Nursing Library
Ravenswood Hospital Med. Center
4550 N. Winchester at Wilson
Chicago, IL 60640
Tel. (312) 878-4300 Ext. 547

Med. Library & Allied Health
Sciences
Resurrection Hospital
7435 Talcott Rd.
Chicago, IL 60631
Tel. (312) 774-8000 Ext. 251

Library
Rush Medical College
1758 W. Harrison St.
Chicago, IL 60612
Tel. (312) 942-5950

Medical Staff Library
St. Anne's Hospital
4950 W. Thomas Street
Chicago, IL 60651
Tel. (312) 378-7100

Luken Health Sciences Library
St. Elizabeth Hospital
1431 N. Claremont Avenue
Chicago, IL 60622
Tel. (312) 278-2000 Ext. 269

Medical Library
St. Joseph Hospital
2900 N. Lake Shore Drive
Chicago, IL 60657
Tel. (312) 975-3038

Joseph G. Stromberg Library
Swedish Covenant Hospital
5145 N. California Ave.
Chicago, IL 60625
Tel. (312) 878-8200 Ext. 258

Library of the Health Sciences
Univ. of Ill. at the Med. Center
1750 W. Polk St.
Chicago, IL 60612
Tel. (312) 966-8974
Twx. IUMEDLIBCG 910-221-1410

Chicago Medical School Library
Univ. of the Health Sciences
2020 W. Ogden Ave.
Chicago, IL 60612
Tel. (312) 226-4100 Ext. 380

Biomedical Libraries
University of Chicago
1100 E. 57th St.
Chicago, IL 60637
Tel. (312) 753-3441

Library
VA Westside Hospital
P.O. Box 8195
Chicago, IL 60680
Tel. (312) 666-6500 Ext. 381

School of Nursing Library
Lake View Memorial Hospital

Major Medical Libraries

812 N. Logan
Danville, IL 61832
Tel. (217) 443-5220

Medical Staff Library
Decatur Memorial Hospital
2300 N. Edward St.
Decatur, IL 62526
Tel. (217) 877-8121 Ext. 662

Medical Library
Alexian Bros. Med. Center
800 Biesterfield Rd.
Elk Grove Village, IL 60007
Tel. (312) 437-5500

Medical-Health Sciences Library
Memorial Hosp. of Dupage County
Avon & Schiller
Elmhurst, IL 60126
Tel. (312) 833-1400 Ext. 591

Webster Medical Library
Evanston Hospital
2650 Ridge Avenue
Evanston, IL 60201
Tel. (312) 492-4585

Memorial Medical Library
St. Francis Hospital
355 Ridge Avenue
Evanston, IL 60202
Tel. (312) 492-4000 Ext. 2456

Medical Library
U.S. Naval Hospital
Building 200

Great Lakes, IL 60088
Tel. (312) 688-4601

Chief Librarian
Veterans Administration Hospital
Building 9
Hines, IL 60141
Tel. (312) 261-6700 Ext. 2514

Andrew J. Sordoni Library
National College of Chiropractic
200 E. Roosevelt Road
Lombard, IL 60148
Tel. (312) 629-2000

Library
Loyola University Medical Center
2160 S. First Avenue
Maywood, IL 60153
Tel. (312) 531-3192

Medical Library
Christ Community Hospital
4440 West 95th Street
Oak Lawn, IL 60453
Tel. 425-8000 Ext. 668

Library
Lutheran General Hospital
1775 Dempster Street
Park Ridge, IL 60068
Tel. (312) 696-2210 Ext. 1465

The Wood Library
Museum of Anesthesiology Inc.
515 Busse Highway
Park Ridge, IL 60068
Tel. (312) 825-5586

Professional Library
George A. Zeller Zone Center
5407 N. University
Peoria, IL 61614
Tel. (309) 691-2200

Medical Library
Methodist Hospital
221 N.E. Glen Oak
Peoria, IL 61603
Tel. (309) 685-6511 Ext. 161

Library of the Health Sciences
Peoria School of Medicine
U. of Ill. at the Medical Center
1400 W. Main Street
Peoria, IL 61606
Tel. (309) 674-8480
Twx. UIMED LIB PEO
910-652-0649

Medical Library
St. Francis Hospital
530 N.E. Glen Oak Ave.
Peoria, IL 61603
Tel. (309) 672-2210

Library of the Health Sciences
University of Illinois
Rockford School of Medicine
1601 Parkview Avenue
Rockford, IL 61101
Tel. (815) 987-7377
Twx. UI 910-631-3416

School of Medicine Library
Southern Illinois University
P.O. Box 3926
Springfield, IL 62708
Tel. (217) 782-7198
Twx. UI 910-242-0523

INDIANA

Biology Library
Indiana University
Jordan Hall 122
Bloomington, IN 47401
Tel. (812) 337-9791

Medical Library
Caylor-Nickel Hospital
311 S. Scott St.
Bluffton, IN 46714
Tel. (219) 824-3500 Ext. 301

The Mc Guire Memorial Library
St. Catherine Hospital
4321 Fir Street
East Chicago, IN 46312
Tel. (219) 397-3080 Ext. 636
Twx. E-CHGO-LBRY
910-697-2008

Library Resources and Services
Miles Laboratories Inc.
1127 Myrtle Street
Elkhart, IN 46514
Tel. (219) 246-8341

Health Sciences Library
Deaconess Hospital
600 Mary Street
Evansville, IN 47747
Tel. (812) 426-3385

Library
Mead Johnson Research Center
Evansville, IN 47721
Tel. (812) 426-6785

Major Medical Libraries

Medical Library
St. Joseph's Hospital
700 Broadway
Fort Wayne, IN 46802
Tel. (219) 423-2614

Memorial Medical Library
St. Margaret Hospital
Hammond, IN 46320
Tel. (219) 932-2300 Ext. 633

Professional Library
Central State Hospital
3000 W. Washington St.
Indianapolis, IN 46222
Tel. (317) 637-5511

Medical Library
Community Hospital of
Indianapolis Inc.
1500 N. Ritter Ave.
Indianapolis, IN 46219
Tel. (317) 353-5591

School of Medicine Library
Indiana University
1100 West Michigan Street
Indianapolis, IN 46202
Tel. (317) 264-7182
Twx. INU-M-INDPLS
810-341-3325

School of Dentistry Library
Indiana University Medical Center
1121 W. Michigan Avenue
Indianapolis, IN 46202
Tel. (317) 264-7204

Medical Library
Larue D. Carter Mem. Hospital

1315 West 10th Street
Indianapolis, IN 46202
Tel. (317) 634-8401 Ext. 248

Professional Library
Marion County General Hospital
960 Locke St.
Indianapolis, IN 46202
Tel. (317) 630-7028

Library Department
Methodist Hospital
1604 N. Capitol Ave.
Indianapolis, IN 46202
Tel. (317) 924-8021

Medical Library
St. Vincent Hospital
2001 West 86th Street
Indianapolis, IN 46260
Tel. (317) 926-3301

VA Medical Library
1481 West 10th Street
Indianapolis, IN 46202
Tel. (317) 635-7401

Pharmacy Library
Purdue University
Lafayette, IN 47907
Tel. (317) 749-2764

Cragmont Medical Library
Madison State Hospital
Madison, IN 47250
Tel. (312) 265-2611

Davis Clinic Medical Library
131 N. Washington St.
Marion, IN 46952
Tel. (317) 664-0511 Ext. 277

Ball Memorial Hospital Library
2401 University Avenue
Muncie, IN 47303
Tel. (317) 747-3204

South Bend Med. Foundation Inc.
Library
531 N. Main Street
South Bend, IN 46601
Tel. (219) 234-4176

KANSAS

Hertzler Research Foundation
Library
Chestnut at 4th
Halstead, KS 67056
Tel. (316) 835-2241 Ext. 63

Clendening Medical Library
University of Kansas Medical Center
39th St. & Rainbow Blvd.
Kansas City, KS 66103
Tel. (913) 831-7166
Twx. KU-MED-CTR-KCK
910-743-6846

Medical Library
Veterans Admin. Center
Leavenworth, KS 66048
Tel. (913) 682-2000 Ext. 223

Rapaport Professional Library
Osawatomie State Hospital

Osawatomie, KS 66064
Tel. (913) 755-3151 Ext. 364

Menninger Clinic Library
P.O. Box 829
Topeka, KS 66601
Tel. (913) 234-9566 Ext. 3601

Professional Library
Topeka State Hospital
2700 W. 6th St.
Topeka, KS 66606
Tel. (913) 296-4411

Dr. Karl A. Menninger Medical Lib.
VA Hospital
2200 Gage Blvd.
Topeka, KS 66622
Tel. (913) 272-3111 Ext. 271

Winfield State Hospital &
Training Center
Winfield, KS 67156
Tel. (316) 221-1200

KENTUCKY

Medical Library
St. Elizabeth Hospital
21 St. and Eastern Ave.
Covington, KY 41014
Tel. (606) 581-1322 Ext. 348

Medical Library
U.S. Army Hospital
Fort Campbell, KY 42223
Tel. (502) 798-6620

Dept. for Human Resources
Library
Kentucky Health Dept.
275 East Main Street
Frankfort, KY 40601
Tel. (502) 564-4530

Medical Center Library
University of Kentucky
Lexington, KY 40506
Tel. (606) 233-5000 Ext. 5762
Twx. KYU-M-LEXTON
510-476-8838

Medical Library
VA Hospital
Lexington, KY 40507

Health Sciences Library
University of Louisville
Louisville, KY 40201
Tel. (502) 582-2211 Ext. 355
Twx. KY 810-535-3135

LOUISIANA

Medical Library
St. Frances Cabrini Hospital
3330 Masonic Dr.
Alexandria, LA 71301
Tel. (318) 443-4571

Medical Library
U.S. Army Hospital
Box 113
Fort Polk, LA 71446
Tel. (318) 578-2545

Health Science Library
Lafayette Charity Hospital
Lafayette, LA 70501
Tel. (318) 233-2525 Ext. 255

Professional Library
Southeast Louisiana Hospital
P.O. Box 3850
Mandeville, LA 70448
Tel. (504) 626-8161 Ext. 326

Sandel Library
Northest Louisiana University
700 University Avenue
Monroe, LA 71201
Tel. (318) 342-2195
Twx. KY 510-977-5373

Library
Alton Ochsner Med. Foundation
1516 Jefferson Hwy.
New Orleans, LA 70121
Tel. (504) 834-7070 Ext. 579

Ambul. Patient Serv. Library
LHSRSA Div. Health Maint.
P.O. Box 60630
New Orleans, LA 70160
Tel. (504) 527-5021

Medical Center Library
Louisiana State University
1542 Tulane Ave.
New Orleans, LA 70112
Tel. (504) 527-5131
Twx. LU-M-NEW-ORL
810-951-6218

Rudolph Matas Medical Library
Tulane University School of

Medicine
1430 Tulane Ave.
New Orleans, LA 70112
Tel. (504) 523-3381 Ext. 537
Twx. LNT-M-NEW-ORL
810-951-5283

Medical Library
Central Louisiana State Hospital
Pineville, LA 71360
Tel. (318) 445-2421 Ext. 429

Medical Library
LSU Medical Center School of
Medicine
P.O. Box 3932
Shreveport, LA 71130
Tel. (318) 425-4421 Ext. 672

MASSACHUSETTS

Medical Staff Library
Sturdy Memorial Hospital
Attleboro, MA 02703
Tel. (617) 222-5200 Ext. 325

Library Service
Bedford VA Hospital
200 Springs Rd.
Bedford, MA 01730
Tel. (275) 750-0534

Francis A. Countway Library of
Medicine
10 Shatuck St.
Boston, MA 02115
Tel. (617) 734-3300 Ext. 104
Twx. MBCO BOSTON 710-338-6702

Lucien Howe Library of
Ophthalmology
243 Charles St.
Boston, MA 02114

Agoos Medical Library
Beth Israel Hospital
330 Brookline Ave.
Boston, MA 02215
Tel. (617) 734-4400 Ext. 225

Boston City Hospital Medical Library
Dept. of Health & Hospitals
818 Harrison Ave.
Boston, MA 02118
Tel. (617) 424-4198

Alumni Medical Library
Boston University School of
Medicine
80 E. Concord St.
Boston, MA 02118
Tel. (617) 262-4200

Joslin Diabetes Foundation Library
170 Pilgrim Rd.
Boston, MA 02215

Library
Mass. College of Optometry
420 Beacon St.
Boston, MA 02115
Tel. (617) 261-3430 Ext. 43

Sheppard Library
Mass. College of Pharmacy
179 Longwood Ave.
Boston, MA 02115
Tel. (617) 734-6700 Ext. 23

Major Medical Libraries

Treadwell Library
Massachusetts General Hospital
Fruit St.
Boston, MA 02114
Tel. (617) 726-2250
Twx. MBMGHTR BOSTON
710-321-6523

Gilbert Horrax Mem. Library
New England Deaconess Hospital
185 Pilgrim Rd.
Boston, MA 02215
Tel. (617) 734-7000 Ext. 2203

Medical & Dental Library
Tufts University
136 Harrison Ave.
Boston, MA 02111
Tel. (617) 423-4600 Ext. 217
Twx. MB 710-321-6333

Medical Library
U.S. Veterans Admin. Hospital
150 S. Huntington Ave.
Boston, MA 02130

Medical Library
St. Elizabeth's Hospital
736 Cambridge St.
Brighton, MA 02135
Tel. (617) 782-7000 Ext. 551

Brockton Hospital Library
Brockton, MA 02402
Tel. (617) 586-2600 Ext. 378

Medical Staff Library
Cardinal Cushing General Hospital
235 Pearl St.

Brockton, MA 02401
Tel. (617) 588-4000 Ext. 612

Medical Library
VA Hospital
Brockton, MA 02401
Tel. (617) 583-4500 Ext. 321

Medical & Nursing Library
Mount Auburn Hospital
330 Mount Auburn St.
Cambridge, MA 02138
Tel. (617) 876-5680 Ext. 315

Sancta Maria Hospital Medical
Library
799 Concord Ave.
Cambridge, MA 02136
Tel. (617) 868-2200 Ext. 264

Nursing Library
Youville Hospital
1575 Cambridge St.
Cambridge, MA 02138

School of Nursing Library
Boston College
Cushing Hall
Chestnut Hill, MA 02167
Tel. (617) 969-0100 Ext. 437
Twx. MCHBCHSTNTHL
710-335-0856

Ida S. Charleton Medical Library
Truesdale Hospital Inc.
1820 Highland Ave.
Fall River, MA 02720
Tel. (617) 674-8411 Ext. 263

Medical Library
Foxborough State Hospital
Chestnut St.
Foxborough, MA 02035
Tel. 543-5351

Framingham Union Hospital Lib.
Evergreen St.
Framingham, MA 01701
Tel. (617) 873-3535 Ext. 334

Medical Library
Cutler Army Hospital
Ft. Devens, MA 01433
Tel. (617) 797-2031

Health Sciences Library
Lakeville Hospital
Main St.
Lakeville, MA 02346
Tel. (617) 947-1231 Ext. 361

Medical Library
Medfield State Hospital
P.O. Box 276
Medfield, MA 02052
Tel. (617) 359-4312 Ext. 212

Medical Library
Bon Secours Hospital
70 East St.
Methuen, MA 01844
Tel. 683-8781

Medical Library
Leonard Morse Hospital
67 Union Street
Natick, MA 01760
Tel. (617) 653-3400 Ext. 658

Newton-Wellesley Hospital Library
2014 Washington St.
Newton Lower Falls, MA 02162
Tel. (617) 244-2800

VA Hospital Library
North Main St.
Northampton, MA 01060
Tel. (413) 584-4040

Medical Library
Berkshire Medical Center
725 North St.
Pittsfield, MA 01201
Tel. (413) 443-5641 Ext. 332

Worchester Foundation For
Experimental Biology Inc.
222 Maple Ave.
Shrewsbury, MA 01545
Tel. (617) 842-8921 Ext. 302

The Library
Springfield Hospital Med. Center
759 Chestnut St.
Springfield, MA 01107
Tel. (413) 787-4293
Twx. MSSH SPRINGFLD
710-350-1484

Hennessey Memorial Library
Goddard Memorial Hospital
909 Sumner Street
Stoughton, MA 02072
Tel. (617) 344-5100 Ext. 395

Worcester Medical Library Inc.
57 Cedar St.
Worcester, MA 01609

Library
Mason Research Institute
23 Harvard Street
Worcester, MA 01608
Tel. (617) 791-0931 Ext. 47

Medical School Library
University of Massachusetts
55 N. Lake Ave.
Worcester, MA 01605
Tel. (617) 791-7851 Ext. 273

George L. Banay Med. Library
Worcester State Hospital
305 Belmont St.
Worcester, MA 01613
Tel. (617) 752-4681 Ext. 276

MARYLAND

Harrison Library
Baltimore City Hospitals
4940 Eastern Ave.
Baltimore, MD 21224
Tel. 342-5400 Ext. 345

Medical Staff Library
Greater Baltimore Med. Center
6701 N. Charles St.
Baltimore, MD 21204

John F. Kennedy Library
John F. Kennedy Institute
707 N. Broadway

Baltimore, MD 21205
Tel. (301) 955-4240

Welch Medical Library
Johns Hopkins Univ. School of Med.
1900 E. Monument St.
Baltimore, MD 21205
Tel. (301) 955-3411
Twx. MOBJ W BALTO
710-234-246

Charles G. Reingner Doctors Lib.
Lutheran Hospital of Maryland
730 Ashburton St.
Baltimore, MD 21216
Tel. (301) 945-1600 Ext. 2240

Library
Medical & Chirurgical Faculty
of the State of Maryland
1211 Cathedral St.
Baltimore, MD 21201
Tel. (301) 539-0872

Mc Glannan Memorial Library
Mercy Hospital
301 St. Paul Place
Baltimore, MD 21202
Tel. (301) 727-5400

Staff Library
Sinai Hospital of Baltimore
Beledere and Greenspring Aves.
Baltimore, MD 21215
Tel. (301) 367-7800 Ext. 8551

Medical Library
St. Joseph Hospital
7620 York Rd.

Baltimore, MD 21204
Tel. (301) 828-5800

Health Sciences Library
University of Maryland
111 So. Greene St.
Baltimore, MD 21201
Tel. (301) 528-7545
Twx. UM HLTH SCI BA
710-234-1610

Medical Library
US Public Health Service Hospital
Wyman Park Dr. & 31st St.
Baltimore, MD 21211
Tel. (301) 338-1100 Ext. 232

Technical Reference Library
NMRI
National Naval Med. Center
Bethesda, MD 20014

Library
National Institutes of Health
9000 Rockville Pike Bldg 10
Bethesda, MD 20014
Tel. (301) 496-2447

Public Health Library
Prince Georges City Health Dept.
Cheverly, MD 20785
Tel. (301) 773-1400 Ext. 450

The Library
Memorial Hospital
Easton, MD 21601
Tel. (301) 822-1000 Ext. 450

FDA Bureau Drugs Library
5600 Fishers Lane Rm. 118-30

Rockville, MD 20852
Tel. (301) 443-3180

Kubie Medical Library
Sheppard & Enoch Pratt Hospital
P.O. Box 6815
Towson, MD 21204
Tel. (301) 823-8200

MAINE

Health Sciences Library
Bangor State Hospital
Bangor, ME 04401
Tel. 947-7386

Health Sciences Library
Eastern Maine Med. Center
Bangor, ME 04401
Tel. 942-6351 Ext. 348

Research Library
The Jackson Laboratory
Bar Harbor, ME 04609
Tel. (207) 288-3373 Ext. 208

Health Science Library
Maine Medical Center
22 Bramhall St.
Portland, ME 04102
Tel. (207) 871-2201
Twx. MEPMC LIB PORT
710-221-6421

Medical Library
VA Center
Togus, ME 04330
Tel. (207) 623-8411 Ext. 278

Health Sciences Library
Thayer Hospital
North St.
Waterville, ME 04901
Tel. (207) 775-5454

MICHIGAN

Medical Library
St. Joseph Mercy Hospital
326 N. Ingalls
Ann Arbor, MI 48104
Tel. (313) 665-4141 Ext. 377

Medical Center Library
The University of Michigan
4400 Kresge Research Building
Ann Arbor, MI 48104
Tel. (313) 764-1210
Twx. MCL UMAA 810-223-6016

McLouith Memorial Medical Library
Oakwood Hospital
18101 Oakwood Boulevard
Dearborn, MI 48124
Tel. (313) 565-1000 Ext. 203

Evangelical Deaconess Hospital Lib.
3245 E. Jefferson Ave.
Detroit, MI 48207
Tel. (313) 568-2000 Ext. 285

Health Science Library
Art Centre Hospital
5435 Woodward Ave.
Detroit, MI 48202
Tel. (313) 831-6660

Kresge Center for Medical Education
Children's Hospital of Michigan
3901 Beaubien
Detroit, MI 48201
Tel. (313) 494-5322

Medical Library
Detroit General Hospital
1326 St. Antoine
Detroit, MI 48226
Tel. (313) 224-0281

Medical Library
Detroit Osteopathic Hospital
12523 Third Ave.
Detroit, MI 48203
Tel. (313) 869-1200 Ext. 380

Doctors Library
Detroit Psychiatric Institute
1151 Taylor Avenue
Detroit, MI 48202
Tel. (313) 872-1540 Ext. 326

Oscar Le Seure Prof. Library
Grace Hospital
4160 John R. Street
Detroit, MI 48201
Tel. (313) 494-6109 Ext. 4946110

Department of Libraries
Harper Hospital
3825 Brush St.
Detroit, MI 48201
Tel. (313) 494-8265

Library
Henry Ford Hospital

2799 W. Grand Blvd.
Detroit, MI 48202
Tel. (313) 875-2900 Ext. 645

Medical Library
Hutzel Hospital
432 East Hancock
Detroit, MI 48201
Tel. (313) 494-7179

Lafayette Clinic Library
951 East Lafayette
Detroit, MI 48207
Tel. (313) 963-5400 Ext. 346

Medical Library
Metropolitan Hospital
1800 Tuxedo Ave.
Detroit, MI 48206
Tel. (313) 869-3600 Ext. 410

Medical Library
Mount Carmel Mercy Hospital
6071 Outer Drive
Detroit, MI 48235
Tel. (313) 864-5400 Ext. 333

Research Library
Parke Davis & Company
Joseph Campau at the River
Detroit, MI 48232
Tel. (313) 663-7585 Ext. 203

Mc Pherson Browning Mem. Library
Rehabilitation Institute Inc.
261 Mack Boulevard
Detroit, MI 48201
Tel. (313) 494-9759

Medical Library
Saint John Hospital
22101 Moross Road
Detroit, MI 48236
Tel. (313) 881-8200 Ext. 257

Samuel Frank Medical Library
Sinai Hospital of Detroit
6767 West Outer Drive
Detroit, MI 48235
Tel. (313) 272-6000 Ext. 8286

Dental Library
University of Detroit
2931 E. Jefferson Ave.
Detroit, MI 48207
Tel. (313) 567-3380 Ext. 10

Vera Shiffman Medical Library
Wayne State University
4325 Brush Street
Detroit, MI 48201
Tel. (313) 577-1168
Twx. MC 810-221-5163

Medical Library
Wayne County General Hospital
Eloise, MI 48132
Tel. (313) 274-3000 Ext. 6048

Medical Library
Flint Osteopathic Hospital
3921 Beecher Rd.
Flint, MI 48504
Tel. (313) 235-8511 Ext. 217

Medical Library
Hurley Hospital
6th & Begole Streets

Major Medical Libraries

Flint, MI 48502
Tel. (313) 232-1161 Ext. 437

Medical Library
Garden City Hospital
4245 N. Inkster Rd.
Garden City, MI 48135

St. Mary's Hospital Library
200 Jefferson SE
Grand Rapids, MI 49502
Tel. (616) 774-6243

Medical Library
Bon Secours Hospital
468 Cadieux Rd.
Grosse Pointe, MI 48230
Tel. 884-8500

Medical Library
Burgess Hospital
1521 Gull Street
Kalamazoo, MI 49001
Tel. (616) 349-1581

Library
Bronson Methodist Hospital
252 Lovell St.
Kalamazoo, MI 49006
Tel. (616) 382-2000

Medical Library
St. Joseph Hospital
20 Parkview
Mt. Clemens, MI 48043
Tel. (313) 463-8611

Hackley Hospital Medical Library
1700 Clinton St.
Muskegon, MI 49443
Tel. (616) 726-3511

Medical Library
Hawthorne Center
18471 Haggerty Rd.
Northville, MI 48167
Tel. (313) 349-3000

Kresge Library-Serials Dept.
Oakland University
Rochester, MI 48063
Tel. (313) 377-2486

Medical Library
William Beaumont Hospital
3601 West Thirteen Mile Rd.
Royal Oak, MI 48072
Tel. (313) 549-7000 Ext. 237

Medical Library
St. Mary's Hospital
830 S. Jefferson Ave.
Saginaw, MI 48601
Tel. (517) 754-2411

Panzner Memorial Library
Providence Hospital
16001 Nine Mile Road
Southfield, MI 48076
Tel. (313) 353-3000 Ext. 297

Medical Library
Ypsilanti State Hospital
P.O. Box A
Ysilanti, MI 48197
Tel. (313) 434-3400

MINNESOTA

Health Science Library
University of Minnesota-Duluth
2400 Oakland
Duluth, MN 55812
Tel. (218) 726-7578
Twx. MN DULL 910-561-0057

Hennepin County Medical
Society Library
2000 Medical Arts Building
Minneapolis, MN 55402
Tel. (612) 333-8367

Health Sciences Library
Fairview Hospital
2312 South 6th St.
Minneapolis MN 55406
Tel. (612) 332-0282 Ext. 371

Medical Library
Hennepin County Med. Hospital
5th & Portland
Minneapolis, MN 55415
Tel. (612) 348-2339
Twx. MN910-576-2954

Kenny Rehabilitation Institute
1800 Chicago Avenue
Minneapolis, MN 55404
Tel. (612) 871-7331 Ext. 397

Medical Library
North Mem. Hospital
3220 Lowry Ave. N.
Minneapolis, MN 55422
Tel. (612) 588-0616 Ext. 432

Bio Medical Library
University of Minnesota
Diehl Hall
Minneapolis, MN 55455
Tel. (612) 373-5585
Twx. MNU-B-MPLS 910-576-287:

Library
Veterans Admin. Hospital
54th Street & 48th Ave. So.
Minneapolis, MN 55417
Tel. (612) 721-7512

DPW Medical Library
Glen Lake State Sanatorium
Oak Terrace Nursing Home
Minnetonka, NM 55343
Tel. (612) 938-7621

Mayo Clinic Library
200 First Ave.
Rochester, MN 55901
Tel. (507) 282-2511 Ext. 2061
Twx. MAYO CLIN LIB
910-565-2480

Boeckmann Library
Ramsey County Medical Society
1500 Lowry Medical Arts Bldg.
Saint Paul, MN 55102
Tel. (612) 224-3346

Medical Library
Veterans Admin. Hospital
St. Cloud, MN 56301
Tel. (612) 252-1670

Medical-Nursing Library
St. Paul-Ramsey Hospital
St. Paul, MN 55101
Tel. (612) 222-4260 Ext. 544

MISSOURI

Library
Logan Chiropractic College
Box 100-430 Schoettler Road
Chestefield, MO 63017
Tel. (314) 383-8941

Medical Library
University of Missouri
Room M 210-Med. Sciences Bldg.
Columbia, MO 65201
Tel. (314) 882-8086
Twx. MOU M COLUMBIA
910-760-1449

Dr. Charles F. Grabske Sr. Library
Independence Sanitarium & Hosp.
1509 W. Truman Rd.
Independence, MO 64050
Tel. 252-4700

ANA Library
American Nurses Association
2420 Pershing Rd.
Kansas City, MO 64108
Tel. (816) 474-5720

Learing Resources Center
Baptist Mem. Hospital
6601 Rockhill Rd.
Kansas City, MO 64131
Tel. (816) 361-3500

Lockwood Memorial Library
Research Hosp. & Medical Center
Meyer Blvd. at Prospect
Kansas City, MO 64132
Tel. (816) 276-4159

Medical Library
The Children's Mercy Hospital
24th at Gillham Rd.
Kansas City, MO 64108
Tel. (816) 471-0626 Ext. 298

Medical Library
Trinity Lutheran Hospital
31st & Wyandotte
Kansas City, MO 64108
Tel. (816) 753-4600 Ext. 637/638

School of Dentistry Library
Univ. of Missouri-Kansas City
5100 Rockhill Rd.
Kansas City, MO 64110
Tel. (816) 276-1526

Medical Library
University of Missouri-Kansas City
515 E. 24th St.
Kansas City MO 64110
Tel. (816) 421-8060
Twx. UMKC MED LIB
910-771-3009

A.T. Still Memorial Library
Kirksville College of
Osteopathic Medicine
212 W. Jefferson
Kirksville, MO 63501
Tel. (816) 626-2345

Professional Library
St. Joseph State Hospital

Box 263
St. Joseph, MO 64502
Tel. (816) 232-8431 Ext. 462

Medical Library
Incarnate Word Hospital
1640 S. Grand
St. Louis, MO 63104
Tel. (314) 664-6500 Ext. 210

Robert J. Brockman Memorial
Library
Malcom Bliss Mental Health
Center,
1420 Grattan
St. Louis, MO 63104
Tel. (314) 241-7600 Ext. 391

Hospital Library
Normandy Osteopathic Hospital
Library
7840 Natural Bridge Road
St. Louis, MO 63121
Tel. (314) 389-0015 Ext. 296

John Young Brown Memorial
Library
St. John's Mercy Medical Center
621 South New Ballas Road
St. Louis, MO 63141
Tel. (432) 650-0276

Library
St. Louis Medical Society
3839 Lindell Court
St. Louis, MO 63108
Tel. (314) 371-5225 Ext. 6

Medical Center Library
St. Louis University
1402 South Grand Boulevard
St. Louis, MO 63104
Tel. (314) 664-9800
Twx. SLU MED LIB STL
910-761-0434

Rothschild Medical Library
The Jewish Hospital
216 S. Kings Highway
St. Louis, MO 63110
Tel. (314) 367-8060

University of Missouri
Missouri Institute of Psychiatry
5400 Arsenal St.
St. Louis, MO 63139
Tel. (314) 644-2400 Ext. 2317
Twx. MIP LIB STL
910-761-0429

School of Dentistry Library
Washington University
4559 Scott Ave.
St. Louis, MO 63110
Tel. (314) 361-4700 Ext. 66

Medical Library
Washington University
School of Medicine
4580 Scott Avenue
St. Louis, MO 63110
Tel. (314) 454-3711
Twx. WASHU MED LIB STL
910-761-2165

MISSISSIPPI

Medical Library
Veterans Admin. Center

Biloxi, MS 39531
Tel. (601) 432-1541 Ext. 221

Health Science Library
Mississippi Baptist Hospital
1190 North State Street
Jackson, MS 39201
Tel. (601) 948-5211 Ext. 225

Mississippi State Board
of Health Library
P.O. Box 1700
Jackson, MS 39205
Tel. (601) 354-6614

Rowland Medical Library
University of Mississippi
Medical Center
N. State St.
Jackson, MS 39216
Tel. (601) 362-4411 Ext. 711
Twx. MSU-M JACKSON
810-966-2739

Medical Library
Keesler Air Force Base
AFM 3010 Rm Ab-1
Keesler AFB, MS 39534
Medical Supply Officer

Austin A. Dodge Pharmacy Library
University of Mississippi
School of Pharmacy
Faser Hall,
University, MS 38677
Tel. (601) 232-7381

Street Memorial Medical Library
Mercy Hospital
P.O. Box 271

Vicksburg, MS 39180
Tel. (601) 636-212

NEBRASKA

Medical Library
Creighton Mem. St. Joseph's Hosp.
2305 South 10th Street
Omaha, NB 68108
Tel. (402) 348-2196

Health Sciences Library
Creighton University
2500 California Street
Omaha, NB 68178
Tel. (402) 536-2908

Library of Medicine
University of Nebraska Medical
Center
42nd Street & Dewey Avenue
Omaha, NB 68105
Tel. (402) 541-4006
Twx. NBU-M OMAHA
910-622-8353

NEVADA

Elko Clinic Library
762 - 14th St.
Elko, NV 89801

Medical Library
Southern Nevada Memorial Hospital
1800 W. Charleston Blvd.
Las Vegas, NV 89102
Tel. (702) 385-2000 Ext. 470
Twx. SO-NV-HOSP-LIB
910-397-6861

Max C. Fleischman Medical
Library
St. Mary's Hospital
235 West 6th St.
Reno, NV 89503
Tel. (702) 323-2041

Life & Health Sciences Library
University of Nevada   Reno
Reno, NV 89507
Tel. (702) 784-6616

NEW HAMPSHIRE

Dana Biomedical Library
Dartmouth College
Hanover, NH 03755
Tel. (603) 646-2858
Twx. NHD D HANOVER
710-366-1828

NEW JERSEY

Medical Library
Institute for Medical Research
Copewood St.
Camden, NJ 08103

Reuben L. Sharp Health-Science
Library
The Cooper Hospital
6th & Stevens Streets
Camden, NJ 08103
Tel. (609) 964-6600 Ext. 487

Medical Library
VA Hospital
East Orange, NJ 07019
Tel. (201) 676-1000 Ext. 388

Medical Library
Raritan Valley Hospital-CmdNJ
275 Green Brook Road
Greenbrook, JN 08812
Tel. (201) 968-6000 Ext. 240

School of Dentistry Library
Fairleigh Dickinson University
110 Fuller Place
Hackensack, NJ 07601
Tel. (201) 836-6300 Ext. 578

Medical Library
Hackensack Hospital
Hackensack, NJ 07601
Tel. (201) 487-4000 Ext. 344

Medical Staff Library
Saint Barnabas Medical Center
Old Short Hills Rd.
Livingstone, NJ 07039
Tel. (201) 992-5500 Ext. 208

Medical Library
VA Hospital
Lyons, NJ 07939
Tel. (201) 647-0180

Research & Engineering Library
Personal Products Corp.
Milltown, NJ 08850
Tel. (201) 524-7544

Medical Library
Mountainside Hospital
Bay & Highland Aves.

Montclair, NJ 07042
Tel. (201) 746-6000 Ext. 517

Library
Warner-Lambert Research
Institute
170 Taborf Road
Morris Plains, NJ 07950
Tel. (201) 285-2875

Medical Library
Morristown Memorial Hospital
100 Madison Ave.
Morristown, NJ 07960
Tel. (201) 538-4500 Ext. 494

Medical Library
Jersey Shore Medical Center
1945 Corlies Avenue
Neptune, NJ 07753
Tel. (201) 755-5500 Ext. 346/474

Middlesex Gen. Hospital Library
180 Somerset St.
New Brunswick, NJ 08901
Tel. (201) 828-3000

Library of Science & Medicine
Rutgers the State University
New Brunswick, NJ 08903
Tel. (201) 247-1766 Ext. 6207

Medical Library
St. Peter's General Hospital
Easton Avenue
New Brunswick, NJ 08903
Tel. (201) 545-8000 Ext. 210

Library
College of Medicine & Dentistry
100 Bergen Street
Newark, NJ 07103
Tel. (201) 877-4358
Twx. NJN CM 710-995-4526

Allied Health Div. Library
Essex County College
375 Osborne Terrace
Newark, NJ 07112

Aquinas Medical Library
St. Michael Medical Center
306 High St.
Newark, NJ 07102
Tel. (201) 623-8200 Ext. 340

Library
Bergen Pines County Hospital
Paramus, NJ 07652
Tel. (201) 261-9000

Medical Library
St. Joseph Hospital
703 Main St.
Paterson, NJ 07503
Tel. (201) 684-7500 Ext. 270

Glass Memorial Library
Muhlenberg Hospital
Plainfield, NJ 07061
Tel. (201) 753-2000 Ext. 340

Carl G. Hartman Library
Ortho Research Foundation
Raritan, NJ 08869
Tel. (201) 524-2236

New Jersey Dept. of Health Library
P.O. Box 1540
Trenton, NJ 08625
Tel. (609) 292-5693

NEW MEXICO

Lovelace Foundation Library
5200 Gibson Boulevard S.E.
Albuquerque, NM 87108
Tel. (505) 842-7158
Twx. NMAL LOVELACE
910-989-1158

Library of the Medical
Sciences
University of New Mexico
School of Medicine
Albuqueruqe, NM 87131
Tel. (505) 277-2311
Twx. NM U-M-Albuq 910-989-1695

Medical Library
Vet. Admin. Hospital
2100 Ridgecrest S.E.
Albuquerque, NM 87108
Tel. (505) 255-1611

NEW YORK

Library
Albany Medical College
47 New Scotland Ave.
Albany, NY 12208
Tel. (518) 462-7521 Ext. 805
Twx. NALA ALB 710-441-8262

New York State Dept. of Health
Library

New Scotland Ave.
Albany, NY 12201
Tel. (518) 474-6172

New York State Medical Library
Washington Ave.
Albany, NY 12224
Tel. (518) 474-7040
Twx. NYS LIB ALBY
710-441-8770

Medical Library
Veterans Admin. Hospital
Albany, NY 12208
Tel. (518) 462-3311 Ext. 342

Medical Library
Binghamton General Hospital
Mitchell Avenue
Binghamton, NY 13903
Tel. (607) 772-1100 Ext. 220

Library
Albert Einstein College of Medicine
Morris Pk. Ave. & Eastchester Rd.
Bronx, NY 10461
Tel. (212) 430-3108
Twx. NN-YU-M-NYC
710-593-2106

The Dr. Ralph L. Dourmashkin
Medical Library
Fordham Hospital
Bronx, NY 10458
Tel. (212) 298-4000 Ext. 240

Medical Library
Lincoln Hospital

333 Southern Blvd.
Bronx, NY 10454
Tel. (212) 960-5616

Medical Library
Veterans Admin. Hospital
130 W. Kingsbridge Road
Bronx, NY 10468
Tel. (212) 584-9000 Ext. 433

Medical Library
Lawrence Hospital
55 Palmer Avenue
Bronxville, NY 10708
Tel. (914) 337-7300 Ext. 306

Brooklyn Coll. of Pharmacy Lib.
600 Lafayette Ave.
Brooklyn, NY 11216
Tel. (212) 622-4040

Harold Fink Mem. Library
Coney Island Hospital
Ocean & Shore Parkways
Brooklyn, NY 11235
Tel. (212) 743-4100

Medical Research Library of
Brooklyn
Downstate Med. Center-Box 14
450 Clarkson Ave.
Brooklyn, NY 11203
Tel. (212) 270-1038
Twx. MED RES BKLYN
710-584-2466

Medical & Nursing Library
Jewish Hospital of Brooklyn
555 Prospect Place
Brooklyn, NY 11238

Tel. (212) 240-1795
Twx. JHMCB LIB NYK
710-584-2410

Hoagland Medical Library
Long Island College Hospital
340 Henry St.
Brooklyn, NY 11201
Tel. (212) 780-1077

The Kingsbrook Jewish Medical
Center Library
86 E. 49th St.
Brooklyn, NY 11203
Tel. (212) 756-9700 Ext. 296

Medical Library
The Methodist Hospital
506 - 6th Street
Brooklyn, NY 11215
Tel. (212) 780-3368 Ext. 3487

Medical Library
VA Hospital Brooklyn
800 Poly Place-Ft. of 7th Ave.
Brooklyn, NY 11209

Medical Library
Wyckoff Heights Hospital
374 Stockholm St.
Brooklyn, NY 11238
Tel. (212) 456-8200

A.H. Aaron Medical Library
Buffalo Gen. Hospital
100 High St.
Buffalo, NY 14203
Tel. (716) 886-5600

Emily Foster Memorial Medical
Library
Children's Hospital
219 Bryant Street
Buffalo, NY 14222
Tel. (716) 878-7304

Medical Library
Edward J. Meyer Memorial Hospital
462 Grider St.
Buffalo, NY 14215
Tel. (716) 894-1212

Medical Library
Mercy Hospital
565 Abbott Road
Buffalo, NY 14220
Tel. (716) 826-7000

Health Sciences Library
Millard Fillmore Hospital
3 Gates Circle
Buffalo, NY 14209
Tel. (716) 882-8000 Ext. 743

Library
Roswell Park Memorial Institute
666 Elm St.
Buffalo, NY 14203

Health Sciences Library
State University of New York
Stockton Kimball Hall
Buffalo, NY 14214
Tel. (716) 831-2441 Ext. 4100
Twx. HSL SUNYAB 710-522-1226

Health Science Library
Central Islip State Hospital

Rehabilitation Bldg.
Central Islip, NY 11722
Tel. (516) 234-6262

Library
Mary Imogene Bassett Hospital
Cooperstown, NY 13326
Tel. (607) 547-6481

Medical Library
Meadowbrook Hospital
2201 Hempstead Tpke.
East Meadow, NY 11554
Tel. (516) 542-2425

Health Sciences Library
SUNY at Stony Brook
P.O. Box 66
East Setauket, NY 11733
Tel. (516) 246-7190
Twx. SUNY LIB STYBK
510-228-7765

Medical Library - A-1-222
Mt. Sinai Hospital Services
City Hospital Center at Elmhurst
79-01 Broadway
Elmhurst, NY 11373
Tel. (212) 830-1538
Twx. ELM NY 710-582-2269

Library
Arnot Ogden Memorial Hospital
Roe Ave. and Grove St.
Elmira, NY 14901
Tel. (607) RE4-5221 Ext. 226

Medical Library
St. Joseph's Hospital

555 East Market St.
Elmira, NY 14902
Tel. (607) 733-6541 Ext. 248

Medical Library
U.S. Naval Medical Research
Unit #3
Fleet Post Office, NY 09527

Medical Library
Booth Memorial Medical Center
Main St. at Booth Memorial Ave.
Flushing, NY 11355
Tel. (212) 445-1000 Ext. 353

Medical Library
Flushing Hospital and Medical
Center
Parsons Blvd. & 45th Ave.
Flushing, NY 11355
Tel. (212) 359-2000

Carl Boettiger Memorial
Library
Medical Society of the County
of Queens
112-25 Queens Blvd.
Forest Hills, NY 11375
Tel. (212) 268-7300 Ext. 6

John N. Shell Library
Nassau Acad. of Medicine
1200 Stewart Ave.
Garden City, NY 11530
Tel. (516) 333-4300

Medical Library
Community Hospital

Glen Cove, NY 11542
Tel. (516) OR6-5000 Ext. 363

Arany Lorand Memorial Library
L I Jewish-Hillside Med. Center
75-59 263rd St.
Glen Oaks, NY 11004
Tel. (212) 343-6700 Ext. 4406

Health Science Library
Suffolk Academy of Medicine
850 Veterans Memorial Highway
Hauppauge, NY 11787
Tel. (516) 724-7970

Doctors Medical Library
St. Luke's Hospital
70 Dubois St.
Newburgh, NY 12550
Tel. (914) 431-4400 Ext. 215

School of Nursing Library
Catholic Medical Center
88-25 153rd Street
Jamaica, NY 11432
Tel. (212) 291-3300 Ext. 230

Central Medical Library
Catholic Medical Center
88-25 153 St.
Jamaica, NY 11432
Tel. (212) 291-3300 Ext. 486

Medical Library
Jamaica Hospital
89th Avenue & Van Wyck Expwy.
Jamaica, NY 11418
Tel. (212) 526-7500

Medical Library Bldg. B
Queens Hospital Center
82-68 164th St.
Jamaica, NY 11432
Tel. (212) 526-8600

Medical Library
Charles S. Wilson Mem. Hospital
3357 Harrison St.
Johnson City, NY 13790
Tel. (607) 773-6030

Kings Park Psychiatric Center
Library
Box A
Kings Park, L.I., NY 11754
Tel. (516) 269-6600 Ext. 671

Daniel Carroll Payson Medical
Library
North Shore University
Hospital
Manhasset, NY 11030
Tel. (516) 562-2420

Library
Nassau County Dept. of Health
240 Old Country Rd.
Mineola, NY 11501

Medical Library
VA Hospital
Montrose, NY 10548
Tel. (914) 737-4400 Ext. 429

Medical-Nursing Library
The Mount Vernon Hospital
Valentine St.
Mount Vernon, NY 10050
Tel. (914) 664-8000 Ext. 877

Medical Library
Northern Westchester Hospital
Mt. Kisco, NY 10549
Tel. (914) 666-6777 Ext. 427

Central New York Academy of
Medicine
210 Clinton Road
New Hartfod, NY 13413
Tel. (315) 735-2204

Medical Library
Long Island Jewish Medical Center
New Hyde Park, NY 11040
Tel. 343-6700 Ext. 2673

J. Marshall Perley Medical Library
New Rochelle Hospital
P.O. Box 501
New Rochelle, NY 10802

Medical Library
American Cancer Society Inc.
219 East 42nd St.
New York, NY 10017

Sophia F. Palmer Library
American Journal of Nursing Co.
10 Columbus Circle
New York, NY 10019
Tel. (212) 582-8820 Ext. 276

Elisha Walker Staff Library
Beekman Downtown Hospital
170 William St.
New York, NY 10038
Tel. (212) 233-5300

Major Medical Libraries

Medical Library
Bellevue Hospital
28th St. & 1st Ave.
New York, NY 10016
Tel. (212) 561-4780

Dept. of Psychiatry Library
Beth Israel Medical Center
Morris J. Bernstein Institute
307 Second Ave.
New York, NY 10003
Tel. (212) 677-2300

Medical Library
Cabrini Health Care Center
Columbus Hospital Division
227 East 19th Street
New York, NY 10003
Tel. (212) 677-4700

Medical Library
Columbia University
630 W. 168th St.
New York, NY 10032
Tel. (212) 579-3688
Twx. NNC-M NYC 710-581-4157

Samuel J. Wood Library
Cornell University Medical College
1300 York Ave.
New York, NY 10021
Tel. (212) 879-9000 Ext. 564
Twx. NN CORM NYC 710-581-4053

John M. Wheeler Library
Edward S. Harkness Eye Institute
635 W. 165th St.

New York, NY 10032
Tel. (212) 579-2916

Medical Library
Equitable Life Assurance Society
1285 Avenue of the Americas
New York, NY 10019
Tel. (212) 554-2936

Haven Emerson Public Health
Library
125 Worth St. Room 223
New York, NY 10013
Tel. (212) 566-5169

Medical Library
Hospital for Joint Diseases
1919 Madison Ave.
New York, NY 10035
Tel. (212) 876-7000 Ext. 271

Medical Library
Hospital for Special Surgery
535 East 70th Street
New York, NY 10021
Tel. (212) 535-5500 Ext. 210

Hunter-Bellevue Nursing
Education Library
440 E. 26th St.
New York, NY 10010
Tel. (212) 686-6800 Ext. 181

The Library
Institute for Muscle Disease Inc.
515 East 71st Street
New York, NY 10021
Tel. (212) 988-6800

Jerome S. Leopold Med. Library
Lenox Hill Hospital
100 East 77th Street
New York, NY 10021
Tel. (212) 794-4266

Library
M.D. Publications Incorporated
30 East 60th St.
New York, NY 10022
Tel. (212) 355-5432

Medical Library
M.J. Lewi College of Podiatry
53-55 E. 124th St.
New York, NY 10035
Tel. (212) 427-8400 Ext. 26

Lee Coombe Memorial Library
Memorial Sloan-Kettering
Cancer Center
1275 York Avenue
New York, NY 10021
Tel. (212) 879-3000 Ext. 2351
Twx. NN MSK NYC 710-581-4161

Library
Metropolitan Life Insurance
1 Madison Ave.
New York, NY 10010
Tel. (212) 578-3700

Medical Library
Montefiore Hospital
210th Street & Bainbridge Ave.
New York, NY 10467
Tel. (212) 920-4666
Twx. NN MH NYC 593-2160

Jacobi Library
Mount Sinai Hospital
Fifth Ave & 100th St.
New York, NY 10029
Tel. (212) 876-1000 Ext. 8150
Twx. NN MTS NYC 710-581-4240

N.Y. Academy of Medicine Library
2 E. 103rd St.
New York, NY 10029
Tel. (212) 876-8200
Twx. NY ACAD MED
710-581-6131

Payne Whitney Psychiatric
Clinic Library
New York Hospital
525 East 68th St.
New York, NY 10021

Frederick M. Dearborn Library
New York Medical College
Metropolitan Hospital
1901 1st Ave.
New York, NY 10029

L.M. Hetrick Library
New York Medical College
Fifth Ave. & 106th Street
New York, NY 10029
Tel. (212) 876-5500
Twx. NN NM NYC 710-581-4040

Medical Library
New York Polyclinic Hospital
345 West 50th Street
New York, NY 10019
Tel. (212) 265-8000 Ext. 205

The Abraham A. Brill Library
New York Psychoanalytic
Institute
247 East 82nd St.
New York, NY 10028
Tel. (212) 287-9690

New York State Psychiatric
Institute Library
722 West 168th Street
New York, NY 10032
Tel. (212) 568-4000 Ext. 229

College of Dentistry Library
New York University
421 First Avenue
New York, NY 10010
Tel. (212) 598-7057

Medical Library
New York University Medical
Center
550 First Avenue
New York, NY 10016
Tel. (212) 679-3200
Twx. NN-U-M-NYC 710-581-4167

Library
Postgraduate Center for Mentaı
Health
124 East 28th Street
New York, NY 10016
Tel. (212) 689-7700 Ext. 710

William Hallock Park Mem.
Library
Public Health Research Institute
of the City of New York
455 First Ave.

New York, NY 10016
Tel. (212) 340-4512

Medical Library
Roosevelt Hospital
428 West 59th Street
New York, NY 10019
Tel. (212) 554-6872

Medical Library
St. Clare's Hospital & Health Center
415 W. 51st St.
New York, NY 10019
Tel. (212) 586-1500

Richard Walker Bolling
Memorial Library
St. Luke's Hospital
421 West 113th Street
New York, NY 10025
Tel. (212) 870-6861

The Medical Library Center of
New York
17 E. 102nd St.
New York, NY 10029
Tel. (212) 427-1630
Twx. NN MLC NYC 710-581-4079

Bio-Medical Library
The Population Council
Rockefeller University
York Ave. and 66th St.
New York, NY 10021
Tel. (212) 360-1706

Medical Library
Veterans Administration Hospital

First Ave. at East 24th St.
New York, NY 10010
Tel. (212) 686-7500 Ext. 445

Medical Library
William Douglas Mc Adams Inc.
110 E. 59th St.
New York, NY 10022
Tel. (212) 759-6300 Ext. 277

Medical Library
VA Hospital
Northport, L.I., NY 11768
Tel. (516) 261-4400 Ext. 226

Library
Norwich Pharmacal Company
Post Office Box 191
Norwich, NY 13815
Tel. (607) 344-9911 Ext. 7-217

Medical Library
Creedmoor State Hospital
80-45 Winchester Blvd. Bldg. 51
Queens Village, NY 11427
Tel. (212) 464-7500 Ext. 1321

Ely and Parnall Memorial
Library
Rochester General Hospital
1425 Portland Avenue
Rochester, NY 14621
Tel. (716) 266-4000 Ext. 267

Edward G. Miner Library
University of Rochester
School of Medicine & Dentistry
601 Elmwood Avenue
Rochester, NY 14662

Tel. (716) 275-3364
Twx. UNV ROCH ML 510-253-2295

Medical Library
Mercy Hospital
1000 North Village Avenue
Rockville Centre, NY 11570
Tel. (516) 255-2255

Medical Library
St. Francis Hospital
Port Washington Blvd.
Roslyn, NY 11576
Tel. (516) 627-6200

C.P. Rhoads Memorial Library
Sloan-Kettering Institute
Walker Lab for Cancer Research
145 Boston Post Rd.
Rye, NY 10580
Tel. (212) 879-3000 Ext. 7277

Trudeau Institute Inc.
P.O. Box 59
Saranac Lake, NY 12983
Tel. (518) 891-3080

Montague Memorial Library
and Study Centre
Will Rogers Hospital
Saranac Lake, NY 12983
Tel. (518) 891-3131 Ext. 20

Medical Nursing Library
Ellis Hospital
1101 Nott St.
Schenectady, NY 12308
Tel. (518) 377-3361

Mental Retardation Library
N.Y.S. Institute for Basic Research
1050 Forest Hill Rd.
Staten Island, Ny 10314
Tel. (212) 698-1122 Ext. 659

Medical Library
St. Vincent's Medical Center
355 Bard Avenue
Staten Island, NY 10310
Tel. (212) 390-1327

Charles Ferguson Medical
Library
U.S.P.H.S. Hospital
Staten Island, NY 10304
Tel. (212) 447-3010 Ext. 505

Medical Library
Community-General of
Greater Syracuse
Broad Road
Syracuse, NY 13215

Medical Library
St. Joseph's School of Nursing
206 Prospect Ave.
Syracuse, NY 13203
Tel. (315) 474-6011 Ext. 344

Russell Sage College Library
46 Ferry St.
Troy, Ny 12180
Tel. (518) 270-2240

Medical Library
Samaritan Hospital
Troy, NY 12180
Tel. (518) 274-3000

Masonic Med. Research Lab Library
Bleecker St.
Utica, NY 13501
Tel. (315) 735-2741

Grasslands Medical Library
Westchester County Medical
Center
Valhalla, NY 10595
Tel. (914) 592-8500 Ext. 2506

Westchester Medical Center Library
Basic Science Bldg.
Valhalla, NY 10595
Tel. (914) 948-4100
Twx. WAML PURCHASE
710-568-1366

Medical Library
MEDDAC
West Point, NY 10996
Tel. (914) 938-3221

Medical Library
White Plains Hospital
41 E. Post Rd.
White Plains, NY 10601
Tel. (914) 949-4500 Ext. 346

Medical Library
Yonkers Gernal Hospital
127 Ashburton Ave.
Yonkers, NY 10701
Tel. 965-8200 Ext. 334-335

NORTH CAROLINA

Library
Buncombe County Medical Society
Mem. Mission Hospital Grounds
Ashville, NC 28801
Tel. 252-5331 Ext. 282

Murdoch Library
John Umstead Hospital
Butner, NC 27509
Tel. (919) 575-7259

Library
Dept of Health Technologies
1990 Beach St.
Winston-Salem, NC 27103
Tel. (919) 727-4987

John C. Whitaker Library
Forsyth Memorial Hospital
3333 Silas Creek Pkwy.
Winston-Salem, NC 27103
Tel. (919) 723-9261

Medical Library
U.S. Naval Hospital
Camp Lejeune, NC 28542

Health Sciences Library
University of North Carolina
North Carolina Mem. Hospital
Chapel Hill, NC 27514
Tel. (919) 966-4433
Twx. NCU-HC HILL 510-920-0761

Med. Library Mecklenbury
County Inc.

Doctors Building
1012 Kings Dr.
Charlotte, NC 28283
Tel. (704) 376-1227

Hunter Library-Serials
Western Carolina University
Cullowhee, NC 28723
Tel. (704) 293-7306

Medical Center Library
Duke University
Durham, NC 27710
Tel. (919) 684-3505
Twx. NCD M DURHAM
510-927-1816

The Coppridge Memorial Library
Watts Hospital
Durham, NC 27705
Tel. (919) 286-1231 Ext. 420

Medical Library
Cherry Hospital
Goldsboro, NC 27530

Helath Affairs Library
East Carolina University
P.O. Box 3315 ECU
Greenville, NC 27834
Tel. (919) 758-6560

Public Health Library
Div. of Health Services
P.O. Box 2091
Raleigh, NC 27602
Tel. (919) 829-7389

Medical Library
Dorothea Dix Hospital

Raleigh, NC 27602
Tel. (919) 832-7581 Ext. 443

Medical Library
Wake County Mem. Hospital
3000 New Bern Ave.
Raleigh, NC 27610
Tel. (919) 755-8336

Library
Burroughs Wellcome Co.
3030 Cornwallis Road
Res Triangle Park, NC 27709
Tel. (919) 779-6000 Ext. 335

Medical Library
Health Sciences Foundation Inc.
2131 South 17th St.
Wilmington, NC 28401
Tel. (919) 763-9021 Ext. 211

Medical Library
Womack Army Hospital
Specialized Treatment Center
Fort Bragg, NC
Tel. (919) 396-0205

Library
Bowman Gray School of Medicine
Winston-Salem, NC 27103
Tel. (919) 727-4693
Twx. NCHG WINSTON
510-931-3386

NORTH DAKOTA

Medical Library
Quain and Ramstad Clinic

Box 1818
Bismarck, ND 58501
Tel. 223-1420 Ext. 210

St. Luke's Hospital
5th Street North at Mills Ave.
Fargo, ND 58102
Tel. (701) 235-3161 Ext. 452

Medical Library
VA Center
Fargo, ND 58102
Tel. (701) 232-3241

United Hospital Library
501 Columbia Rd.
Grand Forks, ND 58201
Tel. (701) 775-5521

Harley E. French Medical Library
University of North Dakota
Grand Forks, ND 58202
Tel. (701) 777-2494

State Hospital Library
Box 476
Jamestown, ND 58401
Tel. (701) 252-2120 Ext. 396

Angus L. Cameron Medical Library
Trinity Professional Bldg
Minot, ND 58701
Tel. (701) 838-3321 Ext. 244

OHIO

Medical Library
Akron City Hospital

525 E. Market St.
Akron, OH 44309
Tel. (216) 726-5131 Ext. 360

J.D. Smith Memorial Library
Akron General Hospital
400 Wabash Ave.
Akron, OH 44307
Tel. (216) 375-6242

Medical Library
The Children's Hospital of Akron
Buchtel Ave. at Bowery St.
Akron, OH 44308

Medical Library
Barberton Citizens Hospital
155-5th Street N.E.
Barberton, OH 44203
Tel. (216) 745-1611

Information Resource Center
Bethesda Hospital
619 Oak Street
Cincinnati, OH 45206
Tel. (513) 559-6337

Research Foundation Library
Children's Hospital
Elland Ave. and Bethesda
Cincinnati, OH 45229
Tel. (513) 861-8000 Ext. 300

Medical Library
Good Samaritan Hospital
Clifton Ave.
Cincinnati, OH 45220
Tel. (513) 872-2434

Medical Library
Jewish Hospital
Burnet Ave.
Cincinnati, OH 45229
Tel. (513) 861-3220 Ext. 375

Occupational Health Library
National Institute of Occupational
Safety & Health
P.O. Bldg. Rm. 503
5th & Walnut St.
Cincinnati, OH 45202
Tel. (513) 684-2695

Medical Center Libraries
University of Cincinnati
Eden & Bethesda Aves.
Cincinnati, OH 45219
Tel. (513) 872-5651
Twx. OCU-M-CIN 810-461-2417

Medical Library
Cleveland Clinic Foundation
9500 Euclid Avenue
Cleveland, OH 44106
Tel. (216) 229-2200 Ext. 326

Cleveland Health Sci. Library
2119 Abington Rd.
Cleveland, OH 44106
Tel. (216) 368-3426

Harold H. Brittingham Mem. Lib.
Cleveland Metro Gen. Hospital
3395 Scranton Road
Cleveland, OH 44109
Tel. (216) 398-6000 Ext. 4313

Medical Library
Fairhill Mental Health Center
12200 Fairhill Rd.
Cleveland, OH 44120
Tel. (216) 421-1340

Medical Library
Fairview General Hospital
18101 Lorain
Cleveland, OH 44111
Tel. (216) 252-1222

Medical Staff Library
Huron Road Hospital
13951 Terrace Rd.
Cleveland, OH 44112
Tel. (216) 851-7000 Ext. 306

Lutheran Medical Center Library
2609 Franklin Blvd.
Cleveland, OH 44113
Tel. (216) 696-4300

George H. Hays Memorial Library
Mt. Sinai Hospital of Cleveland
University Circle
Cleveland, OH 44106
Tel. (216) 795-6000 Ext. 249

Library
Ohio College of Podiatry
2057 Cornell Rd.
Cleveland, OH 44106

Medical Staff Library
St. Luke's Hospital
11311 Shaker Blvd.
Cleveland, OH 44104
Tel. (216) 791-1000 Ext. 313

Medical Library
St. Vincent Charity Hospital
2351 East 22nd St.
Cleveland, OH 44115
Tel. (216) 861-6200 Ext. 229

Medical Library
Doctor's Hospital
1087 Dennison Avenue
Columbus, OH 43210
Tel. 421-4113

Health Center Library
Ohio State University
101 Hamilton Hall
Columbus, OH 43210

Medical Library
Green Cross General Hospital
1900 23rd St.
Cuyahoga Falls, OH 44223
Tel. (216) 929-2911

Shank Memorial Library
Good Samaritan Hospital
1425 W. Fairview Ave.
Dayton, OH 45406
Tel. (513) 278-2612 Ext. 460

Medical Library
Grandview Hospital
405 Grand Ave.
Dayton, OH 45405
Tel. (513) 228-4000 Ext. 209

Memorial Medical Library
Miami Valley Hospital
1 Wyoming St.
Dayton, OH 45409
Tel. (513) 223-6192 Ext. 219

Health Sciences Library
St. Elizabeth Medical Center
601 Miami Blvd. W.
Dayton, OH 45408
Tel. (513) 223-3141 Ext. 564

Library
Kettering Memorial Hospital
3535 Southern Blvd.
Kettering, OH 45429
Tel. (513) 298-4331 Ext. 328

Medical Library
Lakewood Hospital
14519 Detroit Ave.
Lakewood, OH 44107
Tel. (216) 521-4200 Ext. 231

Medical Library
St. Rita's Hospital
730 W. Market St.
Lima, OH 45801
Tel. (419) 255-2010 Ext. 331

Ada Leonard Memorial Library
Middletown Hospital Assn.
105 McKnight Dr.
Middletown, OH 45042
Tel. (513) 422-5411 Ext. 318

Medical Library
Medical College of Ohio
P.O. Box 6190

Toledo, OH 43614
Tel. (419) 385-7461 Ext. 522

Library
St. Vincent Hospital & Med. Center
2213 Cherry St.
Toledo, OH 43608
Tel. (419) 241-8161 Ext. 218

Toledo Hospital Medical Library
2142 North Cove Blvd.
Toledo, OH 43606
Tel. (419) 479-8281 Ext. 627

Toledo Medical Library Assn.
3101 Collingwood Ave.
Toledo, OH 43610
Tel. (419) 246-3601 Ext. 18

Wean Medical Library
Trumbull Memorial Hospital
1350 E. Market St.
Warren, OH 44482
Tel. (216) 399-6461

Medical Library
St. Elizabeth Hospital
1044 Belmont Ave.
Youngstown, OH 44505
Tel. (216) 746-7231 Ext. 215

OKLAHOMA

Biomedical Division Library
S.R. Noble Foundation Inc.
Route One
Ardmore, OK 73401
Tel. (405) 223-5810

Medical Library
Reynolds Army Hospital
Fort Sill, OK 73503
Tel. (405) 351-6029

Presbyterian Hospital Library
300 N.W. 12th St.
Oklahoma City, OK 73103
Tel. (405) 236-0681 Ext. 33

O'Donoghue Medical Library
St. Anthony Hospital
601 N.W. 9th Street
Oklahoma City, OK 73102
Tel. (405) 231-1811 Ext. 2197

Health Sciences Center Library
University of Oklahoma
P.O. Box 26901
Oklahoma City, OK 73190
Tel. (405) 271-4285
Twx. OC 910-831-3179

Ivo A. Nelson Medical Library
St. John's Hospital
1923 South Utica
Tulsa, OK 74104
Tel. (918) 743-3311 Ext. 651

Health Sciences Library
St. Francis Hospital
6161 S. Yale Ave.
Tulsa, OK 74136
Tel. (918) 627-2200

Library
Tulsa County Medical Society
1623 East 12th St.
Tulsa, OK 74114

Tel. (918) 587-1461
Twx. TULCMSL 910-845-2106

Library
Southwestern State College
Weatherford, OK 73096
Tel. (405) 772-5511 Ext. 2242

OREGON

Library
Oregon Reg. Primate Research Center
505 N.W. 185th Ave.
Beaverton, OR 97005
Tel. (503) 645-1141

Library Services
Sacred Heart General Hospital
1200 Alder St.
Eugene, OR 97401
Tel. (503) 686-6837

Medical Library
Emanuel Hospital
2801 N. Gantenbein
Portland, OR 97227
Tel. (503) 280-4696

Good Samaritan Medical Library
Good Samaritan Hospital &
Medical Center
1015 N.W. 22nd Ave.
Portland, OR 97210
Tel. (503) 229-7336

U. of Oregon Health Sci. Library
P.O. Box 573
Portland, OR 97207

Tel. (503) 225-8026
Twx. ORU M PORTLAND
810-464-8063

Dental Library
University of Oregon
611 S.W. Campus Drive
Portland, OR 97201
Tel. (503) 225-8822

Health Sciences Library
Salem Hospital Memorial Unit
665 Winter S.E.
Salem, OR 97301
Tel. 370-5377

PENNSYLVANIA

Wilmer Memorial Medical Library
Abington Memorial Hospital
Abington, PA 19001
Tel. (215) 885-4000 Ext. 417

Medical Library
Allentown Hospital
17th and Chew St.
Allentown, PA 18102
Tel. (215) 434-7161

Health Service Library
Sacred Heart Hospital
Allentown, PA 18102
Tel. (215) 821-3280

S.P. Glover Memorial Library
Altoona Hospital
7th St. and Howard Ave.
Altoona , PA 16603
Tel. (814) 946-2318

Medical Library
Medical Center of Beaver County
Beaver Falls Unit
Beaver Falls. PA 15010
Tel. (412) 843-6000 Ext. 229

Medical Library
St. Luke's Hospital
Bethlehem, PA 18015
Tel. (215) 867-3991

Professional Library
Mayview State Hospital
Bridgeville, PA 15017

Medical Library
The Bryn Mawr Hospital
Bryn Mawr, PA 19010
Tel. (215) 527-0600 Ext. 6346

Medical Library
VA Hospital
Butler, PA 16001
Tel. (412) 287-4781

Professional Library
Woodville State Hospital
Box 456
Carnegie, PA 15106
Tel. (412) 279-2000 Ext. 487

Crozer-Chester Medical
Center Library
15 St. and Upland Ave.
Chester, PA 19013
Tel. (874) 961-1279

Major Medical Libraries

Medical Library
George F. Geisinger Mem. Hospital
Danville, PA 17821
Tel. (717) 275-1000 Ext. 463

Medical Library
Hamot Medical Center
P.O. Box 339
Erie, PA 16512
Tel. 455-6711 Ext. 353

Med. Staff Library &
Nursing School Library
Westmoreland Hospital
532 W. Pittsburgh St.
Greensburg, PA 15601
Tel. (412) 837-0100 Ext. 880

Hospital Library
Harrisburg Hospital
S. Front St.
Harrisburg, PA 17101
Tel. (717) 782-5510

Medical Staff Library
Harrisburg Polyclinic Hospital
Third St. & Polyclinic Ave.
Harrisburg, PA 17105
Tel. (717) 782-4292

Library
Pennsylvania Dept. of Health
P.O. Box 90 Rm. 816
Harrisburg, PA 17120
Tel. (717) 787-3900

M.S. Hershey Med. Center Library
Pennsylvannia State University
Hershey, PA 17033
Tel. (717) 534-8626
Twx. PHEN-HERSHEY
510-657-4011

Mueller Health Sciences Library
Lancaster General Hospital
555 N. Duke Street
Lancaster, PA 17604
Tel. (717) 393-5801

Medical Library
Latrobe Area Hospital
West 2nd Ave.
Latrobe, PA 15650
Tel. (412) 539-9711

Medical Library
McKeesport Hospital
1500 Fifth Avenue
McKeesport, PA 15132
Tel. (412) 466-4000

Medical Library-Darrott Div.
Albert Einstein Medical Center
1429 S. Fifth Street
Philadelphia, PA 19147
Tel. (215) 465-1100 Ext. 386

Luria Medical Library
Albert Einstein Medical Center
Northern Division
York and Tabor Roads
Philadelphia, PA 19141
Tel. (215) 329-0700 Ext. 276

Medical Library
Children's Hospital of Philadelphia

1740 Bainbredge St.
Philadelphia, PA 19146
Tel. (215) 546-2700 Ext. 414

College of Physicians Phila. Library
19 South 22 St.
Philadelphia, PA 19103
Tel. (215) 561-6050
Twx. COL-PHYS-PHILA
710-670-1646

Directorate of Med. Mtrl. Library
Defense Personnel Support Center
Bldg. 9 3-F
2800 So. 20th Street
Philadelphia, PA 19101
Tel. (215) 271-2110

Library
Eastern Penn. Psychiatric Institute
Henry Ave. and Abbottsford Rd.
Philadelphia, PA 19129
Tel. (215) 842-4510

Medical Library
Episcopal Hospital
Front Street & Lehigh Avenue
Philadelphia, PA 19125
Tel. (215) 426-8000 Ext. 316

Library
Hahnemann Med. College & Hospital
245 N. 15th Street
Philadelphia, PA 19102
Tel. (215) 448-7184

Institute for Cancer Research Library
7701 Burholme Ave. Fox Chase
Philadelphia, PA 19111
Tel. (215) 342-1000

Medical Library
Institute of Penn. Hospital
111 N. 49th St.
Philadelphia, PA 19139
Tel. (215) 829-2765

Library
Medical College of Pennsylvania
3300 Henry Ave.
Philadelphia, PA 19129
Tel. (215) 849-0400 Ext. 4401-04

Medical Library
Misericordia Hospital
54th St. and Cedar Ave.
Philadelphia, PA 19143
Tel. (215) 747-7600 Ext. 293

Charles E. Krausz Library
Pennsylvania College of
Podiatric Medicine
Race at Eighth Street
Philadelphia, PA 19107
Tel. (215) 629-0300

Medical Library
Pennsylvania Hospital
8th & Spruce Sts.
Philadelphia, PA 19107
Tel. (215) 892-3531

Library
Philadelphia College of
Pharmacy & Science
43rd St. & Woodland Ave.
Philadelphia, PA 19104
Tel. (215) 386-5800 Ext. 260

Major Medical Libraries

C.J. Marshall Memorial Library
School of Veterinary Medicine
University of Pennsylvania
3800 Spruce Street
Philadelphia, PA 19174
Tel. (215) 594-8874

Library
Smith, Kline & French Labs
1530 Spring Garden St.
Philadelphia, PA 19101
Tel. (215) 564-2400 Ext. 7786-87

Doctors Library
St. Agnes Hospital
1900 S. Broad St.
Philadelphia, PA 19145
Tel. (215) 465-2500 Ext. 1213

Health Sciences Center Library
Temple Univ.-Kresge Science Hall
Broad & Tioga Sts.
Philadelphia, PA 19140
Tel. (215) 221-4034

Scott Memorial Library
Thomas Jefferson University
11th & Walnut Sts.
Philadelphia, PA 19107
Tel. (215) 829-6994

Tri-Institutional Library
420 Service Rd.
Philadelphia, PA 19104
Tel. (215) 823-8503

Medical Library
U.S. Naval Hospital
Broad & Pattison Ave.
Philadelphia, PA 19145
Tel. (215) 755-8314

Medical School Library
University of Pennsylvania
Philadelphia, PA 19104
Tel. (215) 595-5815

Hospital Library
University of Pennsylvania
Philadelphia, PA 19104
Tel. (215) 662-2577

Falk Library Health Professions
University of Pittsburgh
De Soto & Terrace Sts.
Pittsburgh, PA 15213
Tel. (412) 683-1620 Ext. 345
Twx. PGH FALK LIB 710-664-4267

Western Psychiatric Institute
& Clinic Library
University of Pittsburgh
3811 O'Hara St.
Pittsburgh, PA 15213
Tel. (412) 683-1620 Ext. 2215
Twx. PGH RALK LIB
710-664-4262

Hospital Library
VA Hospital
University Drive C
Pittsburgh, PA 15240
Tel. (412) 683-3000 Ext. 260

Medical Library
Western Pennsylvania Hospital
4800 Friendship Ave.
Pittsburgh, PA 15224
Tel. (412) 682-4200 Ext. 373

Medical Library
Pottsville Hospital & Warne Clinic
Pottsville, PA 17901
Tel. (717) 622-6120 Ext. 222

Library
St. Joseph's Hospital
Reading, PA 19603
Tel. (215) 376-4901 Ext. 273

Guthrie Clinic Library
Robert Packer Hospital
Wilbur Ave.
Sayre, PA 18840
Tel. (717) 883-9251 Ext. 312

Medical Library
Tri-County Hospital
Sproul & Thomson Rds.
Springfield, PA 19064
Tel. (215) 328-9200 Ext. 245

Library
Farview State Hospital
Waymart, PA 18472
Tel. (717) 488-6111

Professional Library
Wernersville State Hospital
Wernersville, PA 19565
Tel. (215) 678-3411

Library School of Dental Medicine
University of Pennsylvania
4001 Spruce St.
Philadelphia, PA 19174
Tel. (215) 594-8969

Medical Staff &
School of Nursing Library
265 46th St.
Pittsburgh, PA 15201
Tel. (412) 683-7500 Ext. 312

Medical Library
Allegheny General Hospital
320 E. North Ave.
Pittsburgh, PA 15212
Tel. (412) 322-0100 Ext. 522

Blaxter Memorial Library
Children's Hospital of Pittsburgh
125 De Soto Street
Pittsburgh, PA 15213
Tel. (412) 681-7700 Ext. 560

Howard Anderson Power
Mem. Library
Magee-Woman's Hospital
Forbes & Halket St.
Pittsburgh, PA 15213
Tel. (412) 681-5700

Staff Library
Mercy Hospital
Pride and Locust Sts.
Pittsburgh, PA 15219
Tel. (412) 391-8800

Medical Library
Montefiore Hospital
3459 Fifth Ave.
Pittsburgh, PA 15213
Tel. (412) 683-1100 Ext. 344

Staff Library
Presbyterian-University Hospital
230 Lothrop St.
Pittsburgh, PA 15213
Tel. (412) 682-8100 Ext. 719

Health Sciences Library
Shadyside Hospital
5230 Centre Ave.
Pittsburgh, PA 15232
Tel. (412) 622-2415
Twx. CO 250-969-485N

Medical Library
St. Francis General Hospital
45th Street
Pittsburgh, PA 15201
Tel. (412) 622-4110

Library
Luzerne Co. Medical Society
130 S. Franklin St.
Wilkes-Barre, PA 18701
Tel. (717) 822-5218

Medical Library
Mercy Hospital
196 Hanover Street
Wilkes-Barre, PA 18703
Tel. (717) 822-8101

Medical Library
VA Hospital

Wilkes-Barre PA 18703
Tel. (717) 824-3521 Ext. 292

Hospital Library
Wilkes-Barre Gen. Hospital
Corner of Auburn & River Sts.
Wilkes-Barre, PA 18702
Tel. (717) 823-1121

York Hospital Library
1001 S. George St.
York, PA 17405
Tel. (717) 771-2495

PUERTO RICO

College of Pharmacy Library
Univ. of Puerto Rico
Rio Piedras, PR 00926

RHODE ISLAND

Medical Library Admin. Bldg.
Institute of Mental Health
Box 8281
Cranston, RI 02920
Tel. (401) 463-7900 Ext. 295

Medical Library
Memorial Hospital
Prospect and Pond St.
Pawtucket, RI 02860
Tel. (401) 722-6000

Biological Sciences Library
Brown University
P.O. Box 1839

Providence, RI 02912
Tel. (401) 863-2112

The Medical Library
Miriam Hospital
164 Summit Avenue
Providence, RI 02906
Tel. (401) 274-3700 Ext. 220

Medical Library
Providence Lying-In Hospital
50 Maude St.
Providence, RI 02908
Tel. (401) 521-1000 Ext. 313

Library
Rhode Island Medical Society
106 Francis St.
Providence, RI 02903
Tel. (401) 331-3208

Medical Libraries
St. Joseph's Hospital
Peace and Broad Sts.
Providence, RI 02907
Tel. (401) 331-2700 Ext. 208

Levy Library
Emma Pendleton Bradley Hospital
1011 Veterans Memorial Pkwy.
Riverside, RI 02915
Tel. (401) 434-3400 Ext. 252-265

SOUTH CAROLINA

Library
Anderson Memorial
Hospital
800 N. Fant St.

Anderson, SC 29621
Tel. (224) 341-1275

Library
Medical Univ. of S. Carolina
80 Barre St.
Charleston, SC 29401
Tel. (803) 723-9411 Ext. 585
Twx. SCMC CHLSTON
810-881-1829

Medical Library
Naval Regional Medical Center
Charleston, SC 29408
Tel. (803) 743-5573

Medical Library
VA Hospital
Columbia SC 29201
Tel. (803) 776-4000 Ext. 251

Professional Library
Wm. S. Hall Psychiatric Institute
P.O. Drawer 119
Columbia, SC 29202
Tel. (803) 758-7448

Medical Library
Moncrief Army Hospital
Box 499
Ft. Jackson, SC 29207
Tel. (803) 765-5818

Medical Library
Greenville General Hospital
P.O. Box 2760
Greenville, SC 29602
Tel. (803) 242-8597

Medical Library
Spartanburg General Hospital
101 E. Wood St.
Spartanburg, SC 29303
Tel. (803) 582-1213 Ext. 263

SOUTH DAKOTA

Medical Library
Sioux Valley Hospital
1100 S. Euclid
Sioux Falls, SD 57105
Tel. (605) 336-3440 Ext. 343

Medical Library
University of South Dakota
Clarke St.
Vermillion, SD 57069
Tel. (605) 677-5348

TENNESSEE

Medical Library
Baroness Erlanger Hospital
261 Wiehl St.
Chattanooga, TN 37403
Tel. (615) 265-4261 Ext. 647

Hospital Library
Memorial Hospital
2500 Citico Avenue
Chattanooga, TN 37404
Tel. (615) 698-8751 Ext. 697

Learning Center
Jackson-Madison County
Gen. Hospital
708 W. Forest Ave.

Jackson, TN 38301
Tel. (901) 424-0424

Preston Medical Library
University of Tennessee
1924 Alcoa Highway
Knoxville, TN 37920
Tel. (615) 971-3237

John Brister Library Serials Dept.
Memphis State University
Memphis, TN 38152
Tel. (901) 321-1201

William P. Mac Cracken Jr. Library
Southern College of Optometry
1245 Madison Ave.
Memphis, TN 38104
Tel. (901) 725-0180

Medical Library
St. Jude's Children's Res. Hospital
332 N. Lauderdale
Memphis, TN 38101
Tel. (525) 838-1326

Center for the Health Sciences
University of Tennessee
800 Madison Ave.
Memphis, TN 38163
Tel. (901) 528-5638
Twx. TU-M MEMPHIS
810-591-1466

Medical Library
VA Center
Johnson City
Mountain Home, TN 37684
Tel. (615) 928-0281 Ext. 273

Meharry Alumni Library
Meharry Medical College
1005-18th Ave. North
Nashville, TN 37208
Tel. (615) 327-6318
Twx. TU 810-371-1747

Health Science Library
Nashville General Hospital
72 Hermitage Ave.
Nashville, TN 37210
Tel. (615) 255-6311 Ext. 311

Health Sciences Library
St. Thomas Hospital
Box 380
Nashville, TN 37202
Tel. (615) 244-5151 Ext. 312

Medical Center Library
Vanderbilt University
Nashville, TN 37232
Tel. (615) 322-2292
Twx. TN VAND MED LIB
810-371-1097

VA Hospital
1310 24th Ave. South
Nashville, TN 37203
Tel. (615) 327-4751 Ext. 7615

Medical Library
Oak Ridge Associated University
P.O. Box 117
Oak Ridge, TN 37830
Tel. (615) 483-8411 Ext. 208

TEXAS

ASH Medical Library
Austin State Hospital
4110 Guadalupe St.
Austin, TX 78751
Tel. (512) 465-6521 Ext. 315

Memorial Library
Texas Med. Assn.
1801 Lamar Blvd.
Austin, TX 78701
Tel. (512) 477-6704

Library
Texas State Dept. of Health
1100 West 49th Street
Austin, TX 78756

College of Pharmacy Library
University of Texas
Austin, TX 78712

Memorial Library
St. Elizabeth Hospital
P.O. Box 5405
Beaumont, TX 77702
Tel. (713) 892-7171 Ext. 226

Carswell Medical Library
USAF Regional Hospital
Carswell AFB, TX 76127
Tel. (817) 738-3511 Ext. 7579

Veterinary Medical Library
Texas A&M Univ. College of Vet.
  Med.
College Station, TX 77843
Tel. (713) 846-6111

Major Medical Libraries

Health Sciences Library
Memorial Medical Center
P.O. Box 5280
Corpus Christi, TX 78405
Tel. (512) 884-4511

Med-Nursing-Dental Library
Baylor University
3402 Gaston Ave.
Dallas, TX 75246
Tel. (214) 824-5410 Ext. 373

Library
University of Texas
Health Sci. Center at Dallas
5323 Harry Hines Blvd.
Dallas, TX 75235
Tel. (214) 631-3220
Twx. TXDAS 910-861-4946

Library
North Texas State University
Denton, TX 76203

Medical Library Bldg 7777
William Beaumont General Hospital
El Paso, TX 79920
Tel. (915) 568-3596

Medical Library
U.S. Darnall Army Hospital
Fort Hood, TX 76544
Tel. (817) 685-4237

Academy Library
Academy of Health Sciences
Ft. Sam Houston, TX 78234
Tel. (512) 221-5932

Medical Library
Brooke General Hospital
Ft. Sam Houston, TX 78234
Tel. (512) 221-4119

Stimson Library
Medical Field Service School
Ft. Sam Houston, TX 78234
Tel. (512) 221-5932

Medical Library
John Peter Smith Hospital
1500 S. Main St.
Ft. Worth, TX 76104
Tel. (817) 926-5191 Ext. 424

Library
Texas College of Osteopathic
    Medicine
3516 Camp Bowie Blvd.
Ft. Worth, TX 76107
Tel. (817) 731-2183

Moody Medical Library
Univ. of Texas Medical Branch
912 Mechanic St.
Galveston, TX 77550
Tel. (713) 765-2371
Twx. TXGUM 910-885-5225

Library
M.D. Anderson Hospital &
Tumor Institute
University of Texas
Houston, TX 77025
Tel. (713) 526-5411 Ext. 228
Twx. TXHMD 910-881-3756

Health Sciences Library
St. Joseph Hospital

1919 La Branch
Houston, TX 77002
Tel. (713) 225-3131

Texas Medical Center Library
6401 W. Cullen St.
Houston, TX 77025
Tel. (713) 529-3808
Twx. TXHMC 910-881-3662

University of Houston
Libraries Serials Department
Cullen Blvd.-L Fleming Bldg # 221
Houston, TX 77004
Tel. (713) 748-6600 Ext. 1335

Wilford Hall USAF Hospital
Aerospace Medical Division
Air Force Systems Command
Lackland AFB, TX 78236
Tel. (512) OR1-7455

Health Science Information Center
Texas Tech University
School of Medicine
Box 4569
Lubbock, TX 79409
Tel. (806) 742-5245
Twx. TX 910-896-4329

Mae Hilty Memorial Library
Texas Chiropractic College
5912 Spencer Hwy.
Pasadena, TX 77505
Tel. (713) 487-1170

Southwest Foundation for
Research and Education Library
P.O. Box 28147

San Antonio, TX 78284
Tel. (512) 674-1410

Health Science Center Library
San Antonio
University of Texas
7703 Floyd Curl Dr.
San Antonio, TX 78284
Tel. (512) 696-6271
Twx. TXSAS 910-870-1871

Medical Library
USAF Regional Hospital
Sheppard AFB, TX 76311

Medical Library
Scott & White Memorial Hospital
Temple, TX 76501
Tel. (817) PR8-4451 Ext. 228

Medical Library
Wichita Falls State Hospital
P.O. Box 300
Wichita Falls, TX 76307
Tel. (817) 692-1220

UTAH

Spencer S. Eccles Med. Sci. Library
University of Utah
Salt Lake City, UT 84112
Tel. (801) 581-8771
Twx. W W MED LIB
SL 910-925-5175

Medical Library
VA Hospital
Salt Lake City, UT 84113
Tel. (801) 582-1565 Ext. 306

VERMONT

Medical Library
University of Vermont
Colchester Ave.
Burlington, VT 05401
Tel. (802) 864-4511 Ext. 255
Twx. VTU-M BRLNGTON
710-224-6774

VIRGINIA

School of Medicine Library
University of Virginia
Charlottesville, VA 22901
Tel. (703) 924-2279
Twx. VIU-CHLTVL 510-587-5459

Medical Library
Kenner Army Hospital
Fort Lee, VA 23801
Tel. 734-2989

Medical Library
Mem. Hospital of Martinsville &
Henry County
Commonwealth Blvd.
Martinsville, VA 24112

Boone Memorial Library
De Paul Hospital
Granby & Kingsley Lane
Norfolk, VA 23505
Tel. (703) 489-5270

Norfolk Co. Med. Soc. Library
10th Fl.-Medical Tower

400 Gresham Dr.
Norfolk, VA 23507
Tel. (703) 622-1421

Health Sciences Library
Norfolk General Hospital
600 Gresham Dr.
Norfolk, VA 23507
Tel. (703) 441-3693

Medical Library
U.S. Naval Hospital
Portsmouth, VA 23708
Tel. (703) 397-6581 Ext. 536

Tompkins-Mc Caw Library
Medical College of Va.
Virginia Commonwealth University
Box 667 MCV Station
Richmond, VA 23298
Tel. (804) 770-2033
Twx. VI 710-956-0255

Medical Library
Richmond Memorial Hospital
1300 Westwood Ave.
Richmond, VA 23227
Tel. (804) 359-6961 Ext. 347

Library Service
Veterans Administration Hospital
Broad Rock Rd. & Belt Blvd.
Richmond, VA 23249
Tel. (804) 233-9631 Ext. 458

Medical Library
Winchester Memorial Hospital

S. Stewart St.
Winchester, VA 22601

WASHINGTON

Medical Library
Naval Regional Med. Center
Bremerton, WA 98314
Tel. (206) 478-4269

Library
Atomic Bomb Casualty Comm.
U.S. Marine Corps Air Station
FPO Seattle, WA 98764

Washington State Library
Serials Section
Olympia, WA 98504
Tel. (206) 753-5592

Health Sciences Library
University of Washington
Seattle, WA 98195
Tel. (206) 543-5530
Twx. WAUM SEATTLE
910-444-1385

Health Sciences Library
Sacred Heart Med. Center
W. 101 Eighth Ave.
Spokane, WA 99204
Tel. (509) 455-3904

Spokane, Medical Library
280 B. Paulsen Med-Dental Bldg.
Spokane, WA 99201
Tel. (509) 747-5777

Medical Library
Veterans Administration Hospital
N4815 Assembly
Spokane, WA 99208
Tel. (509) 328-4521

Medical Library
Madigan Army Medical Center
Box 375
Tacoma, WA 98431
Tel. (206) 967-6782

WEST VIRGINIA

Medical Center Library
West Virginia University
Morgantown, WV 26506
Tel. (304) 293-2113

WISCONSIN

Medical Library
Luther Hospital
310 Chestnut St.
Eau Claire, WI 54701
Tel. (715) 832-6611 Ext. 351

Health Science Library
La Crosse Lutheran Hospital
1910 South Ave.
La Crosse, WI 54601
Tel. (608) 785-0530 Ext. 451

Health Sciences Library
St. Francis Hospital
615 S. 10th St.
La Crosse, WI 54601
Tel. (608) 782-8022 Ext. 418

Major Medical Libraries

Primate Library
University of Wisconsin
1223 Capitol Court
Madison, WI 53706
Tel. (608) 263-3512

Medical School Library
University of Wisconsin
1305 Linden Dr.
Madison, WI 53706
Tel. (608) 262-6594
Twx. UWH MED LIB 910-286-2278

F.B. Power Pharmaceutical Library
University of Wisconsin
School of Pharmacy
425 N. Charter St.
Madison, WI 53706
Tel. (608) 262-2894

Marshfield Clinic Library
630 S. Central
Marshfield, WI 54449
Tel. (715) 387-5183

Research Library
Lakeside Laboratories
1707 E. North Ave.

Milwaukee, WI 53201
Tel. (414) 271-9400 Ext. 316

Medical-Dental Library
Medical College of Wisconsin
560 North 16th Street
Milwaukee, WI 53233
Tel. (414) 272-5450 Ext. 240
Twx. WMM MED MILW
910-262-1178

Library
Milwaukee Blood Center Inc.
763 N. 18th St.
Milwaukee, WI 53233

Medical Library
St. Luke's Hospital
2900 W. Oklahoma Ave.
Milwaukee, WI 53215
Tel. (414) 671-2900 Ext. 200

Medical Library
Veterans Administration Center
Wood, WI 53193
Tel. (414) 384-2000 Ext. 2354

Canada

ALBERTA

Calgary Assoc. Clinic Library
214-6 Ave. S.W.
Calgary, AB
Canada
Tel. (403) 263-7120

Medical-Dental Library
Calgary General Hospital
841 Centre Avenue East
Calgary, AB
Canada
Tel. (403) 266-7541 Ext. 382

Medical Division
University of Calgary Library
Medical Division
Foothills Hospital
Calgary, AB
Canada
Tel. (403) 283-0751 Ext. 503

Health Sciences Library
Edmonton General Hospital
11111 Jasper Ave.
Edmonton, AB
Canada
Tel. (403) 482-4421 Ext. 359

Weinlos Library
Misericordia Hospital
16940 87th Ave.
Edmonton, AB
Canada
Tel. (403) 425-8903 Ext. 291

University Library
University of Alberta
Edmonton, AB
Canada

BRITISH COLUMBIA

Woodward Biomedical Library
Serials Department
Univ. of British Columbia
Vancouver 8, BC
Canada
Tel. (604) 228-2762

British Columbia Medical
Library Service
College of Physicians and
Surgeons
1807 W. 10 Ave.
Vancouver 9, BC
Canada
Tel. (604) 736-5551

Victoria Med. Society Library
2334 Trent St.
Victoria, BC
Canada
Tel. (604) 386-2535

MANITOBA

Faculty of Medicine Library
Univ. of Manitoba
Bannatyne Ave.
Winnipeg, MB
Canada
Tel. (204) 786-3621

Dental Library
University of Manitoba
Winnipeg 3, MB
Canada
Tel. (204) 786-3635

NEWFOUNDLAND

Faculty of Medicine Library
Memorial Univ. of Newfoundland
St. Johns, NF
Canada
Tel. (709) 753-1200 Ext. 2687

Medical Library
St. Johns General Hospital
St. Johns, NF
Canada
Tel. (709) 726-3010 Ext. 410

NOVA SCOTIA

W.K. Kellogg Health Sciences
Library
Dalhousie University
Carleton and College St.
Halifax, NS
Canada
Tel. (902) 424-2482

ONTARIO

Health Sciences Library
St. Lawrence College
20 Parkedale Avenue
Brockville, ON

Canada
Tel. (613) 345-0660 Ext. 256

Ontario Veterinary College
Library
University of Guelph
Guelph, ON
Canada
Tel. 824-4120 Ext. 2518

Health Sciences Library
Mc Master University
1200 Main Street West
Hamilton, ON
Canada
Tel. (416) 525-9140 Ext. 2320

The Hamilton Academy of
Medicine Library
286 Victoria Ave. N.
Hamilton, ON
Canada
Tel. 528-1611

Medical Library
Kingston Psychiatric Hospital
Box 603
Kingston, ON
Canada
Tel. 546-1101 Ext. 216

Health Sciences Library
Queens University
Kingston, ON
Canada
Tel. (613) 547-5753

Medical Library
Children's Psychiatric Research

Institute
P.O. Box 2460 Terminal A
London, ON
Canada
Tel. (519) 471-2540 Ext. 255

Period. Dept. General Library
Univ. of Western Ontario
London 72, ON
Canada
Tel. (519) 679-3912

Departmental Library
Dept. of Natl. Health & Welfare
Ottawa, ON
Canada
Tel. (613) 992-5743

George Williamson Medical Library
Ottawa Civic Hospital
1053 Carling Ave.
Ottawa 3, ON
Canada
Tel. (613) 725-4450

Library
Canadian Nurses Association
50 The Driveway
Ottawa 4, ON
Canada
Tel. (613) 237-2133 Ext. 38

Medical Library
St. Joseph Hospital
Mackenzie St.
Sudbury, ON
Canada
Tel. (705) 674-3101

William Boyd Library
Academy of Medicine Toronto
288 Bloor St. West
Toronto, ON
Canada
Tel. (416) 964-7088

Medical Library
St. Michael's Hospital
30 Bond St.
Toronto, ON
Canada
Tel. (416) 360-4941

Fudger Medical Library
Toronto General Hospital
101 College Street
Toronto, ON
Canada
Tel. (416) 595-3549

Dental Library & The Harry R.
   Abbott Memorial Library
University of Toronto
124 Edward Street
Toronto, ON
Canada
Tel. (416) 928-8921

Science and Medicine Library
University of Toronto
   Kings College Circle
Toronto, ON
Canada
Tel. (416) 928-6434

Medical Library
Toronto Western Hospital

399 Bathurst St.
Toronto 130, ON
Canada

Medical Library
Hospital for Sick Children
555 University Ave.
Toronto 2, ON
Canada
Tel. (416) 366-7242 Ext. 1446

Farrar Library
Clarke Institute of Psychiatry
250 College St.
Toronto 28, ON
Canada
Tel. (416) 924-6811 Ext. 467

Medical Library
Sunnybrook Hospital
2075 Bayview Ave.
Toronto 315, ON
Canada
Tel. (416) 486-3880

Sydney Wood Bradley Mem.
   Library
Canadian Dental Assoc.
234 St. George St.
Toronto 5, ON
Canada
Tel. (416) 927-3261

Ontario Cancer Institute Library
500 Sherbourne St.
Toronto 5, ON
Canada
Tel. (416) 924-0671

The Medical Library
Wellesley Hospital

160 Wellesley St. E.
Toronto 5, ON
Canada
Tel. (416) 966-6617

Library
Connaught Laboratories Ltd.
1755 Steeles Ave. West
Willowdale, ON
Canada
Tel. (416) 635-2704

QUEBEC

Library
Constance Lethbridge Centre
7005 De Maisonneve W.
Montreal, PQ
Canada
Tel. (514) 487-1770

Bibliotheque Medicale
Hospital De La Mesericorde
1051 Rue St. Hubert
Montreal, PQ
Canada
Tel. (514) 842-7181 Ext. 207

Medical Library
Mc Gill University
3655 Drummond St.
Montreal, PQ
Canada
Tel. (514) 392-3059

Bibliotheque Medicale
Universite De Montreal
G.P. 6128
Montreal, PQ

Canada
Tel. (514) 343-6908
Twx. WM 610-421-3102

Medical Library
Jewish General Hospital
3755 Cote St. Catherine Rd.
Montreal 26, PQ
Canada
Tel. (514) 342-3111 Ext. 325

Bibliotheque Medicale
Hospital Jean-Talon
1365 Est Rue Jean-Talon
Montreal 329, PQ
Canada
Tel. (514) 273-5151

Bibliotheque Documentation
Hospital Du Sacre-Coeur
5400 Gouin Ouest
Montreal 390, PQ
Canada
Tel. (514) 333-2166

Bibliotheque
Hospital St-Jean-De-Dieu
7401 Rue Hochelaga
Montreal-Gamelin, PQ
Canada
Tel. (514) 254-8381

Bibliotheque Generale
Universite De Sherbrooke
Sherbrooke, PQ
Canada
Tel. (819) 569-7431

SASKATCHEWAN

Medical Library
Regina General Hospital
14th Ave. & St. John St.
Regina, SK
Canada
Tel. (306) 522-1811

Medical Library
University of Saskatchewan
Saskatoon, SK
Canada

Foreign

ARGENTINA

Inst. De Oncologia Bibl. A.H.
Roffo
A.V. San Martin 5481
Buenos Aires,
Argentina

Facultad De Ciencias Medicas
Universidad Nacional De
Cordoba Bibioteca
Estafa 32-Ciudad Universitaria
Cordoba,
Argentina

Centro Medico De Mar Del Plata
Bibl.
San Luis 1978
Mar Del Plata
Argentina,

Biblioteca Biomedica
Universidad Nacional Del Nor
Las Heras 727
Resistecia,
Argentina

AUSTRALIA

Medical Library
Monash University
Post Office Box 92
Clayton,
Australia

Brownless Medical Library
Univ. of Melbourne

Central Med. Lib. Org.
Parkville,
Australia

Hospital Library
Royal Perth Hospital
Wellington St.
Perth 6000,
Australia

Repatriation Dept. Libraries
Central Office Furzer St.
Phillip,
Australia

New South Wales Branch Library
Australian Med. Association
135 Macquarie St.
Sydney,
Australia

Fisher Library
University of Sydney
Gift and Exchange Section
Sydney,
Australia

BELGIUM

Bibliotek Aedes Medicorum
Universiteitskinieken St.
Rafael
Minderbroererstraat 12
Leuven,
Belgium

Bibliotheque De La Faculte De
Medecine

L'Univ. Catholique De Louvain
4 Av.Chapelle-Aux-Champs
1200 Brussels,
Belgium

Biblioteca Medica
Universidad De Antioquia
Apartado Postal 2038
Medellin,
Colombia

BRAZIL

Biblioteca
Fac. De Odontologia De Bauru
Caixa Postal # 73 17100 Bauru
Est Sao Paulo,
Brazil

Regional De Medicina
Vila Clementino
Caixa Clementino
Sao Paulo,
Brazil

Faculdade De Odontologia
Universidade De Sao Paulo
Rua Tres Rios 363 C.P. 8216
Sao Paulo,
Brazil

COLOMBIA

Departmento De Bibliotecad
Universidad Del Valle
Apartado Aero 2188 Nal 439
Cali,
Colombia

ENGLAND

The Barnes Library The Med.
   School
Univ. of Birmingham
Birmingham B15 2TJ,
England

The Library
The Medical School
University Walk
Bristol 8,
England

Medical Library
University of Leeds School of
Medicine
Thoresby Pl.
Leeds 2,
England

The University Library
University Road
Leicester,
England

Library
University of Liverpool
P.O. Box 123
Liverpool L693DA,
England

The Wellcome Institute of the
History of Medicine
183 Euston Rd.
London, N.W.,
England

Chester Beatty Research Institute
Institute of Cancer Research
Fulham Rd.
London S.W.3.,
England

London School of Hygiene &
Tropical Medicine Library
Keppel St.
London W.C.1.,
England

Royal Society of Medicine
Library
1 Wimpole St.
London W.1,
England

Pharmaceutical Society of
Great Britain Library
17 Bloomsbury Square
London WC1,
England

Medical Library
Royal College of Surgery of England
35/43 Lincolns Inn Fields
London WC2A 3PN,
England

Medical School Library
Charing Cross Hospital
Fulham Place Rd.
London W6 8RF,
England

University Library/Medicine
NewCastle Upon Tyne,
England

Med./Sci. Library
University of Nottingham
Nottingham,
England

FINLAND

Library
University of Kuopio
Kuopio,
Finland

GUATEMALA

Instituto De Nutricion De
Centro America Y Panama Library
Carretera Roosevelt
Guatemala City-11,
Guatemala

GUYANA

Guyana Med. Science Library
Georgetown Hospital Compound
New Market Street
Georgetown,
Guyana

HOLLAND

Medical Library
Erasmus University
P.O. Box 1738
Rotterdam,
Holland

HONG KONG

Medical Library
University of Hong Kong
Sassoon Road
Hong Kong,
Hong Kong

INDIA

Library
St. John's Medical College
Johnnagara
Bangalore-34,
India
Twx. SAINJOHNS

Dodd Memorial Library
Christain Med. Coll. Hospital

Tamil Nadu
Vellore-4,
India

IRAN

Medical School Library
Pahlavi University
Shiraz,
Iran

The A. Torab Mehra Med. Library
Shiraz Medical Center
Nemazee Hospital
Shiraz,
Iran

ISRAEL

Jewish National & University
Library
P.O.B. 503
Jerusalem,
Israel

Medical Library
Beilinson Hospital
P.O. Box 85
Petach Tikwah,
Israel

JAPAN

Kawasaki Med. College Library
577 Matsushima Kurashiki

Okayama,
Japan

Library
Sapporo Medical College
South 1 West 17 Chuo-Ku
Sapporo,
Japan

Showa University Library
Hatanodai-1 Shinagaw-Ku
Tokyo,
Japan

Medical Library
University of Tokyo
Hongo Bunkyo-Ku
Tokyo,
Japan

Library
Yamanouchi Pharmaceutical Co.
   Ltd.
1-8 Azusawa-1-Chome
Tokyo,
Japan

National Cancer Center Library
Tsukiji 5-Chome Chuo-Ku
Tokyo 104,
Japan

Int. 1 Medical Information Center
   Inc.
30 Daikyocho Shinjuku-Ku
Tokyo 160,
Japan

Medical Library
Keio University
35 Shinanomachi Shinjuku-Ku
Tokyo 160,
Japan

LEBANON

Medical Library
American University of Beirut
Bliss St.
Beirut,
Lebanon

MALAYSIA

National Univ. of Malaysia Library
Jalan Pantai Baru
Peti Surat 124
Kuala Lumpur,
Malaysia

MALTA

University Medical Library
Medical School
Guardamangia,
Malta

MEXICO

Departamento De Biblioteca
Instututo Nacional De
Cardiologia
Avenida Cuauhtemoc 300
Mexico D.F.,
Mexico

Bibiloteca Central I.M.S.S.
Instituto Mexicano Del Segura
Social
Apartado Postal 73-065
Mexico 12 D.F.,
Mexico

NEW ZEALAND

Earnest & Marion Davis Library
Auckland Hospital
Park Road
Auckland 3,
New Zealand

NIGERIA

Benin University Library
Private Mail Bag 1191
Benin City,
Nigeria

NORWAY

Universitetsbiblioteket 1 Oslo
Medical Department
Drammensweien 42 B
Oslo,
Norway

PERU

Dereccion De Bibl. Y Pub. of De
Acquis Bibliogr.-Me.

Univ. nac. Mayor De San Marcos
AP 454
Lima,
Peru

Library
Colegio Medico Del Peru
Av. Santa Cruz 315
Lima 18,
Peru

PHILLIPINES

Ramon Magsaysay Memorial
Medical Center
University of the East
Aurora Blvd.
Quezon City,
Phillipines

SOUTH AFRICA

Medical Library
University of Cape Town
Anzio Road Observatory 7900
Cape Town,
South Africa

Witwatersrand Medical Library
Medical School
Hospital St.
Johannesburg,
South Africa

Medical Library
Univ. of Stellenbosch
P.O. Box 91
Tiervlei C.P.,
South Africa

SWEDEN

Bio-Medicinska Biblioteket
Universitets Biblioteket
Fack 400 33
Goteborg 33,
Sweden

SWITZERLAND

Universitatsspital Bibliothek
Ramistrasse 100
Zurich 8006,
Switzerland

Library
World Health Organization
Avenue Appia
1211 Geneva 27,
Switzerland

SYRIA

Faculty of Medicine Library
University of Aleppo
Aleppo,
Syria

THAILAND

Library Faculty of Science
Mahidol University
Rama 6 Road
Bangkok 4,
Thailand

VENEZUELA

Bibl. De La Pac De Odontologia
Univ. Central De Venezuela
Aptd. De Correos 61 351
Caracas,
Venezuela

Instituto De Medicina Exper.
Biblioteca
Univ. Central De Venezuela
Aptd. 50587-Sabana Grade
Caracas,
Venezuela

Bibl. De La Fac. De Medicina
Universidad Del Zulia
Apartado 526
Maracaibo,
Venezuela

WEST GERMANY

Bibliothek
Medizinische Hochschule
Karl-Weichert-Allee 9 PF 180
3 Hannover-Kleefeld,
West Germany

WEST INDIES

Library
University of the West Indies
Mona
Kingston 7, Jamaica,
West Indies

ZAMBIA

Library
Queen Elizabeth Hospital
St. Michail, Barbados,
West Indies

University of Zambia Library
P.O. Box 2379
Lusaka,
Zambia

METRIC—APOTHECARIES' LIQUID MEASURE

Milli-liters	Minims	Milli-liters	Fluidrams	Milli-liters	Fluid ounces
1	16.231	5	1.35	30	1.01
2	32.5	10	2.71	40	1.35
3	48.7	15	4.06	50	1.69
4	64.9	20	5.4	500	16.91
5	81.1	25	6.76	1000 (1 L.)	33.815
		30	7.1		

APOTHECARIES'—METRIC WEIGHT

Grains	Grams
1/150	0.0004
1/120	0.0005
1/100	0.0006
1/80	0.0008
1/64	0.001
1/50	0.0013
1/40	0.0014
1/30	0.0022
1/25	0.0026
1/16	0.004
1/12	0.005
1/10	0.006
1/9	0.007
1/8	0.008
1/7	0.009
1/6	0.01
1/5	0.013

METRIC—APOTHECARIES' WEIGHT

Scruples	Grams
1	1.296 (1.3)
2	2.592 (2.6)
3	3.888 (3.9)

Drams	Grams
1	3.888
2	7.776
3	11.664
4	15.552
5	19.440
6	23.328
7	27.216
8	31.103

Ounces	Grams
1	31.103
2	62.207
3	93.310
4	124.414

APOTHECARIES'– METRIC WEIGHT		METRIC– APOTHECARIES' WEIGHT	
1/4	0.016	5	155.517
1/3	0.02	6	186.621
1/2	0.032	7	217.724
1	0.065	8	248.828
1½	0.097 (0.1)	9	279.931
2	0.12	10	311.035
3	0.20	11	342.138
4	0.24	12 (1 lb.)	373.242
5	0.30	Milligrams	Grains
6	0.40	1	0.015432
7	0.45	2	0.030864
8	0.50	3	0.046296
9	0.60	4	0.061728
10	0.65	5	0.077160
15	1.00	6	0.092592
20	1.30		
30	2.00		

OBSTETRICAL TABLE TO DETERMINE DATE OF CONFINEMENT

Numbers shown on the top lines in each section represent the first day of the last menstrual period. Those appearing directly below indicate the probable date of the parturition.

| Jan. | 1 | 2 | 3 | 4 | 5 | 6 | 7 | 8 | 9 | 10 | 11 | 12 | 13 | 14 | 15 | 16 | 17 | 18 | 19 | 20 | 21 | 22 | 23 | 24 | 25 | 26 | 27 | 28 | 29 | 30 | 31 | |
| Oct. | 8 | 9 | 10 | 11 | 12 | 13 | 14 | 15 | 16 | 17 | 18 | 19 | 20 | 21 | 22 | 23 | 24 | 25 | 26 | 27 | 28 | 29 | 30 | 31 | 1 | 2 | 3 | 4 | 5 | 6 | 7 | Nov. |

| Feb. | 1 | 2 | 3 | 4 | 5 | 6 | 7 | 8 | 9 | 10 | 11 | 12 | 13 | 14 | 15 | 16 | 17 | 18 | 19 | 20 | 21 | 22 | 23 | 24 | 25 | 26 | 27 | 28 | |
| Nov. | 8 | 9 | 10 | 11 | 12 | 13 | 14 | 15 | 16 | 17 | 18 | 19 | 20 | 21 | 22 | 23 | 24 | 25 | 26 | 27 | 28 | 29 | 30 | 1 | 2 | 3 | 4 | 5 | Dec. |

| Mar. | 1 | 2 | 3 | 4 | 5 | 6 | 7 | 8 | 9 | 10 | 11 | 12 | 13 | 14 | 15 | 16 | 17 | 18 | 19 | 20 | 21 | 22 | 23 | 24 | 25 | 26 | 27 | 28 | 29 | 30 | 31 | |
| Dec. | 6 | 7 | 8 | 9 | 10 | 11 | 12 | 13 | 14 | 15 | 16 | 17 | 18 | 19 | 20 | 21 | 22 | 23 | 24 | 25 | 26 | 27 | 28 | 29 | 30 | 31 | 1 | 2 | 3 | 4 | 5 | Jan. |

| April | 1 | 2 | 3 | 4 | 5 | 6 | 7 | 8 | 9 | 10 | 11 | 12 | 13 | 14 | 15 | 16 | 17 | 18 | 19 | 20 | 21 | 22 | 23 | 24 | 25 | 26 | 27 | 28 | 29 | 30 | |
| Jan. | 6 | 7 | 8 | 9 | 10 | 11 | 12 | 13 | 14 | 15 | 16 | 17 | 18 | 19 | 20 | 21 | 22 | 23 | 24 | 25 | 26 | 27 | 28 | 29 | 30 | 31 | 1 | 2 | 3 | 4 | Feb. |

| May | 1 | 2 | 3 | 4 | 5 | 6 | 7 | 8 | 9 | 10 | 11 | 12 | 13 | 14 | 15 | 16 | 17 | 18 | 19 | 20 | 21 | 22 | 23 | 24 | 25 | 26 | 27 | 28 | 29 | 30 | 31 | |
| Feb. | 5 | 6 | 7 | 8 | 9 | 10 | 11 | 12 | 13 | 14 | 15 | 16 | 17 | 18 | 19 | 20 | 21 | 22 | 23 | 24 | 25 | 26 | 27 | 28 | 1 | 2 | 3 | 4 | 5 | 6 | 7 | Mar. |

| June | 1 | 2 | 3 | 4 | 5 | 6 | 7 | 8 | 9 | 10 | 11 | 12 | 13 | 14 | 15 | 16 | 17 | 18 | 19 | 20 | 21 | 22 | 23 | 24 | 25 | 26 | 27 | 28 | 29 | 30 | |
| Mar. | 8 | 9 | 10 | 11 | 12 | 13 | 14 | 15 | 16 | 17 | 18 | 19 | 20 | 21 | 22 | 23 | 24 | 25 | 26 | 27 | 28 | 29 | 30 | 31 | 1 | 2 | 3 | 4 | 5 | 6 | April |

July 1 2 3 4 5 6 7 8 9 10 11 12 13 14 15 16 17 18 19 20 21 22 23 24 25 26 27 28 29 30 31

April 7 8 9 10 11 12 13 14 15 16 17 18 19 20 21 22 23 24 25 26 27 28 29 30 1 2 3 4 5 6 7 May

Aug. 1 2 3 4 5 6 7 8 9 10 11 12 13 14 15 16 17 18 19 20 21 22 23 24 25 26 27 28 29 30 31

May 8 9 10 11 12 13 14 15 16 17 18 19 20 21 22 23 24 25 26 27 28 29 30 31 1 2 3 4 5 6 7 June

Sept. 1 2 3 4 5 6 7 8 9 10 11 12 13 14 15 16 17 18 19 20 21 22 23 24 25 26 27 28 29 30

June 8 9 10 11 12 13 14 15 16 17 18 19 20 21 22 23 24 25 26 27 28 29 30 1 2 3 4 5 6 7 July

Oct. 1 2 3 4 5 6 7 8 9 10 11 12 13 14 15 16 17 18 19 20 21 22 23 24 25 26 27 28 29 30 31

July 8 9 10 11 12 13 14 15 16 17 18 19 20 21 22 23 24 25 26 27 28 29 30 31 1 2 3 4 5 6 7 Aug.

Nov. 1 2 3 4 5 6 7 8 9 10 11 12 13 14 15 16 17 18 19 20 21 22 23 24 25 26 27 28 29 30

Aug. 8 9 10 11 12 13 14 15 16 17 18 19 20 21 22 23 24 25 26 27 28 29 30 31 1 2 3 4 5 6 Sept.

Dec. 1 2 3 4 5 6 7 8 9 10 11 12 13 14 15 16 17 18 19 20 21 22 23 24 25 26 27 28 29 30 31

Sept. 7 8 9 10 11 12 13 14 15 16 17 18 19 20 21 22 23 24 25 26 27 28 29 30 1 2 3 4 5 6 7 Oct.

179 Commonly Misspelled Medical Words

ab'scess
ac''e tab'u lum
ach''a la'si a
al''o pe'ci a
am''y loi do'sis
an''a phy lax'ia
an'eu rysm
ar''rhe no blas to'ma
ath''er o scle ro'sis
ba cil'li form
bac te'ri o phage
bar''bi'tu rate
bleph'a ron
bron''chi ec'ta sis
bron'chi ole
buc'ca
ca chex'i a
cal ca'ne us
cal'lus
ca'lyx
cap''i tel'lum
car'ci no gen
ca'se ous
cau'dad
cha la'zion
cho re'i form
chyle
cir rho'sis
coc'cyx
con''tre coup'
co ry'za
cul-de-sac
cy a no'sis
de cid'u a
de his'cence
di''a pho re'sis
di u re'sis

dys cra'si a
dys''men or rhe'a
dys to'ci a
ec''chy mo'sis
ec'ze ma
em''phy se'ma
en ceph''a li'tis
en''do me''tri o'sis
e piph'y sis
er''y sip'e las
ex san'gui nate
fa'ci es
fen''es tra'tion
fim'bri a
fis'tu la
flat'u lence
fol'li cle
fu'run cle
gan'gli on
gas''tro en''ter i'tis
gas''tro en''ter os'to my
gin'gi vae
glo mer'u lus
glu te'ol
gyn''e co mas'ti a
hal'lux
he man''gi o'ma
he''ma tem'e sis
he ma tu'vi a
hem''i an op'si a
he mop'ty sis
her ne or'rhaphy
ho''me os'ta sis
hor de o'lum
hy'dro cele
hy per em'e sis
hys''ter ec'to my

488

i at"ro gen'ic
id"i o syn'cra sy
il"e i'tis
il'e us
in cip'i ent
in ner va'tion
in sid'i ous
in si'tu
in"tus sus cep'tion
is che'mi a
is'chi um
jaun'dice
je ju'num
ker nic'ter us
ke"to gen'e sis
ke"to nu'ri a
ky pho'sis
la'bile
lab"y rin thi'tis
lam"i nec'to my
lar'ynx
leu"ko pe'ni a
lin'gual
li thi'a sis
lym phad"e ni'tis
lym phad"e nop'a thy
mal le'o lus
mas"toid ec'to my
me a'tus
me"di as ti'num
meg"a kar'y o cyte
me nin'ge al
me nin"go en ceph"a li'tis
men"or rha'gi a
me"tror rha'gi a
my"as the'ni a
nar cis'sism
ne phri'tis
neph"ro li thi'a sis

neph"ro scle ro'sis
neu ri'tis
nys tag'mus
ol"i ge'mia
ol"i gu'ri a
om phal'ic
o"o pho rec'to my
oph"thal mol'o gist
or"chi ec'to my
os"te o my"e li'tis
pach"y men"in gi'tis
pal'pe bra
pan"cre a ti'tis
pa pil"le de'ma
par"a cen te'sis
par"a ple'gi a
par"o nych'i a
per"i or"te ri'tis
per"i stal'sis
pe te'chi a
phe"o chro"mo cy to'ma
phle bi'tis
pit"y ri'a sis
pneu"mo en ceph"a log'ra phy
pneu"mo tho'rax
pol"y cy the'mi a
pop"li te'al
pres"by o'pi a
proc"i den'ti a
pro"te in u'ri a
pseu"do cy e'sis
pto'sis
pu"er pe'ri um
py"e lo ne phri'tis
quad"ri ple'gi a
ra chi'tic
ra"di o pague'
re"cru des'cence
re sus"ci ta'tion

rheu′ma tism
rhi ni′tis
ron″geur′
scir′rhous
scle′ro sis
se″ro san guin′e ous
si″al ad″e ni′tis
sphe′noid
spon″dy li′tis
ster″e og no′sis
stra bis′mus
syn′cope
syn o′vi a

tach″y car′di a
tel an″gi ec′ta sis
tho″ra cen te′sis
throm bo phle bi′tis
tin ni′tus
ty′pa num
ur″ti ca′ri a
u′vu la
var′i co cele″
ver ru′ca
xan″tho chro′mi a
xiph′oid
zy′go ma